Respiratory Disorders
SOURCEBOOK
FIFTH EDITION

Respiratory Disorders
SOURCEBOOK

FIFTH EDITION

Basic Consumer Health Information about the Risk Factors, Symptoms, Diagnosis, and Treatment of Lung and Respiratory Disorders, Including Asthma, Bronchitis, Chronic Obstructive Pulmonary Disease (COPD), Influenza, Lung Cancer, Pneumonia, and Other Infectious and Inflammatory Pulmonary Diseases

Along with Information about Pediatric Respiratory Disorders, Tips on Preventing Respiratory Problems and Living with Chronic Lung Disease, a Glossary of Related Terms, and a Directory of Resources for Additional Help and Information

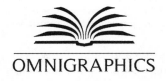

OMNIGRAPHICS
615 Griswold, Ste. 520, Detroit, MI 48226

Bibliographic Note
Because this page cannot legibly accommodate all the copyright notices, the Bibliographic
Note portion of the Preface constitutes an extension of the copyright notice.

* * *

OMNIGRAPHICS
Angela L. Williams, *Managing Editor*
* * *

Copyright © 2019 Omnigraphics

ISBN 978-0-7808-1723-4
E-ISBN 978-0-7808-1724-1

Library of Congress Cataloging-in-Publication Data

Names: Williams, Angela L., 1963- editor.

Title: Respiratory disorders sourcebook / Angela Williams, editor.

Description: Fifth edition. | Detroit, MI: Omnigraphics, Inc., [2019] | Series: Health
reference series | Includes bibliographical references and index. | Summary:
"Provides basic consumer health information about prevention, symptoms, diagnosis,
and treatment of respiratory disorders, along with tips for coping with chronic lung
disease. Includes index, glossary of related terms, and other resources"-- Provided by
publisher.

Identifiers: LCCN 2019023385 (print) | LCCN 2019023386 (ebook) | ISBN
9780780817234 (library binding) | ISBN 9780780817241 (ebook)

Subjects: LCSH: Respiratory organs--Diseases.

Classification: LCC RC731.R468 2019 (print) | LCC RC731 (ebook) | DDC 616.2--
dc23

LC record available at https://lccn.loc.gov/2019023385

LC ebook record available at https://lccn.loc.gov/2019023386

Table of Contents

Part II: Infectious Respiratory Disorders

Part III: Inflammatory Respiratory Disorders

Part IV: Other Conditions That Affect Respiration

Part VII: Living with Chronic Respiratory Problems

Part VIII: Additional Help and Information

Preface

About This Book

A person can take in, on average, 12 to 16 breaths a minute, or approximately 17,000 to 23,000 breaths a day. When the respiratory system is working properly, most of this work is done automatically; however, for millions of people with respiratory disorders, meeting the body's vital need to take in life-sustaining oxygen and remove carbon dioxide becomes a challenge. Infections can cause mucus that narrows the airways and asthma triggers can cause muscles around the airways to tighten, restricting airflow. In addition, long-term exposure to toxins, such as cigarette smoke, air pollution, and chemical fumes, can lead to a condition called "chronic obstructive pulmonary disease" (COPD), a progressive disease that affects millions of Americans and is the third leading cause of death in the United States.

Respiratory Disorders Sourcebook, Fifth Edition provides updated information about the causes, triggers, and treatments of infectious and inflammatory diseases of the respiratory system, including asthma, COPD, influenza, pneumonia, sinusitis, and tuberculosis. It also discusses other conditions that impair a person's ability to breathe, such as cystic fibrosis, lung cancer, and traumatic lung disorders. Lab and imaging tests used to diagnose respiratory disorders are explained, and a separate part deals with breathing problems in children. The book also offers tips for living with chronic lung conditions, a glossary of related terms, and a directory of helpful organizations.

How to Use This Book

This book is divided into parts and chapters. Parts focus on broad areas of interest. Chapters are devoted to single topics within a part.

Part I: Understanding and Preventing Respiratory Problems describes the components of the respiratory system and how they work together to facilitate healthy breathing. It discusses factors that can impact respiratory functioning, including genetics, allergies, hormonal changes, the aging process, and exposure to toxins and irritants. The part concludes with statistical information about common respiratory disorders in the United States.

Part II: Infectious Respiratory Disorders discusses bacterial, viral, and fungal agents that lead to such illnesses as the common cold, bronchitis, influenza, ear infections, pertussis (whooping cough), pneumonia, sinusitis, tonsillitis, strep throat, aspergillosis, histoplasmosis, and inhalation anthrax. The part also offers tips for preventing the transmission of communicable respiratory diseases.

Part III: Inflammatory Respiratory Disorders begins with information about the most common chronic respiratory disorder—asthma. The part also describes other respiratory disorders that are characterized by inflammation. These include chronic obstructive pulmonary disease (COPD) and occupational lung diseases, such as those related to exposure to asbestos, silica, and mold.

Part IV: Other Conditions That Affect Respiration offers information about disorders and diseases that impact lung function and the ability to breath normally, including cystic fibrosis (CF), lung cancer, lymphangioleiomyomatosis (LAM), amyotrophic lateral sclerosis (ALS), and muscular dystrophy. This part also discusses lung trauma and lung-related emergencies that can be life threatening, such as pulmonary embolism, pulmonary hypertension, and pneumothorax. The part concludes with information on how travel conditions can impact respiratory function.

Part V: Pediatric Respiratory Disorders discusses the effect of specific respiratory disorders on children. These include asthma, croup, respiratory syncytial virus (bronchiolitis), and sudden infant death syndrome (SIDS).

Part VI: Diagnosing and Treating Respiratory Disorders explains how pulmonologists and respiratory therapists treat and work with patients, and it describes common diagnostic tests, including pulmonary function tests, bronchoscopy, blood gas test, chest scans and x-rays, sweat test, and others. Information about commonly used medications, surgical procedures, and pulmonary rehabilitation therapies is also included.

Part VII: Living with Chronic Respiratory Problems offers tips about minimizing triggers that contribute to asthma and other respiratory disorders, and it talks about emergency action plans. Strategies for using common medical devices associated with respiratory care—including inhalers, peak flow monitors, and nebulizers—are also included.

Part VIII: Additional Help and Information provides a glossary of important terms related to respiratory disorders and a directory of organizations that offer information to patients with respiratory disorders and their families and caregivers.

Bibliographic Note

This volume contains documents and excerpts from publications issued by the following U.S. government agencies: Agency for Healthcare Research and Quality (AHRQ); Agency for Toxic Substances and Disease Registry (ATSDR); Centers for Disease Control and Prevention (CDC); Clinical Center; Effective Health Care Program; *Eunice Kennedy Shriver* National Institute of Child Health and Human Development (NICHD); Genetic and Rare Diseases Information Center (GARD); Genetics Home Reference (GHR); National Cancer Institute (NCI); National Heart, Lung, and Blood Institute (NHLBI); National Institute of Environmental Health Sciences (NIEHS); National Institute of Neurological Disorders and Stroke (NINDS); National Institute on Deafness and Other Communication Disorders (NIDCD); National Institutes of Health (NIH); *NIH News in Health*; Occupational Safety and Health Administration (OSHA); Office of Disease Prevention and Health Promotion (ODPHP); Office on Women's Health (OWH); Rehabilitation Research & Development Service (RR&D); U.S. Department of Energy (DOE); U.S. Department of Health and Human Services (HHS); U.S. Department of Veterans Affairs (VA); U.S. Environmental Protection Agency (EPA); and U.S. Food and Drug Administration (FDA).

It may also contain original material produced by Omnigraphics and reviewed by medical consultants.

About the Health Reference Series

The *Health Reference Series* is designed to provide basic medical information for patients, families, caregivers, and the general public.

Each volume takes a particular topic and provides comprehensive coverage. This is especially important for people who may be dealing with a newly diagnosed disease or a chronic disorder in themselves or in a family member. People looking for preventive guidance, information about disease warning signs, medical statistics, and risk factors for health problems will also find answers to their questions in the *Health Reference Series*. The *Series*, however, is not intended to serve as a tool for diagnosing illness, in prescribing treatments, or as a substitute for the physician/patient relationship. All people concerned about medical symptoms or the possibility of disease are encouraged to seek professional care from an appropriate healthcare provider.

A Note about Spelling and Style

Health Reference Series editors use *Stedman's Medical Dictionary* as an authority for questions related to the spelling of medical terms and the *Chicago Manual of Style* for questions related to grammatical structures, punctuation, and other editorial concerns. Consistent adherence is not always possible, however, because the individual volumes within the *Series* include many documents from a wide variety of different producers, and the editor's primary goal is to present material from each source as accurately as is possible. This sometimes means that information in different chapters or sections may follow other guidelines and alternate spelling authorities. For example, occasionally a copyright holder may require that eponymous terms be shown in possessive forms (Crohn's disease vs. Crohn disease) or that British spelling norms be retained (leukaemia vs. leukemia).

Medical Review

Omnigraphics contracts with a team of qualified, senior medical professionals who serve as medical consultants for the *Health Reference Series*. As necessary, medical consultants review reprinted and originally written material for currency and accuracy. Citations including the phrase "Reviewed (month, year)" indicate material reviewed by this team. Medical consultation services are provided to the *Health Reference Series* editors by:

Dr. Vijayalakshmi, MBBS, DGO, MD
Dr. Senthil Selvan, MBBS, DCH, MD
Dr. K. Sivanandham, MBBS, DCH, MS (Research), PhD

Our Advisory Board

Health Reference Series *Update Policy*

The inaugural book in the *Health Reference Series* was the first edition of *Cancer Sourcebook* published in 1989. Since then, the *Series* has been enthusiastically received by librarians and in the medical community. In order to maintain the standard of providing high-quality health information for the layperson the editorial staff at Omnigraphics felt it was necessary to implement a policy of updating volumes when warranted.

Medical researchers have been making tremendous strides, and it is the purpose of the *Health Reference Series* to stay current with the most recent advances. Each decision to update a volume is made on an individual basis. Some of the considerations include how much new information is available and the feedback we receive from people who use the books. If there is a topic you would like to see added to the update list, or an area of medical concern you feel has not been adequately addressed, please write to:

Managing Editor
Health Reference Series
Omnigraphics
615 Griswold, Ste. 520
Detroit, MI 48226

Part One

Understanding and Preventing Respiratory Problems

Chapter 1

How the Lungs and Respiratory System Work

What Are the Lungs?

Your lungs are organs in your chest that allow your body to take in oxygen from the air. They also help remove carbon dioxide (a waste gas that can be toxic) from your body. The lungs' intake of oxygen and removal of carbon dioxide is called "gas exchange." Gas exchange is part of breathing. Breathing is a vital function of life; it helps your body work properly.

Other organs and tissues also help make breathing possible.

The Respiratory System

The respiratory system is made up of organs and tissues that help you breathe. The main parts of this system are the airways, the lungs and linked blood vessels, and the muscles that enable breathing.

Airways

The airways are pipes that carry oxygen-rich air to your lungs. They also carry carbon dioxide, a waste gas, out of your lungs.

This chapter includes text excerpted from "How the Lungs Work," National Heart, Lung, and Blood Institute (NHLBI), November 20, 2018.

The airways include your:

- Nose and linked air passages (called "nasal cavities")
- Mouth
- Larynx, or voice box
- Trachea, or windpipe
- Tubes called "bronchial tubes" or "bronchi," and their branches

Air first enters your body through your nose or mouth, which wets and warms the air. (Cold, dry air can irritate your lungs.) The air then travels through your voice box and down your windpipe. The windpipe splits into two bronchial tubes that enter your lungs.

A thin flap of tissue called the "epiglottis" covers your windpipe when you swallow. This prevents food and drinks from entering the air passages that lead to your lungs.

Except for the mouth and some parts of the nose, all of the airways have special hairs called "cilia" that are coated with sticky mucus. The cilia trap germs and other foreign particles that enter your airways when you breathe in air.

These fine hairs then sweep the particles up to the nose or mouth. From there, they are swallowed, coughed, or sneezed out of the body. Nose hairs and mouth saliva also trap particles and germs.

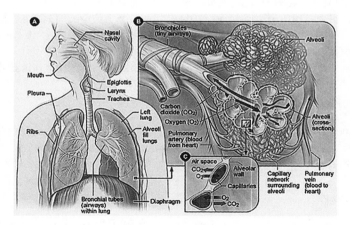

Figure 1.1. *The Human Respiratory System*

Figure A shows the location of the respiratory structures in the body. Figure B is an enlarged view of the airways, alveoli (air sacs), and capillaries (tiny blood vessels). Figure C is a closeup view of gas exchange between the capillaries and alveoli. CO_2 is carbon dioxide, and O_2 is oxygen.

4

Lungs and Blood Vessels

Your lungs and linked blood vessels deliver oxygen to your body and remove carbon dioxide from your body. Your lungs lie on either side of your breastbone and fill the inside of your chest cavity. Your left lung is slightly smaller than your right lung to allow room for your heart.

Within the lungs, your bronchi branch into thousands of smaller, thinner tubes called "bronchioles." These tubes end in bunches of tiny round air sacs called "alveoli."

Each of these air sacs is covered in a mesh of tiny blood vessels called "capillaries." The capillaries connect to a network of arteries and veins that move blood through your body.

The pulmonary artery and its branches deliver blood rich in carbon dioxide (and lacking in oxygen) to the capillaries that surround the air sacs. Inside the air sacs, carbon dioxide moves from the blood into the air. At the same time, oxygen moves from the air into the blood in the capillaries.

The oxygen-rich blood then travels to the heart through the pulmonary vein and its branches. The heart pumps the oxygen-rich blood out to the body.

The lungs are divided into five main sections called "lobes." Some people need to have a diseased lung lobe removed. However, they can still breathe well using the rest of their lung lobes.

Muscles Used for Breathing

Muscles near the lungs help expand and contract (tighten) the lungs to allow breathing. These muscles include the:

- Diaphragm
- Intercostal muscles
- Abdominal muscles
- Muscles in the neck and collarbone area

The diaphragm is a dome-shaped muscle located below your lungs. It separates the chest cavity from the abdominal cavity. The diaphragm is the main muscle used for breathing.

The intercostal muscles are located between your ribs. They also play a major role in helping you breathe. Beneath your diaphragm are abdominal muscles. They help you breathe out when you are breathing fast (for example, during physical activity).

5

Muscles in your neck and collarbone area help you breathe in when other muscles involved in breathing do not work well, or when lung disease impairs your breathing.

What Happens When You Breathe
Breathing In

When you breathe in, or inhale, your diaphragm contracts (tightens) and moves downward. This increases the space in your chest cavity, into which your lungs expand. The intercostal muscles between your ribs also help enlarge the chest cavity. They contract to pull your rib cage both upward and outward when you inhale.

As your lungs expand, air is sucked in through your nose or mouth. The air travels down your windpipe and into your lungs. After passing through your bronchial tubes, the air finally reaches and enters the alveoli (air sacs).

Through the very thin walls of the alveoli, oxygen from the air passes to the surrounding capillaries (blood vessels). A red blood cell protein called "hemoglobin" helps move oxygen from the air sacs to the blood.

At the same time, carbon dioxide moves from the capillaries into the air sacs. The gas has traveled in the bloodstream from the right side of the heart through the pulmonary artery.

Oxygen-rich blood from the lungs is carried through a network of capillaries to the pulmonary vein. This vein delivers the oxygen-rich blood to the left side of the heart. The left side of the heart pumps the blood to the rest of the body. There, the oxygen in the blood moves from blood vessels into surrounding tissues.

Breathing Out

When you breathe out, or exhale, your diaphragm relaxes and moves upward into the chest cavity. The intercostal muscles between the ribs also relax to reduce the space in the chest cavity. As the space in the chest cavity gets smaller, air rich in carbon dioxide is forced out of your lungs and windpipe, and then out of your nose or mouth.

Breathing out requires no effort from your body unless you have a lung disease or are doing physical activity. When you are physically active, your abdominal muscles contract and push your diaphragm against your lungs even more than usual. This rapidly pushes air out of your lungs.

What Controls Your Breathing

A respiratory control center at the base of your brain controls your breathing. This center sends ongoing signals down your spine and to the muscles involved in breathing. These signals ensure your breathing muscles contract (tighten) and relax regularly. This allows your breathing to happen automatically, without you being aware of it.

To a limited degree, you can change your breathing rate, such as by breathing faster or holding your breath. Your emotions also can change your breathing. For example, being scared or angry can affect your breathing pattern. Your breathing will change depending on how active you are and the condition of the air around you. For example, you need to breathe more often when you do physical activity. In contrast, your body needs to restrict how much air you breathe if the air contains irritants or toxins.

To adjust your breathing to changing needs, your body has many sensors in your brain, blood vessels, muscles, and lungs.

- Sensors in the brain and in two major blood vessels (the carotid artery and the aorta) detect carbon dioxide or oxygen levels in your blood and change your breathing rate as needed.

- Sensors in the airways detect lung irritants. The sensors can trigger sneezing or coughing. In people who have asthma, the sensors may cause the muscles around the airways in the lungs to contract. This makes the airways smaller.

- Sensors in the alveoli (air sacs) can detect fluid buildup in the lung tissues. These sensors are thought to trigger rapid, shallow breathing.

- Sensors in your joints and muscles detect movement of your arms or legs. These sensors may play a role in increasing your breathing rate when you are physically active.

Lung Diseases and Conditions

Breathing is a complex process. If injury, disease, or other factors affect any part of the process, you may have trouble breathing. For example, the fine hairs (cilia) that line your upper airways may not trap all of the germs you breathe in. These germs can cause an infection in your bronchial tubes (bronchitis) or deep in your lungs (pneumonia). These infections cause a buildup of mucus or fluid that narrows the airways and limits airflow in and out of your lungs.

If you have asthma, breathing in certain substances that you are sensitive to can trigger your airways to narrow. This makes it hard for air to flow in and out of your lungs. Over a long period, breathing in cigarette smoke or air pollutants can damage the airways and air sacs. This can lead to a disease called "chronic obstructive pulmonary disease (COPD)." COPD prevents proper airflow in and out of your lungs and can hinder gas exchange in the air sacs.

An important step to breathing is the movement of your diaphragm and other muscles in your chest, neck, and abdomen. This movement lets you inhale and exhale. Nerves that run from your brain to these muscles control their movement. Damage to these nerves in your upper spinal cord can cause breathing to stop, unless a ventilator or a respirator is used to help you breathe.

A steady flow of blood in the small blood vessels that surround your air sacs is vital for gas exchange. Long periods of inactivity or surgery can cause a blood clot called a "pulmonary embolism" (PE) to block a lung artery. A pulmonary embolism can reduce or block the flow of blood in the small blood vessels and hinder gas exchange.

Chapter 2

Improving Physical Activity and Lung Function

What Is Physical Activity?

Physical activity is any body movement that works your muscles and requires more energy than resting. Walking, running, dancing, swimming, yoga, and gardening are a few examples of physical activity.

According to the U.S. Department of Health and Human Services' (HHS) *2008 Physical Activity Guidelines for Americans* physical activity generally refers to movement that enhances health.

Exercise is a type of physical activity that is planned and structured. Lifting weights, taking an aerobics class, and playing on a sports team are examples of exercise.

Physical activity is good for many parts of your body. This chapter focuses on the benefits of physical activity for your heart and lungs. The chapter also provides tips for getting started and staying active. Physical activity is one part of a heart-healthy lifestyle. A heart-healthy lifestyle also involves following a heart-healthy eating regimen, aiming for a healthy weight, managing stress, and quitting smoking.

This chapter includes text excerpted from "Older Adults and Alcohol," National Heart, Lung, and Blood Institute (NHLBI), November 8, 2013. Reviewed August 2019.

Types of Physical Activity

The four main types of physical activity are aerobic, muscle-strengthening, bone-strengthening, and stretching. Aerobic activity is the type that benefits your heart and lungs the most.

Aerobic Activity

Aerobic activity moves your large muscles, such as those in your arms and legs. Running, swimming, walking, bicycling, dancing, and doing jumping jacks are examples of aerobic activity. Aerobic activity also is called "endurance activity."

Aerobic activity makes your heart beat faster than usual. You also breathe harder during this type of activity. Over time, regular aerobic activity makes your heart and lungs stronger and able to work better.

Other Types of Physical Activity

The other types of physical activity—muscle-strengthening, bone strengthening, and stretching—benefit your body in other ways.

Muscle-strengthening activities improve the strength, power, and endurance of your muscles. Doing pushups and situps, lifting weights, climbing stairs, and digging in the garden are examples of muscle-strengthening activities.

With bone-strengthening activities, your feet, legs, or arms support your body's weight, and your muscles push against your bones. This helps make your bones strong. Running, walking, jumping rope, and lifting weights are examples of bone-strengthening activities.

Muscle-strengthening and bone-strengthening activities can also be aerobic, depending on whether they make your heart and lungs work harder than usual. For example, running is both an aerobic activity and a bone-strengthening activity.

Stretching helps improve your flexibility and your ability to fully move your joints. Touching your toes, doing side stretches, and doing yoga exercises are examples of stretching.

Levels of Intensity in Aerobic Activity

You can do aerobic activity with light, moderate, or vigorous intensity. Moderate- and vigorous-intensity aerobic activities are better for your heart than light-intensity activities. However, even light-intensity activities are better than no activity at all.

The level of intensity depends on how hard you have to work to do the activity. To do the same activity, people who are less fit usually have to work harder than people who are more fit. So, for example, what is light-intensity activity for one person may be moderate-intensity for another.

Light- and Moderate-Intensity Activities

Light-intensity activities are common daily activities that do not require much effort. Moderate-intensity activities make your heart, lungs, and muscles work harder than light-intensity activities do.

On a scale of 0 to 10, moderate-intensity activity is a 5 or 6 and produces noticeable increases in breathing and heart rate. A person doing moderate-intensity activity can talk but not sing.

Vigorous-Intensity Activities

Vigorous-intensity activities make your heart, lungs, and muscles work hard. On a scale of 0 to 10, vigorous-intensity activity is a 7 or 8. A person doing vigorous-intensity activity cannot say more than a few words without stopping for a breath.

Examples of Aerobic Activities

Below are examples of aerobic activities. Depending on your level of fitness, they can be light, moderate, or vigorous in intensity:

- Pushing a grocery cart around a store
- Gardening, such as digging or hoeing that causes your heart rate to go up
- Walking, hiking, jogging, and running
- Water aerobics or swimming laps
- Bicycling, skateboarding, rollerblading, and jumping rope
- Ballroom dancing and aerobic dancing
- Tennis, soccer, hockey, and basketball

Benefits of Physical Activity

Physical activity has many health benefits. These benefits apply to people of all ages and races and both sexes. For example, physical activity helps you maintain a healthy weight and makes it easier to do daily tasks, such as climbing stairs and shopping.

Physically active adults are at lower risk for depression and decline in cognitive function as they get older. (Cognitive function includes thinking, learning, and judgment skills.) Physically active children and teens may have fewer symptoms of depression than their peers.

Physical activity also lowers your risk for many diseases, such as coronary heart disease (CHD), diabetes, and cancer. Many studies have shown the clear benefits of physical activity for your heart and lungs.

Physical Activity Strengthens Your Heart and Improves Lung Function

When done regularly, moderate- and vigorous-intensity physical activity strengthens your heart muscle. This improves your heart's ability to pump blood to your lungs and throughout your body. As a result, more blood flows to your muscles, and oxygen levels in your blood rise.

Capillaries, your body's tiny blood vessels, also widen. This allows them to deliver more oxygen to your body and carry away waste products.

Physical Activity Reduces Coronary Heart Disease Risk Factors

When done regularly, moderate- and vigorous-intensity aerobic activity can lower your risk for coronary heart disease. Coronary heart disease is a condition in which a waxy substance called "plaque" builds up inside your coronary arteries. These arteries supply your heart muscle with oxygen-rich blood.

Plaque narrows the arteries and reduces blood flow to your heart muscle. Eventually, an area of plaque can rupture (break open). This causes a blood clot to form on the surface of the plaque. If the clot becomes large enough, it can mostly or completely block blood flow through a coronary artery. Blocked blood flow to the heart muscle causes a heart attack.

Certain traits, conditions, or habits may raise your risk for CHD. Physical activity can help control some of these risk factors because it:

- Can lower blood pressure and triglyceride. Triglycerides are a type of fat in the blood.

- Can raise high-density lipoprotein (HDL) cholesterol levels. High-density lipoprotein is sometimes called "good cholesterol."

- Helps your body manage blood sugar and insulin levels, which lowers your risk for type 2 diabetes

- Reduces levels of C-reactive protein (CRP) in your body. This protein is a sign of inflammation. High levels of CRP may suggest an increased risk for CHD.

- Helps reduce overweight and obesity when combined with a reduced-calorie diet. Physical activity also helps you maintain a healthy weight over time once you have lost weight.

- May help you quit smoking. Smoking is a major risk factor for CHD.

Inactive people are more likely to develop CHD than people who are physically active. Studies suggest that inactivity is a major risk factor for CHD, just like high blood pressure, high blood cholesterol, and smoking.

Recommendations for Physical Activity

The U.S. Department of Health and Human Services has released physical activity guidelines for all Americans aged 6 and older.

The *2008 Physical Activity Guidelines for Americans* explain that regular physical activity improves health. They encourage people to be as active as possible. The guidelines recommend the types and amounts of physical activity that children, adults, older adults, and other groups should do. The guidelines also provide tips for how to fit physical activity into your daily life.

The information below is based on the HHS guidelines.

Guidelines for Children and Youth

The guidelines advise that:

- Children and youth do 60 minutes or more of physical activity every day. Activities should vary and be a good fit for their age and physical development. Children are naturally active, especially when they are involved in unstructured play (such as recess). Any type of activity counts toward the advised 60 minutes or more.

- Most physical activity should be moderate-intensity aerobic activity. Examples include walking, running, skipping, playing on the playground, playing basketball, and biking.

- Vigorous-intensity aerobic activity should be included at least 3 days a week. Examples include running, doing jumping jacks, and fast swimming.

- Muscle-strengthening activities should be included at least 3 days a week. Examples include playing on playground equipment, playing tug-of-war, and doing pushups and pullups.

- Bone-strengthening activities should be included at least 3 days a week. Examples include hopping, skipping, doing jumping jacks, playing volleyball, and working with resistance bands.

Children and youth who have disabilities should work with their doctors to find out what types and amounts of physical activity are safe for them. When possible, these children should meet the recommendations in the guidelines.

Some experts also advise that children and youth reduce screen time because it limits time for physical activity. They recommend that children aged two and older should spend no more than two hours a day watching television or using a computer (except for school work).

Guidelines for Adults

The guidelines advise that:

- Some physical activity is better than none. Inactive adults should gradually increase their level of activity. People gain health benefits from as little as 60 minutes of moderate-intensity aerobic activity per week.

- For major health benefits, do at least 150 minutes (2 hours and 30 minutes) of moderate-intensity aerobic activity or 75 minutes (1 hour and 15 minutes) of vigorous-intensity aerobic activity each week. Another option is to do a combination of both. A general rule is that 2 minutes of moderate-intensity activity counts the same as 1 minute of vigorous-intensity activity.

- For even more health benefits, do 300 minutes (5 hours) of moderate-intensity aerobic activity or 150 minutes (2 hours and 30 minutes) of vigorous-intensity activity each week (or a combination of both). The more active you are, the more you will benefit.

- When doing aerobic activity, do it for at least 10 minutes at a time. Spread the activity throughout the week.

Muscle-strengthening activities that are moderate or vigorous intensity should be included 2 or more days a week. These activities should work all of the major muscle groups (legs, hips, back, chest, abdomen, shoulders, and arms). Examples include lifting weights, working with resistance bands, and doing situps and pushups, yoga, and heavy gardening.

Guidelines for Adults Aged 65 or Older

The guidelines advise that:

- Older adults should be physically active. Older adults who do any amount of physical activity gain some health benefits. If inactive, older adults should gradually increase their activity levels and avoid vigorous activity at first.

- Older adults should follow the guidelines for adults, if possible. Do a variety of activities, including walking. Walking has been shown to provide health benefits and a low risk of injury.

- If you cannot do 150 minutes (2 hours and 30 minutes) of activity each week, be as physically active as your abilities and conditions allow.

- You should do balance exercises if you are at risk for falls. Examples include walking backward or sideways, standing on one leg, and standing from a sitting position several times in a row.

- If you have a chronic (ongoing) condition—such as heart disease, lung disease, or diabetes—ask your doctor what types and amounts of activity are safe for you.

Guidelines for Women during Pregnancy and Soon after Delivery

The guidelines advise that:

- You should ask your doctor what physical activities are safe to do during pregnancy and after delivery.

- If you are healthy but not already active, do at least 150 minutes (2 hours and 30 minutes) of moderate-intensity aerobic activity each week. If possible, spread this activity across the week.

- If you are already active, you can continue being active as long as you stay healthy and talk with your doctor about your activity level throughout your pregnancy.

15

- After the first three months of pregnancy, you should not do exercises that involve lying on your back.

- You should not do activities, such as horseback riding, downhill skiing, soccer, and basketball, in which you might fall or hurt yourself,

Guidelines for Other Groups

The HHS guidelines also have recommendations for other groups, including people who have disabilities and people who have chronic conditions such as osteoarthritis (OA), diabetes, and cancer.

Getting Started and Staying Active

Physical activity is an important part of a heart-healthy lifestyle. To get started and stay active, make physical activity part of your daily routine, keep track of your progress, be active and safe, and talk to your doctor if you have a chronic (ongoing) health condition.

Make Physical Activity Part of Your Daily Routine

You do not have to become a marathon runner to get all of the benefits of physical activity. Do activities that you enjoy, and make them part of your daily routine.

If you have not been active for a while, start low and build slow. Many people like to start with walking and slowly increase their time and distance. You also can take other steps to make physical activity part of your routine.

Personalize the Benefits

People value different things. Some people may highly value the health benefits from physical activity. Others want to be active because they enjoy recreational activities or they want to look better or sleep better.

Some people want to be active because it helps them lose weight or it gives them a chance to spend time with friends. Identify which physical activity benefits you value. This will help you personalize the benefits of physical activity.

Be Active with Friends and Family

Friends and family can help you stay active. For example, go for a hike with a friend. Take dancing lessons with your spouse, or play ball with your child. The possibilities are endless.

Make Everyday Activities More Active

You can make your daily routine more active. For example, take the stairs instead of the elevator. Instead of sending e-mails, walk down the hall to a coworker's office. Rake the leaves instead of using a leaf blower.

Reward Yourself with Time for Physical Activity

Sometimes, going for a bike ride or a long walk relieves stress after a long day. Think of physical activity as a special time to refresh your body and mind.

Keep Track of Your Progress

Consider keeping a log of your activity. A log can help you track your progress. Many people like to wear a pedometer (a small device that counts your steps) to track how much they walk every day. These tools can help you set goals and stay motivated.

Be Active and Safe

Physical activity is safe for almost everyone. You can take steps to make sure it is safe for you too.

- Be active on a regular basis to raise your fitness level.

- Do activities that fit your health goals and fitness level. Start low and slowly increase your activity level over time. As your fitness improves, you will be able to do physical activities for longer periods and with more intensity.

- Spread out your activity over the week and vary the types of activity you do.

- Use the right gear and equipment to protect yourself. For example, use bicycle helmets, elbow and knee pads, and goggles.

- Be active in safe environments. Pick well-lit and well-maintained places that are clearly separated from car traffic.

- Follow safety rules and policies, such as always wearing a helmet when biking.

- Make sensible choices about when, where, and how to be active. Consider weather conditions, such as how hot or cold it is, and change your plans as needed.

Talk to Your Doctor If Needed

Healthy people who do not have heart problems do not need to check with a doctor before beginning moderate-intensity activities.

If you have a heart problem or chronic disease, such as heart disease, diabetes, or high blood pressure, talk to your doctor about what types of physical activity are safe for you.

You also should talk to your doctor about safe physical activities if you have symptoms such as chest pain or dizziness.

Chapter 3

Factors That Affect Respiratory System Function

Chapter Contents

Section 3.1

Do Allergies Cause Asthma?

This section includes text excerpted from "Breathing Easier,"
Centers for Disease Control and Prevention (CDC), 2008.
Reviewed August 2019.

What Is Asthma?

In people with asthma, something causes the airways of the lungs to narrow or become blocked, making it hard to breathe. Normally, the airways to the lungs are fully open when we breathe, so air moves in and out freely. People with asthma have highly sensitive airways that become inflamed easily. They have asthma all the time, but they have asthma episodes or attacks only when something bothers their airways. During an episode, they may cough and wheeze or become short of breath. Sometimes an episode is so severe, they need emergency medical attention to breathe normally again.

What Causes Asthma

The cause of asthma is largely unknown, although sometimes having asthma is linked to a specific trigger, such as having inhaled certain chemicals at work. However, if someone in your family has asthma, you are more likely to have it, so there may be a hereditary component to the disease.

An asthma episode occurs when a person with asthma inhale substances in the air that trigger symptoms at home, work, or school. Asthma triggers lurk indoors and out.

In many people with asthma, the same substances (called "allergens") that cause allergy symptoms can trigger an asthma attack. These allergens may be inhaled, such as pollen, tobacco smoke, or dust, or eaten, such as shellfish. Avoiding or limiting exposure to known allergens can help prevent asthma symptoms.

Air pollution is one of the most underappreciated contributors to asthma episodes. Children with asthma are particularly vulnerable to ozone, even at levels below the Environmental Protection Agency's (EPA) current standard. Pollution from truck and auto exhaust also raises the risk of asthma symptoms.

In addition, an asthma attack can be caused in some people by strenuous physical exercise, certain medicines, and even bad weather such as thunderstorms. No two cases of asthma are exactly alike. Some people react to just a few of these triggers, some to many. Some people need only a single trigger to set off an asthma attack, while for others several triggers must be present at the same time. People with asthma must learn which factors trigger their episodes, and then try to minimize their exposure to them.

Section 3.2

Chronic Obstructive Pulmonary Disease—Its Causes and Risk Factors

This section includes text excerpted from "COPD—Are You at Risk?" National Heart, Lung, and Blood Institute (NHLBI), September 2013. Reviewed August 2019.

Chronic obstructive pulmonary disease (COPD) is a serious lung disease that over time makes it hard to breathe. COPD has other names, such as emphysema or chronic bronchitis. In those who have COPD, the airways, or tubes that carry air in and out of the lungs are partly blocked, making it difficult to breathe.

People who have COPD:

- Become short of breath while doing everyday activities

- Produce excess sputum

- Cough frequently, or constantly. Some call this a "smoker's cough."

- Wheeze

- Feel as if they cannot breathe

- Are unable to take a deep breath

As time goes by, these symptoms get gradually worse. COPD develops slowly, and can worsen over time. Many people with COPD avoid activities they used to enjoy because they become short of breath so easily. When COPD becomes severe, it can get in the way of doing

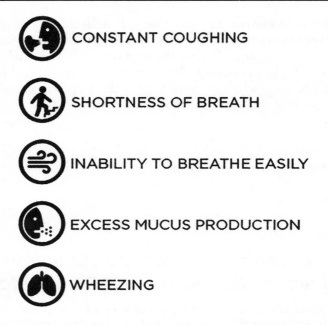

CONSTANT COUGHING

SHORTNESS OF BREATH

INABILITY TO BREATHE EASILY

EXCESS MUCUS PRODUCTION

WHEEZING

Figure 3.1. *Signs and Symptoms of COPD* (Source: "COPD National Action Plan," National Heart, Lung, and Blood Institute (NHLBI).)

even the most basic tasks, such as light housekeeping, taking a walk, bathing, and getting dressed.

Chronic obstructive pulmonary disease is serious, yet many do not know they have it. As we age, it is easy to think that some of the symptoms of COPD are just part of "getting older." But they are not. If you think you have even mild symptoms, tell your doctor or healthcare provider as soon as possible. COPD is the third leading cause of death in the United States, claiming more than 120,000 American lives each year. More than 12 million have been diagnosed, but another 12 million are likely to have COPD and do not know it.

You Could Be at Risk of Chronic Obstructive Pulmonary Disease

You could be at risk for COPD if you:

- **Used to smoke or still do.** COPD most often occurs in people age 40 and over who are current or former smokers. Smoking is the most common cause of COPD, accounting for as many as nine out of ten COPD-related deaths. However, as many as one out of six people who have COPD never smoked.

- **Have long-term exposure to lung irritants.** COPD can also occur in people who have had long-term exposure to things that can irritate your lungs, such as certain chemicals, dust, or fumes in the workplace. Heavy or long-term exposure to secondhand smoke or other air pollutants may also contribute to COPD.

- **Have a genetic condition called "alpha-1 antitrypsin (AAT) deficiency."** As many as 100,000 Americans have AAT deficiency. They can get COPD even if they have never smoked or had long-term exposure to harmful pollutants.

What Is Alpha-1 Antitrypsin Deficiency?*

Alpha-1 antitrypsin deficiency is an inherited condition that causes low levels of, or no, AAT in the blood. AATD occurs in approximately 1 in 2,500 individuals. This condition is found in all ethnic groups; however, it occurs most often in Whites of European ancestry.

Alpha-1 antitrypsin is a protein that is made in the liver. The liver releases this protein into the bloodstream. AAT protects the lungs so they can work normally. Without enough AAT, the lungs can be damaged, and this damage may make breathing difficult.

Everyone has two copies of the gene for AAT and receives one copy of the gene from each parent. Most people have two normal copies of the *AAT* gene. Individuals with AAT deficiency have one normal copy and one damaged copy, or they have two damaged copies. Most individuals who have one normal gene can produce enough AAT to live healthy lives, especially if they do not smoke.

People who have two damaged copies of the gene are not able to produce enough AAT, which leads them to have more severe symptoms.

Text is excerpted from "About Alpha-1 Antitrypsin Deficiency," National Human Genome Research Institute (NHGRI), January 4, 2012.

Are You at Risk of Chronic Obstructive Pulmonary Disease?

Things everyone at risk should do:

- **Quit smoking.** There are many online resources and several new aids available from your healthcare provider. Visit www. smokefree.gov; lungusa.org; or call 800-784-8669.

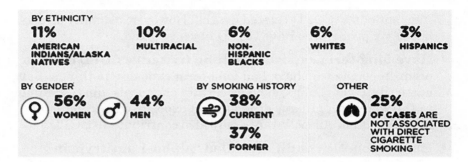

Figure 3.2. *Who Has COPD* (Source: "COPD National Action Plan," National Heart, Lung, and Blood Institute (NHLBI).)

- **Avoid exposure to pollutants.** Stay away from things that could irritate your lungs, such as dust, strong fumes and cigarette smoke.

- **Visit your doctor or healthcare provider regularly.** Make a list of your breathing symptoms, and think about any activities that you can no longer do because of shortness of breath.

- **Protect yourself from the flu.** Do your best to avoid crowds during flu season. It is also a good idea to get a flu shot every year.

Know for Sure. Get a Spirometry Test.

Spirometry is a common, noninvasive lung function test that can detect COPD before symptoms become severe. It measures the amount of air you can blow out of your lungs (volume) and how fast you can blow it out (flow). That way, your doctor or healthcare provider can tell if you have COPD, and how severe it is. The spirometry reading can help determine the best course of treatment.

Section 3.3

Menstrual Cycle, Pregnancy, and Asthma

This section includes text excerpted from "Asthma,"
Office on Women's Health (OWH), U.S. Department of
Health and Human Services (HHS), June 11, 2019.

Asthma is a chronic lung disease that causes episodes of wheezing, breathlessness, tightness in the chest, or coughing. After age 15, asthma is more common in girls and women than in boys and men. Women with asthma may have more symptoms during certain times in the menstrual cycle. Asthma may cause problems during pregnancy. You can help prevent or stop asthma attacks with medicine and by staying away from your asthma triggers, such as pollen, mold, or air pollution.

How Does Menstrual Cycle Affect Asthma?

Changing hormone levels throughout your menstrual cycle may make your asthma symptoms worse during some parts of the cycle.

If your asthma symptoms get worse during certain parts of your cycle every month, track your symptoms and menstrual cycle on a calendar. After a few months, you might be able to predict when your asthma symptoms will flare up based on your menstrual cycle. You can then stay away from other asthma triggers during these times.

Tell your doctor or nurse:

- If your asthma attacks happen during a certain time in your menstrual cycle

- If you take birth control

- If you take any kind of hormones

- About any over-the-counter (OTC) medicines you take. Some common pain medicines that women take to relieve menstrual cramps, such as aspirin and ibuprofen, can trigger asthma attacks in some women.

How Does Asthma Affect Pregnancy?

Many women who have asthma do not have any problems during pregnancy. But asthma can cause problems for you and your baby during pregnancy because of changing hormone levels. Your unborn baby depends on the air you breathe in for oxygen. Asthma attacks during pregnancy can prevent your unborn baby from getting enough oxygen.

Pregnant women with asthma have a higher risk for:

- Preeclampsia

- Gestational diabetes

- Problems with the placenta, including placental abruption

- Premature birth (babies born before 37 weeks of pregnancy)

- Low birth weight baby (less than 5 and a half pounds)

- Cesarean section (C-section)

- Serious bleeding after childbirth (called "postpartum hemorrhage")

Pregnancy may also make asthma symptoms seem worse due to acid reflux or heartburn. If you have asthma and are thinking about becoming pregnant, talk to your doctor or nurse. Having your asthma under control before you get pregnant can help prevent problems during pregnancy.

Section 3.4

Effects of Aging on the Respiratory System

"Effects of Aging on the Respiratory System,"
© 2017 Omnigraphics. Reviewed August 2019.

Respiration, better known as "breathing," is the process of inhaling oxygen from the air and exhaling carbon dioxide from the body. Inhaled air flows through the airways into the lungs, where it fills tiny sacs called "alveoli." Blood vessels surrounding the alveoli carry oxygen into the bloodstream to be circulated among the organs and tissues. At the same time, the blood vessels empty carbon dioxide from the bloodstream into the alveoli to be removed from the body through exhalation.

The natural aging process affects respiration in a number of ways. Since the lungs stop producing new alveoli once people reach the age of about 20, their ability to exchange carbon dioxide and oxygen declines slowly from that point onward. Losses in muscle tone and changes in the nervous system also contribute to a gradual reduction in respiratory function as people age. Older people also face a higher risk of diminished lung capacity due to infections, diseases, and the destructive long-term effects of smoking and air pollution.

Changes in the Respiratory System

The aging process causes a gradual decline in the overall function of the lungs and respiratory tract. Some of the changes that occur during this process include the following:

- The diaphragm, a large muscle in the abdomen that pushes air in and out of the lungs, becomes weaker over time. As a result, the maximum force of inhalation and exhalation decreases with age.

- The intercostal muscles between the ribs grow weaker, decreasing the chest's ability to stretch during breathing.

- Bone mass decreases in the ribcage and spine, further reducing the capacity of the chest to expand and contract while breathing.

- Muscles and tissues in the airways lose elasticity over time, causing the airways to close more easily.

- The lungs' ability to expand and contract declines due to reduced levels of the protein elastin.

- Signals between the brain and the lungs lose strength and clarity, reducing the body's ability to respond to low oxygen levels or high carbon dioxide levels in the blood.

- Nerves in the airways that trigger the coughing reflex become less sensitive, allowing smoke, germs, or other foreign particles to build up and damage the lungs.

- Other bodily defenses designed to protect the lungs grow weaker, leaving the respiratory system more vulnerable to infections and diseases. For instance, the nose secretes fewer IgA antibodies to fight viruses, and the hair-like cilia lining the airways lose their ability to move mucus out of the body.

Effects of Age-Related Respiratory Changes

All of these age-related changes to the lungs cause a gradual decrease in maximum lung function. The rate of airflow declines, and the amount of oxygen in the bloodstream decreases. For some elderly people, low oxygen levels become chronic, causing persistent breathing difficulty, shortness of breath, and tiredness. But most generally healthy people maintain enough lung function to perform daily activities. They are most likely to notice symptoms of the gradual decrease in lung capacity during vigorous aerobic exercise, such as running, biking, or swimming. Other factors may contribute to a reduced ability to exercise as well, however, such as age-related changes in the heart, blood vessels, bones, and muscles.

The age-related changes to the respiratory system also make older people more susceptible to abnormal breathing patterns, such as sleep apnea. People with this condition stop breathing numerous times while they are asleep. Lung changes related to age also make elderly people more susceptible to infections, such as pneumonia and bronchitis, as well as diseases such as emphysema and lung cancer.

Preventing Age-Related Respiratory Problems

There are a number of measures people can take to minimize the impact of aging on the respiratory system. Some tips for maintaining good lung function include the following:

- Avoid smoking, which causes lung damage and speeds up the aging process.

- Exercise regularly to maintain peak lung capacity and function as long as possible.

- Avoid spending prolonged periods in bed during illness or recovery from surgery, which allows mucus to collect in the lungs and increases the risk of lung infections. Instead, get up and move around as much as possible and perform deep-breathing exercises to maintain lung function.

- Get annual vaccines to reduce the risk of respiratory infections such as influenza and pneumococcal pneumonia.

References

1. "Aging Changes in the Lungs," HealthCentral, 2015.

2. Lechtzin, Noah. "Effects of Aging on the Respiratory System," Merck Manuals, 2016.

3. Martin, Laura J. "Aging Changes in the Lungs," MedlinePlus, A.D.A.M Medical Encyclopedia, October 27, 2014.

Section 3.5

Genetics and Lung Cancer

This section includes text excerpted from "Lung Cancer," Genetics Home Reference (GHR), National Institutes of Health (NIH), December 2017.

Lung cancer is a disease in which certain cells in the lungs become abnormal and multiply uncontrollably to form a tumor. Lung cancer may not cause signs or symptoms in its early stages. Some people with lung cancer have chest pain, frequent coughing, blood in the mucus, breathing problems, trouble swallowing or speaking, loss of appetite and weight loss, fatigue, or swelling in the face or neck. Additional symptoms can develop if the cancer spreads (metastasizes) into other tissues. Lung cancer occurs most often in adults in their sixties or seventies. Most people who develop lung cancer have a history of long-term tobacco smoking; however, the condition can occur in people who have never smoked.

Lung cancer is generally divided into two types, small cell lung cancer and nonsmall cell lung cancer, based on the size of the affected cells when viewed under a microscope. Nonsmall cell lung cancer accounts for 85 percent of lung cancer, while small cell lung cancer accounts for the remaining 15 percent.

Frequency of Lung Cancer

In the United States, lung cancer is the second most commonly diagnosed cancer, after breast cancer, accounting for about one-quarter of all cancer diagnoses. It is estimated that more than 222,500 people develop lung cancer each year. Approximately 6.6 percent of individuals will develop lung cancer during their lifetime. An estimated 72 to

80 percent of lung cancer cases occur in tobacco smokers. Lung cancer is the leading cause of cancer deaths, accounting for an estimated 27 percent of all cancer deaths in the United States.

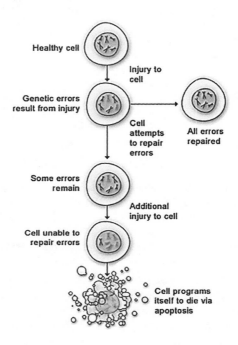

Figure 3.3. *Apoptosis* (Source: U.S. National Library of Medicine (NLM).)

Causes of Lung Cancer

Cancers occur when genetic mutations build up in critical genes, specifically those that control cell growth and division (proliferation) or the repair of damaged deoxyribonucleic acid (DNA). These changes allow cells to grow and divide uncontrollably to form a tumor. In nearly all cases of lung cancer, these genetic changes are acquired during a person's lifetime and are present only in certain cells in the lungs. These changes, which are called "somatic mutations," are not inherited. Somatic mutations in many different genes have been found in lung cancer cells. In rare cases, the genetic change is inherited and is present in all the body's cells (germline mutations).

Somatic mutations in the *TP53*, *EGFR*, and *KRAS* genes are common in lung cancers. The *TP53* gene provides instructions for making a protein, called "p53," that is located in the nucleus of cells throughout

30

the body, where it attaches (binds) directly to DNA. The protein regulates cell growth and division by monitoring DNA damage. When DNA becomes damaged, p53 helps determine whether the DNA will be repaired or the cell will self-destruct (undergo apoptosis).

The *EGFR* and *KRAS* genes each provide instructions for making a protein that is embedded within the cell membrane. When these proteins are turned on (activated) by binding to other molecules, signaling pathways are triggered within cells that promote cell proliferation.

TP53 gene mutations result in the production of an altered p53 protein that cannot bind to DNA. The altered protein cannot regulate cell proliferation effectively and allows DNA damage to accumulate in cells. Such cells may continue to divide in an uncontrolled way, leading to tumor growth. Mutations in the *EGFR* or *KRAS* gene lead to the production of a protein that is constantly turned on (constitutively activated). As a result, cells constantly receive signals to proliferate, leading to tumor formation. When these genetic changes occur in cells in the lungs, lung cancer develops.

Mutations in many other genes have been found to recur in lung cancer cases. Most of these genes are involved in the regulation of gene activity (expression), cell proliferation, the process by which cells mature to carry out specific functions (differentiation), and apoptosis.

Researchers have identified many lifestyle and environmental factors that expose individuals to cancer-causing compounds (carcinogens) and increase the rate at which somatic mutations occur, contributing to a person's risk of developing lung cancer. The greatest risk factor is long-term tobacco smoking, which increases a person's risk of developing lung cancer 25-fold. Other risk factors include exposure to air pollution, radon, asbestos, certain metals, and chemicals, or secondhand smoke; long-term use of hormone replacement therapy (HRT) for menopause; and a history of lung disease, such as tuberculosis (TB), emphysema, or chronic bronchitis. A history of lung cancer in closely related family members is also an important risk factor; however, because relatives with lung cancer are frequently smokers, it is unclear whether the increased risk is the result of genetic factors or exposure to secondhand smoke.

Inheritance Pattern of Lung Cancer

Most cases of lung cancer are not related to inherited genetic changes. These cancers are associated with somatic mutations that occur only in certain cells in the lung.

When lung cancer is related to inherited genetic changes, the cancer risk follows an autosomal dominant pattern, which means one copy of the altered gene in each cell is sufficient to increase a person's chance of developing the disease. It is important to note that people inherit an increased risk of cancer, not the disease itself. Not all people who inherit mutations in these genes will develop lung cancer.

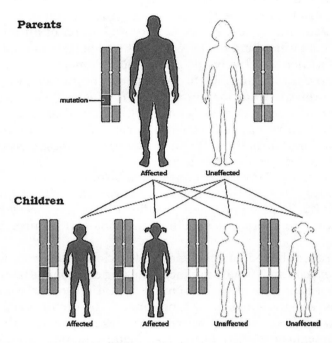

Figure 3.4. *Autosomal Dominant Inheritance* (Source: U.S. National Library of Medicine (NLM).)

Chapter 4

Toxins, Pollutants, and Respiratory Diseases

Chapter Contents

Section 4.1

Smoking and Respiratory Diseases

This section includes text excerpted from "Keep Your Air Clear:
How Tobacco Can Harm Your Lungs," U.S. Food and Drug
Administration (FDA), December 12, 2017.

Every organ in the human body serves an important purpose in keeping it running and in prime condition. Most healthy people are not cognizant of their organs—such as lungs—on a daily basis, because they are able to breathe without difficulty and perform their daily tasks without major effort. But damage to these vital organs can cause serious disease, and sometimes death. Cigarettes can harm the tissue of the lungs, impeding their ability to function properly, and can increase the risk for conditions, such as emphysema, lung cancer, and chronic obstructive pulmonary disease (COPD).

The primary function of your lungs is to deliver oxygen-rich blood to the rest of your body from the air you breathe in and expel carbon dioxide as waste when you exhale. While no tobacco product is safe, combustible products—or those you must light on fire to use, such as cigarettes—are especially damaging to the lungs.

Smoking and Your Lungs

Cigarette smoking can cause immediate damage to your health. Each puff of cigarette smoke contains a mix of over 7,000 chemicals. When you breathe this in, the smoke hits your lungs very quickly, and the blood that is then carried to the rest of your body contains these toxic chemicals. Because tobacco smoke contains carbon monoxide, this deadly gas displaces the oxygen in your blood, depriving your organs of the oxygen they need.

Other chemicals found in cigarette smoke include acrolein, which can cause irreversible lung damage, and even in low amounts, it can cause a sore throat in 10 minutes. Cigarettes may also contain bronchodilators, or chemicals that are meant to open up the airways of the lungs and could increase the amount of dangerous chemicals absorbed by the lungs.

Cigarette smoking can have major consequences on the lungs at all ages. Babies whose mothers smoked during pregnancy may have lungs that develop abnormally, and teens who smoke cigarettes can develop smaller, weaker lungs that never grow to full size and never perform at their peak capacity. In addition, smoking can destroy the cilia—or tiny hairs in your airway that keep dirt and mucus out of your lungs. When these cilia are destroyed, you develop what is known as "smoker's cough," a chronic cough that is often seen in long-term or daily smokers.

Lung damage due to smoking does not end there. On average, 8 out of 10 cases of are caused by smoking. People with COPD experience difficulty breathing and eventually die because of a lack of air. There is no cure for COPD. Furthermore, nearly all lung cancer—the top cause of cancer death in both men and women—is caused by smoking, and smokers are 20 times more likely to develop lung cancer than nonsmokers. In addition to lung cancer, smoking can lead to other respiratory cancers, such as:

- The oropharynx (the back of the mouth, including parts of the tongue, the soft palate, the side and back of the throat, and the tonsils)

- Larynx (the "voice box")

- Trachea (the "windpipe")

- Bronchus (one of two large airways that connect the trachea to the lungs)

Not Just Cigarettes: Other Tobacco Products and Lung Health

While cigarettes—given their high rate of use, addictive nature, and toxic mix of chemicals—are the most dangerous tobacco product, any tobacco product you inhale could cause lung damage. Cigar smoking can increase the risk of COPD, and lead to cancers of the lung, oral cavity, and larynx, among other cancers.

Electronic Nicotine Delivery Systems (ENDS), such as e-cigarettes, are still relatively new tobacco products and are still being evaluated for their impacts on health. But e-cigarette use—or "vaping"—may be harmful to your lungs. Some e-cigarette aerosols have been found to contain some of the same chemicals in cigarettes, including the lung irritant acrolein, and formaldehyde, which may adversely affect the throat. Flavoring chemicals are considered safe for eating, but could be harmful when inhaled. Buttery flavors like caramel, toffee, and chocolate contains chemicals diacetyl and acetoin, which can be harmful to your lungs. Additionally, fruit-flavored e-cigarettes can have higher concentrations of a chemical called "acrylonitrile," which is a known respiratory irritant.

How You Can Protect Your Lungs from Tobacco

Your lungs are one of your body's filtration systems, taking in air from the atmosphere, adding oxygen to the blood for circulation throughout the body, and expelling excess carbon dioxide. When tobacco is inhaled, it interferes with this delicate balance. The best way to ensure lung health is to never start using tobacco, but if you are an addicted smoker, the sooner you quit, the sooner your lungs can begin to heal. Quitting smoking can lower the risk of getting cancer. In fact, when you quit smoking, your risk of:

- Cancer of the larynx is reduced immediately

- Lung cancer drops by 50 percent 10 years after quitting

- Mouth and throat cancers drop by 50 percent five years after quitting

Anyone who quits smoking will experience better overall health. Just 12 hours after quitting, the carbon monoxide level in your blood drops to normal, allowing more oxygen to circulate to your organs.

Section 4.2

Secondhand Smoke and Respiratory Health

This section includes text excerpted from "Health Effects of Secondhand Smoke," Centers for Disease Control and Prevention (CDC), January 17, 2018.

What Is Secondhand Smoke?

Secondhand smoke is the combination of smoke from the burning end of a cigarette and the smoke breathed out by smokers. Secondhand smoke contains more than 7,000 chemicals. Hundreds are toxic and about 70 can cause cancer.

There is no risk-free level of exposure to secondhand smoke.

- Secondhand smoke causes numerous health problems in infants and children, including more frequent and severe asthma attacks, respiratory infections, ear infections, and sudden infant death syndrome (SIDS).

- Smoking during pregnancy results in more than 1,000 infant deaths annually.
- Some of the health conditions caused by secondhand smoke in adults include coronary heart disease, stroke, and lung cancer.

Secondhand Smoke Causes Lung Cancer

Secondhand smoke causes lung cancer in adults who have never smoked.

- Nonsmokers who are exposed to secondhand smoke at home or at work increase their risk of developing lung cancer by 20 to 30 percent.
- Secondhand smoke causes more than 7,300 lung cancer deaths among U.S. nonsmokers each year.
- Nonsmokers who are exposed to secondhand smoke are inhaling many of the same cancer-causing substances and poisons as smokers.
- Even brief secondhand smoke exposure can damage cells in ways that set the cancer process in motion.
- As with active smoking, the longer the duration and the higher the level of exposure to secondhand smoke, the greater the risk of developing lung cancer.

Secondhand Smoke Causes Sudden Infant Death Syndrome

Sudden infant death syndrome (SIDS) is the sudden, unexplained, unexpected death of an infant in the first year of life. It is the leading cause of death in otherwise healthy infants. Secondhand smoke increases the risk for SIDS.

- Smoking by women during pregnancy increases the risk for SIDS.
- Infants who are exposed to secondhand smoke after birth are also at greater risk for SIDS.
- Chemicals in secondhand smoke appear to affect the brain in ways that interfere with its regulation of infants' breathing.

37

- Infants who die from SIDS have higher concentrations of nicotine in their lungs and higher levels of cotinine (a biological marker for secondhand smoke exposure) than infants who die from other causes.

Parents can help protect their babies from SIDS by taking the following three actions:

- Do not smoke when pregnant.
- Do not smoke in the home or around the baby.
- Put the baby down to sleep on its back.

Secondhand Smoke Harms Children

Secondhand smoke can cause serious health problems in children.

- Studies show that older children whose parents smoke get sick more often. Their lungs grow less than children who do not breathe secondhand smoke, and they get more bronchitis and pneumonia.
- Wheezing and coughing are more common in children who breathe secondhand smoke.
- Secondhand smoke can trigger an asthma attack in a child. Children with asthma who are around secondhand smoke have more severe and frequent asthma attacks. A severe asthma attack can put a child's life in danger.
- Children whose parents smoke around them get more ear infections. They also have fluid in their ears more often and have more operations to put in ear tubes for drainage.

Parents can help protect their children from secondhand smoke by taking the following actions:

- Do not allow anyone to smoke anywhere in or near your home.
- Do not allow anyone to smoke in your car, even with the window down.
- Make sure your children's day care centers and schools are tobacco-free.
- If your state still allows smoking in public areas, look for restaurants and other places that do not allow smoking.

"No-smoking sections" do not protect you and your family from secondhand smoke.

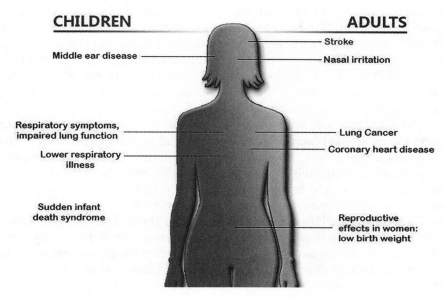

Figure 4.1. *Health Consequences Causally Linked to Exposure to Secondhand Smoke*

Section 4.3

Indoor Air Pollution and Respiratory Health

This section includes text excerpted from "Indoor Air Quality (IAQ)," U.S. Environmental Protection Agency (EPA), January 29, 2018.

Indoor air quality (IAQ) refers to the air quality within and around buildings and structures, especially as it relates to the health and comfort of building occupants. Understanding and controlling common pollutants indoors can help reduce your risk of indoor health concerns.

Health effects from indoor air pollutants may be experienced soon after exposure or, possibly, years later.

Immediate Effects

Some health effects may show up shortly after a single exposure or repeated exposures to a pollutant. These include irritation of the eyes, nose, and throat, headaches, dizziness, and fatigue. Such immediate effects are usually short-term and treatable. Sometimes the treatment is simply eliminating the person's exposure to the source of the pollution, if it can be identified. Soon after exposure to some indoor air pollutants, symptoms of some diseases such as asthma may show up, be aggravated or worsened.

The likelihood of immediate reactions to indoor air pollutants depends on several factors including age and preexisting medical conditions. In some cases, whether a person reacts to a pollutant depends on individual sensitivity, which varies tremendously from person to person. Some people can become sensitized to biological or chemical pollutants after repeated or high-level exposures.

Certain immediate effects are similar to those from colds or other viral diseases, so it is often difficult to determine if the symptoms are a result of exposure to indoor air pollution. For this reason, it is important to pay attention to the time and place symptoms occur. If the symptoms fade or go away when a person is away from the area, for example, an effort should be made to identify indoor air sources that may be possible causes. Some effects may be made worse by an inadequate supply of outdoor air coming indoors or from the heating, cooling, or humidity conditions prevalent indoors.

Long-Term Effects

Other health effects may show up either years after exposure has occurred or only after long or repeated periods of exposure. These effects, which include some respiratory diseases, heart disease and cancer, can be severely debilitating or fatal. It is prudent to try to improve the indoor air quality (IAQ) in your home even if symptoms are not noticeable.

While pollutants commonly found in indoor air can cause many harmful effects, there is considerable uncertainty about what concentrations or periods of exposure are necessary to produce specific health problems. People also react very differently to exposure to indoor air pollutants. Further research is needed to better understand which health effects occur after exposure to the average pollutant concentrations found in homes and which occurs from the higher concentrations that occur for short periods of time.

Section 4.4

Ozone and Health

This section includes text excerpted from "Air
Quality—Ozone and Your Health," Centers for Disease
Control and Prevention (CDC), May 4, 2018.

Outdoor air quality has improved since the 1990s, but many challenges remain in protecting Americans from air quality problems. Ground-level ozone, the main part of smog, and particle pollution are just two of the many threats to air quality and public health in the United States.

How Can Ozone Affect Your Health?

If you have asthma, bronchitis, or emphysema, ozone can make your symptoms worse. Carefully follow your asthma management plan on days when ozone levels are high.

Ozone has also been linked to:

- Coughing and pain when taking a deep breath

- Lung and throat irritation

- Wheezing and trouble breathing during exercise or outdoor activities

Who Is Most at Risk?

Ozone can affect anyone, but it bothers some people more than others. People most likely to experience health effects caused by ozone include:

- People with asthma or other lung diseases

- Older adults

- People of all ages who exercise or work hard outside

- Babies and children

Protect Yourself and Your Family

The good news is there is a lot you can do to protect yourself and your family from the health effects caused by ground-level ozone. Start by learning about the air quality index (AQI) from the U.S. Environmental Protection Agency (EPA).

Take Action

When ground-level ozone levels are high, take steps to limit the amount of air you breathe in while you are outside. For example:

- Think about spending more time indoors, where ozone levels are usually lower.

- Choose easier outdoor activities (such as walking instead of running) so you do not breathe as hard.

- Plan outdoor activities at times when ozone levels are lower (usually in the morning and evening).

Section 4.5

Climate Change and Airway Diseases

This section includes text excerpted from "Health Impacts,"
National Institute of Environmental Health
Sciences (NIEHS), September 25, 2018.

Changes in the greenhouse gas concentrations and other drivers alter the global climate and bring about myriad human health consequences. Environmental consequences of climate change, such as extreme heat waves, rising sea levels, changes in precipitation resulting in flooding and droughts, intense hurricanes, and degraded air quality, affect directly and indirectly the physical, social, and psychological health of humans. For instance, changes in precipitation are creating changes in the availability and quantity of water, as well as resulting in extreme weather events such as intense hurricanes and flooding. Climate change can be a driver of disease migration, and can exacerbate health effects resulting from the release of toxic air pollutants in vulnerable populations such as children, the elderly, and those with asthma or cardiovascular disease.

Certain adverse health effects can be minimized or avoided with sound mitigation and adaptation strategies. Strategies for mitigating and adapting to climate change can prevent illness and death in people now, while also protecting the environment and health of future generations.

Mitigation refers to actions being taken to reduce greenhouse gas emissions and to enhance the sinks that trap or remove carbon from the atmosphere. Adaptation refers to actions being taken to lessen the impact on health and the environment due to changes that cannot be prevented through mitigation. Appropriate mitigation and adaptation strategies will positively affect both climate change and the environment, and thereby positively affect human health. Some adaptation activities will directly improve human health through changes in our public health and healthcare infrastructure.

It is critical that adaptation and mitigation decisions and policies be developed with a sound basis in the best current science on climate change and its effects. There are gaps in our understanding of the relationship between climate change, the environment, and human health.

Chapter 5

Avoiding Smoke Exposure

Chapter Contents

Section 5.1

Where to Get Help to Quit Smoking

This section includes text excerpted from "Ask for Help,"
Smokefree.gov, U.S. Department of Health and
Human Services (HHS), June 8, 2016.

Getting support from the important people in your life can make a big difference when you quit smoking. Friends, family, co-workers, and others can be there for you. You are not alone.

You also can connect with others and grow your support network through Smokefree's social media resources:

- Facebook—SmokefreeUS (www.facebook.com/SmokefreeUS) and Smokefree Women (www.facebook.com/smokefree.women)

- Twitter—SmokefreeUS (twitter.com/SmokefreeUS)

- Instagram—SmokefreeUS (www.instagram.com/smokefreeUS)

- Pinterest—SmokefreeUS (www.pinterest.com/SmokefreeUS)

Give your social circle a boost by connecting with other people who share your interests. Think about the things you like to do. Then start a conversation with someone new. Chances are, you will find you have things in common.

Tips for Getting Support

Here are some tips for getting support, either in person or online.

Ask for Help

You might like to solve problems on your own, but everyone can use a little help from time to time. It does not mean you are weak. If you are not sure how to ask, text a friend or send an email. You might say, "I want to quit smoking. Can you help?" Know an ex-smoker? Ask them why and how they quit.

Be Specific about What You Want

Your friends and family will not always be able to know what help you need as you quit. Be specific about what support you want and do not want. Try to be nice about it. They are just trying to do what is best for you. For example, if you are feeling stressed after a long day at work and craving a cigarette, ask a friend to help plan a smokefree night out to distract you.

Avoid Stressful Situations

Stress can make you feel like you want to smoke. Think about what stresses you most and look for ways to deal with that stress. Ask friends and family to be aware of your stressors. They can help make your life easier as you quit.

Say Thank You

Tell your friends you appreciate them, whether you speak it, text it, or show it with your actions. Saying thanks does not take a lot of time, so do it in the moment before you forget. Got a friend who gave up their last piece of gum to help you beat a cigarette craving? Buy some gum and give it to them with a note that says, "Thanks for helping me stay quit!" And being grateful has benefits for you too. Studies show that being grateful can improve physical health, mental health, and self-esteem. Being grateful also can reduce stress.

Focus on People Who Can Help

If a friendship does not feel right anymore, it might be time to let it go. Do not be afraid to try a little distance with people who are not giving you the support you need. Letting go can be hard, but it is sometimes for the best. Then focus on spending time with people who make you feel good about yourself and want you to succeed.

Invest in Your Relationships

The relationships you encourage and support the most may be the ones that are there for you the most while you quit. You will also feel more comfortable calling on them for support if the relationship is strong. You might go to a movie your friend really wants to see, even if it is not your top choice. Or go out of your way to call a friend just to chat and see how things are going.

Support Others

Support is a two-way street. If you want others to be there for you, you have to be there for them, too. Check in with your friends and help them out when you can. Sometimes small favors mean the most. Do something to brighten someone's day. Make a friend smile by emailing or texting them a joke, get someone a small treat for their birthday, or call a family member to see how they are doing. Got a quit method or quitting tip that worked for you? Post it on social media at Smoke-freeUS (www.facebook.com/SmokefreeUS) or Smokefree Women (www. facebook.com/smokefree.women). Sharing your success can be a great motivator and support for others to become smokefree.

Section 5.2

Smoking Cessation

This section includes text excerpted from "Quitting Smoking," Centers for Disease Control and Prevention (CDC), December 11, 2017.

Tobacco use can lead to tobacco/nicotine dependence and serious health problems. Quitting smoking greatly reduces the risk of developing smoking-related diseases. Tobacco/nicotine dependence is a condition that often requires repeated treatments, but there are helpful treatments and resources for quitting.

Smokers can and do quit smoking. In fact, nowadays, there are more former smokers than current smokers.

Nicotine Dependence

Most smokers become addicted to nicotine, a drug that is found naturally in tobacco. More people in the United States are addicted to nicotine than to any other drug. Research suggests that nicotine may be as addictive as heroin, cocaine, or alcohol.

Quitting smoking is hard and may require several attempts. People who stop smoking often start again because of withdrawal symptoms, stress, and weight gain.

Nicotine withdrawal symptoms may include:

• Feeling irritable, angry, or anxious

- Having trouble thinking
- Craving tobacco products
- Feeling hungrier than usual

Health Benefits of Quitting

Tobacco smoke contains a deadly mix of more than 7,000 chemicals; hundreds are harmful, and about 70 can cause cancer. Smoking increases the risk for serious health problems, many diseases, and death. People who stop smoking greatly reduce their risk for disease and early death. Although the health benefits are greater for people who stop at earlier ages, there are benefits at any age. You are never too old to quit.

Stopping smoking is associated with the following health benefits:

- Lowered risk for lung cancer and many other types of cancer
- Reduced risk for heart disease, stroke, and peripheral vascular disease (narrowing of the blood vessels outside your heart)
- Reduced heart disease risk within one to two years of quitting
- Reduced respiratory symptoms, such as coughing, wheezing, and shortness of breath. While these symptoms may not disappear, they do not continue to progress at the same rate among people who quit compared with those who continue to smoke
- Reduced risk of developing some lung diseases (such as chronic obstructive pulmonary disease, also known as "COPD," one of the leading causes of death in the United States).
- Reduced risk for infertility in women of childbearing age. Women who stop smoking during pregnancy also reduce their risk of having a low birth weight baby.

Smokers' Attempts to Quit

Among all current U.S. adult cigarette smokers, nearly 7 out of every 10 (68.0%) reported in 2015 that they wanted to quit completely. Since 2002, the number of former smokers has been greater than the number of current smokers.

Percentage of adult daily cigarette smokers who stopped smoking for more than 1 day in 2015 because they were trying to quit:

- More than 5 out of 10 (55.4%) of all adult smokers

- Nearly 7 out of 10 (66.7%) smokers aged 18 to 24 years
- Nearly 6 out of 10 (59.8%) smokers aged 25 to 44 years
- More than 4 out of 10 (49.6%) smokers aged 45 to 64 years
- About 4 out of 10 (47.2%) smokers aged 65 years or older

Percentage of high-school cigarette smokers who tried to stop smoking in the past 12 months:

- More than 4 out of 10 (45.5%) of all high-school students who smoke

Ways to Quit Smoking

Most former smokers quit without using one of the treatments that scientific research has shown can work. However, the following treatments are proven to be effective for smokers who want help to quit:

- Brief help by a doctor (such as when a doctor takes 10 minutes or less to give a patient advice and assistance about quitting)
- Individual, group, or telephone counseling
- Behavioral therapies (such as training in problem solving)
- Treatments with more person-to-person contact and more intensity (such as more or longer counseling sessions)
- Programs to deliver treatments using mobile phones

Medications for quitting that have been found to be effective include the following:

- Nicotine replacement products
- Over-the-counter (OTC) (nicotine patch (which is also available by prescription), gum, lozenge)
- Prescription (nicotine patch, inhaler, nasal spray)
- Prescription nonnicotine medications include bupropion SR (Zyban®), varenicline tartrate (Chantix®)

Counseling and medication are both effective for treating tobacco dependence, and using them together is more effective than using either one alone.

- More information is needed about quitting for people who smoke cigarettes and also use other types of tobacco.

Helpful Resources

Call 800-784-8669 if you want help quitting. This is a free telephone support service that can help people who want to stop smoking or using tobacco. Callers are routed to their state quitlines, which offer several types of quit information and services. These may include:

- Free support, advice, and counseling from experienced quitline coaches

- A personalized quit plan

- Practical information on how to quit, including ways to cope with nicotine withdrawal

- The latest information about stop-smoking medications

- Free or discounted medications (available for at least some callers in most states)

- Referrals to other resources

- Mailed self-help materials

Section 5.3

How to Reduce Passive Smoke Exposure

This section includes text excerpted from "Secondhand Smoke," Smokefree.gov, U.S. Department of Health and Human Services (HHS), June 5, 2016.

Smoking harms both you and the ones you love. Quitting smoking will benefit you plus help you protect the people in your life. Quitting will make the people you care about happier and healthier. This may be one of your reasons for quitting.

Dangers of Secondhand Smoke

The main way smoking hurts nonsmokers is through secondhand smoke. Secondhand smoke is the combination of smoke that comes from a cigarette and smoke breathed out by a smoker. When a nonsmoker is around someone smoking, they breathe in secondhand smoke.

Secondhand smoke is dangerous to anyone who breathes it in. It can stay in the air for several hours after somebody smokes. Breathing secondhand smoke for even a short time can hurt your body.

Health Effects of Secondhand Smoke

Over time, secondhand smoke has been associated with serious health problems in nonsmokers:

- Lung cancer in people who have never smoked

- More likely that someone will get heart disease, have a heart attack' and die early

- Breathing problems such as coughing' extra phlegm' wheezing' and shortness of breath

Secondhand smoke is especially dangerous for children, babies, and women who are pregnant:

- Mothers who breathe secondhand smoke while pregnant are more likely to have babies with low birth weight.

- Babies who breathe secondhand smoke after birth have more lung infections than other babies.

- Secondhand smoke causes kids who already have asthma to have more frequent and severe attacks.

- Children exposed to secondhand smoke are more likely to develop bronchitis, pneumonia, and ear infections and are at increased risk for sudden infant death syndrome (SIDS).

The only way to fully protect nonsmokers from the dangers of secondhand smoke is to not allow smoking indoors. Separating smokers from nonsmokers (such as "no smoking" sections in restaurants)' cleaning the air' and airing out buildings does not get rid of secondhand smoke.

Other Ways Smoking Affects Others

Smoking affects the people in your life in other ways, beyond their health. When you smoke, you may miss out on:

- Spending time with family and friends.

- Having more money to spend on the people you love.

- Setting a good example for your children. Children who are raised by smokers are more likely to become smokers themselves.

Steps You Can Take to Protect Your Loved Ones

The best thing you can do to protect your family from secondhand smoke is to quit smoking. Right away, you get rid of their exposure to secondhand smoke in your home and car, and reduce it anywhere else you go together.

Make sure your house and car remain smokefree. Kids breathe in secondhand smoke at home more than any other place. The same goes for many adults. Do not allow anyone to smoke in your home or car. Setting this rule will:

- Reduce the amount of secondhand smoke your family breathes in

- Help you quit smoking and stay smokefree

- Lower the chance of your child becoming a smoker

When you are on the go, you can still protect your family from secondhand smoke:

- Make sure caretakers such as nannies, babysitters, and day care staff do not smoke.

- Eat at smoke-free restaurants.

- Avoid indoor public places that allow smoking.

- Teach your children to stay away from secondhand smoke.

Chapter 6

Preventing Indoor Air Pollution

Chapter Contents

Section 6.1

Indoor Air Quality at Home

This section contains text excerpted from the following sources: Text
in this section begins with excerpts from "Protect Indoor Air Quality
in Your Home," U.S. Environmental Protection Agency (EPA), July
25, 2017; Text under the heading "Steps You Can Take to Protect
Indoor Air Quality" is excerpted from "Take Action for Climate
Readiness and Indoor Air Quality," U.S. Environmental Protection
Agency (EPA), September 13, 2017.

Whether you live in an apartment, townhome, or single-family
home, an old home or are building a new home, there are many ways
to protect and improve your indoor air quality (IAQ).

Indoor pollution sources that release gases or particles into the air
are a primary cause of IAQ problems in homes. Inadequate ventilation
can increase indoor pollutant levels by not bringing in enough fresh
outdoor air to dilute emissions from indoor sources and by not carrying
indoor air pollutants out of the home. High temperature and humidity
levels can also increase concentrations of some pollutants.

Steps You Can Take to Protect Indoor Air Quality

You can take several steps to help maintain a healthy indoor air
environment as we adapt to the challenges of climate change. Good
IAQ starts with the construction and repair of the buildings we live
and work in—good ventilation, reduction of pollutants, energy efficiency—and continues with public awareness of key steps that can be
taken to maintain a healthy indoor environment and prevent exposure
to high levels of indoor contaminants.

Many of the steps you can take to improve IAQ at home will help
resolve multiple problems at once.

- Control moisture and limit mold growth. You can manage indoor
  humidity by venting appliances that produce moisture to the
  outside. Use air conditioners and dehumidifiers when needed,
  and clean up water leaks and spills quickly.

- If you are in the market for a new home, consider a home that
  has earned the ENERGY STAR and the Indoor airPLUS label.
  ENERGY STAR-qualified homes are significantly more energy
  efficient than standard homes. Indoor airPLUS is an additional
  label that only ENERGY STAR homes can earn for including

features to help protect against moisture and mold, pests, combustion gases, and other airborne pollutants.

- Make sure you have proper ventilation in an existing home or a new home you are having built. Consider working with a contractor to determine the best ways to maintain a comfortable indoor environment and improve ventilation in your existing or new home.

Section 6.2

Indoor Air Quality in Schools

This section includes text excerpted from "Why Indoor Air Quality Is Important to Schools," U.S. Environmental Protection Agency (EPA), October 25, 2018.

Most people are aware that outdoor air pollution can impact their health, but indoor air pollution can also have significant and harmful health effects. U.S. Environmental Protection Agency (EPA) studies of human exposure to air pollutants indicate that indoor levels of pollutants may be two to five times—and occasionally more than 100 times—higher than outdoor levels. These levels of indoor air pollutants are of particular concern because most people spend about 90 percent of their time indoors. For the purposes of this guidance, the definition of good indoor air quality (IAQ) management includes:

- Control of airborne pollutants

- Introduction and distribution of adequate outdoor air

- Maintenance of acceptable temperature and relative humidity

Temperature and humidity cannot be overlooked because thermal comfort concerns underlie many complaints about "poor air quality." Furthermore, temperature and humidity are among the many factors that affect indoor contaminant levels.

Outdoor sources should also be considered since outdoor air enters school buildings through windows, doors and ventilation systems.

57

Thus, transportation and grounds maintenance activities become factors that affect indoor pollutant levels as well as outdoor air quality on school grounds.

Why Is Indoor Air Quality of Schools Important?

In recent years, comparative risk studies performed by EPA and its Science Advisory Board (SAB) have consistently ranked indoor air pollution among the top five environmental risks to public health. Good IAQ is an important component of a healthy indoor environment, and can help schools reach their primary goal of educating children.

Failure to prevent or respond promptly to IAQ problems can:

- Increase long- and short-term health problems for students and staff such as:

  - Cough

  - Eye irritation

  - Headache

  - Allergic reactions, and

  - In rarer cases, life-threatening conditions, such as Legionnaire disease, or carbon monoxide (CO) poisoning

- Aggravate asthma and other respiratory illnesses. Nearly 1 in 13 children of school-age has asthma, the leading cause of school absenteeism due to chronic illness. There is substantial evidence that indoor environmental exposure to allergens, such as dust mites, pests, and molds, plays a role in triggering asthma symptoms. These allergens are common in schools. There is also evidence that exposure to diesel exhaust from school buses and other vehicles exacerbates asthma and allergies. These problems can:

  - Impact student attendance, comfort, and performance

  - Reduce teacher and staff performance

  - Accelerate the deterioration and reduce the efficiency of the school's physical plant and equipment

  - Increase potential for school closings or relocation of occupants

  - Strain relationships among school administration, parents, and staff

- Create negative publicity
- Impact community trust
- Create liability problems

Indoor air problems can be subtle and do not always produce easily recognized impacts on health, well-being, or the physical plant. Symptoms, such as:

- Headache
- Fatigue
- Shortness of breath
- Sinus congestion
- Coughing
- Sneezing
- Dizziness
- Nausea
- Irritation of the eye, nose, throat, and skin

Symptoms are not necessarily due to air quality deficiencies, but may also be caused by other factors—poor lighting, stress, noise, and more. Due to varying sensitivities among school occupants, IAQ problems may affect a group of people or just one individual. In addition, IAQ problems may affect people in different ways.

Individuals that may be particularly susceptible to effects of indoor air contaminants include, but are not limited to, people with:

- Asthma, allergies, or chemical sensitivities
- Respiratory diseases
- Suppressed immune systems (due to radiation, chemotherapy, or disease)
- Contact lenses

Certain groups of people may be particularly vulnerable to exposures of certain pollutants or pollutant mixtures. For example:

- People with heart disease may be more adversely affected by exposure to carbon monoxide than healthy individuals.
- People exposed to significant levels of nitrogen dioxide are at higher risk for respiratory infections.

In addition, the developing bodies of children might be more susceptible to environmental exposures than those of adults. Children breathe more air, eat more food and drink more liquid in proportion to their body weight than adults. Therefore, air quality in schools is of particular concern. Proper maintenance of indoor air is more than a "quality" issue; it encompasses safety and stewardship of your investment in students, staff, and facilities.

Section 6.3

Indoor Air Quality in Workplace

This section includes text excerpted from "Indoor Air Quality," Occupational Safety and Health Administration (OSHA), October 20, 2010. Reviewed August 2019.

The quality of indoor air inside offices, schools, and other workplaces is important not only for workers' comfort but also for their health. Poor indoor air quality (IAQ) has been tied to symptoms like headaches, fatigue, trouble concentrating, and irritation of the eyes, nose, throat, and lungs. Also, some specific diseases have been linked to specific air contaminants or indoor environments, like asthma with damp indoor environments. In addition, some exposures, such as asbestos and radon, do not cause immediate symptoms but can lead to cancer after many years.

Many factors affect IAQ. These factors include poor ventilation (lack of outside air), problems controlling temperature, high or low humidity, recent remodeling, and other activities in or near a building that can affect the fresh air coming into the building. Sometimes, specific contaminants like dust from construction or renovation, mold, cleaning supplies, pesticides, or other airborne chemicals (including small amounts of chemicals released as a gas over time) may cause poor IAQ.

The right ventilation and building care can prevent and fix IAQ problems. Although Occupational Safety and Health Administration (OSHA) does not have IAQ standards, it does have standards about ventilation and standards on some of the air contaminants that can be involved in IAQ problems. OSHA responds to questions about standards with letters of interpretation. OSHA's letters of interpretation specifically addressing IAQ issues can be found in Other Resources.

Frequently Asked Questions
What Is "Indoor Air Quality"?

Indoor air quality, also called "indoor environmental quality," describes how inside air can affect a person's health, comfort, and ability to work. It can include temperature, humidity, lack of outside air (poor ventilation), mold from water damage, or exposure to other chemicals. Currently, OSHA has no IAQ standards but it does provide guidelines about the most common IAQ workplace complaints.

What Is Considered Good Indoor Air Quality?

The qualities of good IAQ should include comfortable temperature and humidity, adequate supply of fresh outdoor air, and control of pollutants from inside and outside of the building.

What Are the Most Common Causes of Indoor Air Quality Problems?

The most common causes of IAQ problems in buildings are:

- Not enough ventilation, lack of fresh outdoor air, or contaminated air being brought into the building

- Poor upkeep of ventilation, heating, and air-conditioning systems

- Dampness and moisture damage due to leaks, flooding, or high humidity

- Occupant activities, such as construction or remodeling

- Indoor and outdoor contaminated air

How Can I Tell If There Is an Indoor Air Quality Problem in My Workplace?

People working in buildings with poor IAQ may notice unpleasant or musty odors or may feel that the building is hot and stuffy. Some workers complain about symptoms that happen at work and go away when they leave work, such as having headaches or feeling tired. Fever, cough, and shortness of breath can be symptoms of a more serious problem. Asthma and some causes of pneumonia (for example, Legionnaire Disease and Hypersensitivity Pneumonitis) have been linked to IAQ problems. If you have symptoms that are not going away or are getting worse, talk to your doctor about them. But not all exposures cause symptoms, so there is no substitute for good building management.

Is There a Test That Can Find an Indoor Air Quality Problem?

There is no single test to find an IAQ problem. Your employer should check measurements of temperature, humidity, and air flow. In addition, inspection and testing of ventilation, heating and air conditioning systems (to make sure they are working according to specifications for building use and occupancy) should be performed. A building walk-through to check for odors and look for water damage, leaks, dirt, or pest droppings may be helpful. Leaks need to be eliminated. Standing water in humidifiers, air-conditioning units, on roofs, and in boiler pans can become contaminated with bacteria or fungi and need to be eliminated. In some circumstances, specific testing for radon or asbestos may be required as part of building occupancy. For instance, in schools asbestos needs to be checked every three years and re-inspected every six months (under the Asbestos Hazard Emergency Response Act (AHERA)).

What Should My Employer Be Doing to Prevent Indoor Air Quality Problems?

Employers are required to follow the General Duty Clause of the OSHA Act, which requires them to provide workers with a safe workplace that does not have any known hazards that cause or are likely to cause death or serious injury. The OSHA Act also requires employers to obey occupational safety and health standards created under it. Employers should be reasonably aware of the possible sources of poor air quality, and they should have the resources necessary to recognize and control workplace hazards. It is also their responsibility to inform employees of the immediate dangers that are present. Specific state and local regulations may apply.

Is There Any Specific Information That I Should Keep Track of to Identify Indoor Air Quality Problems at Work?

The following information may be helpful to your doctor or employer to figure out if there is an IAQ problem at your workplace:

- Do you have symptoms that just occur at work and go away when you get home? What are these symptoms?

- Are these symptoms related to a certain time of day, a certain season, or certain location at work?

- Did the symptoms start when something new happened at work, such as renovation or construction projects?

- Are there other people at work with similar complaints?

- Did you already see a doctor for your symptoms, and if so, did the doctor diagnose an illness related to IAQ?

If I Think There Is an Indoor Air Quality Problem at Work or I Think My Office or Building Where I Work Is Making Me Sick, What Can I Do?

If you are concerned about air quality at work, ask your employer to check the ventilation, heating and air conditioning systems and to make sure there is no water damage. If you think that you have symptoms that may be related to IAQ at your work, talk to your doctor about them to see if they could be caused by indoor air pollution.

Under the OSHA Act, you have the right to contact an OSHA Office or to contact OSHA's toll-free number: 800-321-6742 or TTY: 877-889-5627. Workers who would like a workplace inspection should send a written request. A worker can tell OSHA not to let their employer know who filed the complaint. It is against the Act for an employer to fire, demote, transfer, or discriminate in any way against a worker for filing a complaint or using other OSHA rights. States with OSHA-approved state plans provide the same protections to workers as federal OSHA, although they may follow slightly different complaint processing procedures.

You may also request a health hazard evaluation (HHE) from the National Institute of Occupational Safety and Health (NIOSH). At no cost to employers or workers, NIOSH may investigate workplace health hazards in response to requests from employers, employees and their representatives, and federal agencies.

Section 6.4

Using a Respirator at Work

This section contains text excerpted from the following sources: Text beginning with the heading "What Is a Respirator?" is excerpted from "NIOSH—NPPTL—Respirator Trusted-Source Information Page," National Institute for Occupational Safety and Health (NIOSH), Centers for Disease Control and Prevention (CDC), January 29, 2018; Text under the heading "What Does It Mean to be National Institute for Occupational Safety and Health-Approved?" is excerpted from "Respirator Awareness: Your Health May Depend on It," National Institute for Occupational Safety and Health (NIOSH), Centers for Disease Control and Prevention (CDC), June 2013, Reviewed August 2019; Text under the heading "Frequently Asked Questions about Respiratory Protection" is excerpted from "Filtering Out Confusion: Frequently Asked Questions about Respiratory Protection," National Institute for Occupational Safety and Health (NIOSH), Centers for Disease Control and Prevention (CDC), April 2018.

What Is a Respirator?

You may have been told by your employer that you need to wear a respirator to perform some of your workplace tasks. In fact, approximately 5 percent of all U.S. workers in about 20 percent of all work establishments wear respirators at least some of the time while performing their job functions. These workers are employed at approximately 1.3 million establishments nationwide. Approximately 900,000 of these establishments have been determined to be "very small" (i.e., having fewer than 20 employees).

A respirator is a personal protective device that is worn on the face, covers at least the nose and mouth, and is used to reduce the wearer's risk of inhaling hazardous airborne particles (including dust particles and infectious agents), gases or vapors. Respirators should only be used as a "last line of defense" in the Hierarchy of Controls when engineering and administrative controls are not feasible or are in the process of being put in place.

Respirators protect the user in two basic ways. The first type of respirator removes contaminants from the air, and are called "air-purifying respirators" (APRs). APRs include particulate respirators, which filter out airborne particles, and "gas masks," which filter out chemicals and gases. Other respirators protect by supplying clean respirable air from another source. Air-Supplying Respirators (ASRs) comprise this category of respirators. They include airline respirators, which use compressed air from a remote source; and self-contained breathing apparatus (SCBA), which include their own air supply.

The classification of particulate respirators can be further subdivided into three categories:

- **Particulate filtering facepiece respirators.** Sometimes referred to as disposable respirators because the entire respirator is discarded when it becomes unsuitable for further use due to considerations of hygiene, excessive resistance, or physical damage. These are also commonly referred to as "N95s."

- **Elastomeric respirators.** Sometimes referred to as reusable respirators because the facepiece is cleaned and reused but the filter cartridges are discarded and replaced when they become unsuitable for further use.

- **Powered air-purifying respirators (PAPRs).** A battery-powered blower moves the airflow through the filters.

What Is a National Institute for Occupational Safety and Health-Approved N95 Filtering Facepiece Respirator?

Even though you see N95 on the package, it still may not be the right kind of respirator or one that meets National Institute for Occupational Safety and Health (NIOSH) approval requirements.

You may have heard that a NIOSH-approved N95 respirator is recommended for your respiratory protection needs. This is one of the most commonly used respirators. Again, even though you see N95 on the package, it still may not be the right kind of respirator or one that meets NIOSH approval requirements.

Filtering Facepiece respirators are divided into various classes based on their filtration capabilities. "N95 respirator" is a term used to describe the class of respirators which use N95 filters to remove particles from the air that is breathed through them. The NIOSH respirator approval regulation defines the term N95 to refer to a filter class that removes at least 95 percent of airborne particles during "worst-case" testing using a "most-penetrating" sized particle during NIOSH testing. Filters meeting the criteria are given a 95 rating. Many filtering facepiece respirators have an N95 class filter and those meeting this filtration performance are often referred to simply as N95 respirators.

What Does It Mean to be National Institute for Occupational Safety and Health-Approved?

All respirators used in healthcare settings must be approved by NIOSH and are thoroughly evaluated and tested by NIOSH to meet strict federal safety requirements. To receive NIOSH approval, respirators must adhere to established standards of quality and performance. Only then will NIOSH authorize a respirator manufacturer to use the NIOSH name in block letters or a NIOSH logo on the product. Manufacturers must have and maintain an established quality program that ensures that their products meet the NIOSH requirements.

Markings on a NIOSH-approved filtering facepiece respirator may appear on the facepiece itself or on the straps and include the elements shown in Figure 6.1. If a filtering facepiece respirator has approval markings but is not on the NIOSH table of approved filtering facepiece respirators, it is likely to be either a counterfeit product or a respirator that has had its certification revoked or rescinded by NIOSH. If there is no TC number on the respirator's packaging, the user instructions, or the product itself, it is not NIOSH-approved. If you are unsure of your respirator's approval status, you can call NIOSH at 412-386-4000.

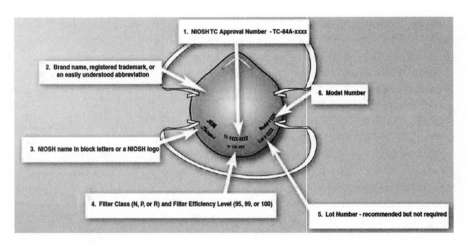

Figure 6.1. *Example of Exterior Markings on a NIOSH-Approved Filtering Facepiece Respirator*

Frequently Asked Questions about Respiratory Protection

Can Filtering Facepiece Respirators Safely be Reused?

Yes, in certain situations. Reuse refers to the practice of using the same respirator multiple times during a work shift. The respirator is stored between uses and put on (donned) again prior to the next potential exposure. In most workplace situations, an filtering facepiece respirator (FFR) can be reused as part of an employer's respiratory protection program. Safe FFR reuse is affected by a number of variables that impact respiratory function and contamination over time. Unless the respirator manufacturer identifies a specified duration of use, for example, "single use only," or the employer's respiratory protection program excludes reuse, users can wear an FFR until it is damaged, soiled, or causing noticeably increased breathing resistance.

Filtering facepiece respirators should only be reused by the same wearer and should be stored in the following ways:

- According to the manufacturer's recommendations

- In a way that protects them from damage, dust, contamination, sunlight, extreme temperatures, excessive moisture, damaging chemicals

- In a way that prevents deformation of the facepiece, straps, and exhalation valve, if present.

Regardless of the setting, the number of times an FFR is reused should be limited. There is no way of determining the maximum possible number of safe respirator reuses as a generic number to be applied in all cases.

When Employees Should Not Reuse Their Filtering Facepiece Respirators?

While limited FFR reuse is practiced safely in many workplaces, extra caution should be taken in workplaces where there are additional risks posed by handling a potentially contaminated respirator. For example, FFRs should not be reused in biosafety and animal biosafety levels two and three laboratories. Pathogens can remain on the respirator surface for extended periods of time and can potentially be transferred by touch to the wearer's hands and thus risk causing infection through subsequent touching of the mucus membranes of the face (i.e., self-inoculation). Similar to other personal protective equipment (PPE) used in these environments, such as gloves, FFRs should be discarded after each use and disposed of with other contaminated laboratory waste. There are also additional considerations when implementing FFR reuse in a healthcare setting.

How Long can Employees Wear the Same Filtering Facepiece Respirator?

Extended use refers to the practice of wearing the same respirator for repeated exposures, without removing (doffing) the respirator. Continuous or extended FFR use of several hours or more is common in many industries. In general, an employee can safely wear the same FFR until it is damaged, soiled, or causing noticeably increased breathing resistance. The maximum length of continuous use in non-dusty workplaces is typically dictated by hygienic concerns (e.g., the respirator was discarded because it became contaminated), or practical considerations that call for automatic removal and break in wearing the respirator (e.g., need to use the restroom, meal breaks, etc.), rather than a predetermined number of hours. However, for dusty workplaces that could result in high filter loading (e.g., 200 mg of material captured by the filter), service time for N-series filters (such as the commonly-used N95) should be limited to 8 hours of use (continuous or intermittent). Extensions should only be granted by performing an evaluation in specific workplace settings that:

- Demonstrates extended use will not degrade the filter efficiency below the efficiency level specified in 42 CFR Part 84, or

- Demonstrates the total mass loading of the filter(s) is less than 200 mg.

The key consideration for safe extended use is that the respirator must maintain its fit and function.

Chapter 7

Outdoor Air Pollution: Minimizing the Effects

Chapter Contents

Section 7.1

Protect Yourself and Your Family from Debris Smoke

This section includes text excerpted from "Protect Yourself and Your Family from Debris Smoke," Centers for Disease Control and Prevention (CDC), October 26, 2005. Reviewed August 2019.

Natural disasters, such as hurricanes and floods, can leave a lot of debris. Some of this debris may be burned during cleanup. Smoke from these outdoor fires is unhealthy for you to breathe.

How Debris Smoke Affects Your Health

Smoke may cause you to cough. It can cause shortness of breath or tightness in the chest. It also can sting your eyes, nose, or throat. These problems can begin a very short time after you breathe the smoke. You may have little warning, especially if you have lung or heart disease. Infants, children, pregnant women, older adults, and people with chronic diseases such as asthma are at greater risk from smoke.

Steps You Can Take to Protect Yourself and Your Family from Debris Smoke

Check with your local health and safety officials to find out when fires are planned in your area. If you smell or see smoke, or know that fires are nearby, you can take the following steps to protect yourself and your family:

- Leave the area if you are at greater risk from breathing smoke.

- Limit your exposure to smoke outdoors and indoors.

- Stay inside and use your air conditioner. If you do not have an air conditioner or smoke is likely to get inside your house, leave the area until the smoke is completely gone.

- Avoid activities that put extra demands on your lungs and heart. These include exercising or physical chores, both outdoors and indoors.

- Make sure you take all your medications according to the doctor's directions. Contact your doctor if your health gets worse.

- Dust masks, bandanas, or other cloths (even if wet) will not protect you from smoke.

Section 7.2

Understanding Urban Air Toxics

This section includes text excerpted from "Urban Air Toxics," U.S. Environmental Protection Agency (EPA), March 17, 2017.

What Are Urban Air Toxics?

Air toxics, also known as "toxic air pollutants" or "hazardous air pollutants," (HAPs) are those pollutants that cause or may cause cancer or other serious health effects, such as reproductive effects or birth defects, or adverse environmental and ecological effects.

The Clean Air Act (CAA), 42 U.S.C. § 7401, identifies 187 hazardous air pollutants HAPs that U.S. Environmental Protection Agency (EPA) is required to control to protect public health. More specifically, to address HAPs in urban areas, section 112(k) of the CAA directs EPA to:

- Identify a subset of 30 HAPs that present the greatest threat to public health in the largest number of urban areas. These 30 HAPs are known as the "30 urban air toxics."

- Identify area sources that represent 90 percent of the combined emissions of the 30 urban air toxics, and subject these sources to regulation. The EPA identified 68 area source categories of urban air toxics.

Health Effects of Urban Air Toxics

Air toxics tend to pose greater risks in urban areas because these areas have large populations and a higher concentration of emission sources. Combined exposures from all sources of air pollution, including major stationary sources, smaller area sources, indoor sources, and mobile sources can increase public health risks from air toxics. Low-income neighborhoods, tribal populations and communities of color that live in urban areas may be disproportionately exposed to air pollution, which is a barrier to economic opportunity and security.

Urban Air Toxic Pollutants

Of the 187 hazardous air pollutants (HAPs) that EPA is required to control, they have identified 30 that pose the greatest potential health threat in urban areas. These HAPs are referred to as the 30 urban air toxics. EPA also identified an additional three HAPs, but these HAPs are not generally emitted by area sources and, as such, were not included as part of the 30 urban air toxics. The three additional HAPs are coke oven emissions, 1,2-dibromoethane, and carbon tetrachloride.

Table 7.1. List of 30 Urban Air Toxics

Acetaldehyde	Dioxin	Mercury Compounds
Acrolein	Propylene dichloride	Methylene chloride (dichloromethane)
Acrylonitrile	1,3-dichloropropene	Nickel compounds
Arsenic compounds	Ethylene dichloride (1,2-dichloroethane)	Polychlorinated biphenyls (PCBs)
Benzene	Ethylene oxide	Polycyclic organic matter (POM)
Beryllium compounds	Formaldehyde	Quinoline
1,3-butadiene	Hexachlorobenzene	1,1,2,2-tetrachloroethane
Cadmium compounds	Hydrazine	Tetrachloroethylene (perchloroethylene)
Chloroform	Lead compounds	Trichloroethylene
Chromium compounds	Manganese compounds	Vinyl chloride

Section 7.3

Air Quality and Your Health

This section includes text excerpted from "Bad Air Day,"
NIH News in Health, National Institutes of Health (NIH),
July 2011. Reviewed August 2019.

In many parts of the country, summer has the worst air quality of any season. When the forecast says it is a code red day for air quality, what does it mean for your health? If you have planned a picnic, a bike ride or even a walk with a friend, should you change your plans?

"The answer depends on a lot of factors. There is no simple 'yes' or 'no' answer for everyone," says Dr. Darryl Zeldin, acting clinical director of environmental health sciences at National Institutes of Health (NIH). He and other NIH-supported researchers have been studying how substances in the air can affect health. Knowing more about air quality and air alerts will help you make smart decisions about spending time outside this summer.

The combination of high temperatures, few winds and breezes, pollution and airborne particles can brew up an unhealthful mixture in the air, just waiting to enter your lungs. These substances can make it hard to breathe and can sap your energy. If the air quality is especially poor, it may take a few days for your body to recover. And if you are regularly exposed to high levels of unhealthy air, the health consequences can linger for months or even years.

One of the most-studied pollutants in summertime air is an invisible gas called "ozone." It is created when sunlight triggers a chemical reaction between oxygen-containing molecules and pollution that comes from cars, power plants, factories, and other sources.

"Ozone is produced only when you have sunlight and high temperatures or stagnant air, which is why ozone is generally not a problem in the winter," says Dr. Frank Gilliland, an expert in environmental health at the University of Southern California. "High levels of ozone reduce lung function and lead to inflammation, or swelling, in the airways. When the levels are high enough, you can get symptoms such as coughing or throat irritation. Your eyes might water. Your chest might hurt when you breathe."

Ozone is a highly reactive molecule that can irritate the lining of your airways and lungs. If you have a lung condition like asthma, the damage can be more harmful. "When people with poorly controlled asthma are exposed to just a little bit of ozone, the amount of inflammation in the lungs goes way up, and the airways become more twitchy," says Zeldin. "As a result, air passages narrow, which makes it harder to breathe."

Ozone's effects can come on quickly and linger or even worsen with time. "When people hear it will be a bad-air day, most expect their breathing will be affected that day. But in fact, they often feel the effects most strongly the next day or the day after," says Dr. David Peden, an environmental medicine researcher at the University of North Carolina at Chapel Hill. "This is especially true for people with asthma. When there is a bump in ozone levels, asthma usually gets worse or out of control a day or two after exposure. We often see an increase in emergency room visits, hospitalizations, and use of asthma 'rescue' medications."

Researchers have also been studying particulates—the fine and coarse particles that spew from things that burn fuel, such as cars, power plants, and wildfires. Particulates, unlike ozone, can cause health problems year-round. Like ozone, particulates have been linked to a worsening of lung problems, especially asthma. Particulates and ozone also are associated with increased cardiovascular events, such as stroke and heart attack.

Studies by Gilliland and his colleagues have found that children living near busy roadways—surrounded by particulate air pollution— are more likely to develop asthma and other breathing disorders. "We have found it can affect lung development substantially in children," Gilliland says. "We also found that particulate pollution can affect the development of atherosclerosis in adults, and it is associated with cognitive decline in the elderly."

Several NIH-funded research teams have found that genes may affect your response to air pollution. At least one gene seems to protect against the harmful effects of ozone. Unfortunately, up to 40 percent of the population lacks a working copy of this helpful gene, so they are more susceptible to ozone damage. "About 24 hours after exposure to ozone, these people have much more inflammation in the airways compared to those who have a working copy of the gene," says Peden. Researchers are now looking for ways to protect these susceptible people from the damage caused by ozone.

Fortunately, air quality monitors have been set up at over a thousand locations across the country to measure the levels of major pollutants. These daily and sometimes hourly measurements are widely reported in newspapers and on TV, radio, and the Internet. To help make sense of the data, the U.S. Environmental Protection Agency (EPA) has developed a tool called the "Air Quality Index" (AQI). The

AQI can tell you how clean or polluted the air is in your area so you can make informed decisions about the best way to protect your health.

The AQI assesses different types of air pollution, including ozone, particulates, and sulfur dioxide. Depending on the levels, each pollutant is assigned a color-coded AQI category ranging from 0, which is green or "good," up to 300, which is purple or "very unhealthy." Usually, the pollutant with the highest levels is reported as the AQI value for that day.

In general, any time the AQI is forecast to hit above 100—that means code orange, red or purple—consider adjusting your activities to reduce exposure to air pollution. "On orange days you should limit prolonged outdoor activities if you have an underlying lung condition like asthma or are in a sensitive group, including children and older adults," says Zeldin. "On red alert days, you should avoid being active outdoors during peak ozone hours, even if you are in pretty good health. If you can, put off mowing the yard or going for a run until later in the evening—or even go first thing in the morning before sunrise and all the traffic starts." Ozone levels tend to peak between mid-afternoon and early evening.

If you want to exercise outside on days when you are at risk, consider reducing the time and intensity of your workout. If you usually jog for 45 minutes, try walking for a half-hour instead. Avoid jogging or biking on roads with heavy traffic. Of course, the best way to reduce exposure to outdoor air is to exercise indoors, at home or in a gym.

If you plan to be outside, track air quality in your area by checking newspapers, listening to the radio, or visiting online sites such as www.airnow.gov. If you have asthma or other lung conditions, you need to be extra cautious when air quality is poor.

Chapter 8

Statistics on Respiratory Disorders

Chapter Contents

Section 8.1

Overview of Respiratory Disease Statistics

This section includes text excerpted from "Respiratory Diseases,"
Office of Disease Prevention and Health Promotion (ODPHP), U.S.
Department of Health and Human Services (HHS), June 19, 2019.

Asthma and chronic obstructive pulmonary disease (COPD) are significant public-health burdens. Specific methods of detection, intervention, and treatment exist that may reduce this burden and promote health.

Asthma is a chronic inflammatory disorder of the airways characterized by episodes of reversible breathing problems due to airway narrowing and obstruction. These episodes can range in severity from mild to life-threatening. Symptoms of asthma include wheezing, coughing, chest tightness, and shortness of breath. Daily preventive treatment can prevent symptoms and attacks and enable individuals who have asthma to lead active lives.

Chronic obstructive pulmonary disease is a preventable and treatable disease characterized by airflow limitation that is not fully reversible. The airflow limitation is usually progressive and associated with an abnormal inflammatory response of the lungs to noxious particles or gases (typically from exposure to cigarette smoke). Treatment can lessen symptoms and improve quality of life for those with COPD.

Why Are Respiratory Diseases Important?

As of now more than 25 million people in the United States have asthma. Approximately 14.8 million adults have been diagnosed with COPD, and approximately 12 million people have not yet been diagnosed. The burden of respiratory diseases affects individuals and their families, schools, workplaces, neighborhoods, cities, and states. Because of the cost to the healthcare system, the burden of respiratory diseases also falls on society; it is paid for with tax dollars, higher health insurance rates, and lost productivity. Annual healthcare expenditures for asthma alone are estimated at $20.7 billion.

Asthma

The prevalence of asthma has increased since 1980. However, deaths from asthma have decreased since the mid-1990s. The causes of asthma are an active area of research and involve both genetic and environmental factors.

Risk factors for asthma currently being investigated include:

- Having a parent with asthma
- Sensitization to irritants and allergens
- Respiratory infections in childhood
- Overweight

Asthma affects people of every race, sex, and age. However, significant disparities in asthma morbidity and mortality exist, particularly for low-income and minority populations. Populations with higher rates of asthma include:

- Children
- Women (among adults) and boys (among children)
- African Americans
- Puerto Ricans
- People living in the northeastern United States
- People living below the federal poverty level
- Employees with certain exposures in the workplace

While there is currently no cure for asthma, there are diagnosis and treatment guidelines that are aimed at ensuring that all people with asthma live full and active lives.

Chronic Obstructive Pulmonary Disease

Chronic obstructive pulmonary disease is the fourth leading cause of death in the United States. In 2014, approximately 142,000 individuals died from COPD, and almost as many died from lung cancer (approximately 155,500) in the same year. In nearly 8 out of 10 cases, COPD is caused by exposure to cigarette smoke. Other environmental exposures (such as those in the workplace) may also cause COPD.

Genetic factors strongly influence the development of the disease. For example, not all smokers develop COPD. Quitting smoking may slow the progression of the disease. Women and men are affected equally, yet more women than men have died of COPD since 2000.

Section 8.2

Asthma Stats

This section includes text excerpted from "Asthma Facts,"
U.S. Environmental Protection Agency (EPA), May 2018.

Asthma continues to be a serious public-health problem in the
United States.

According to the Centers for Disease Control and Prevention's
(CDC) 2015 and 2016 *National Health Interview Surveys* (NHIS):

- An estimated 24.6 million people, including 6.1 million children,
  have asthma.

- More than 11.5 million people with asthma, including nearly 3
  million children, report having had one or more asthma attacks
  in 2015.

Uncontrolled asthma is a common reason people seek medical
attention.

- The 2010 *National Hospital Ambulatory Medical Care Survey*
  (NHAMCS) reported 1.3 million outpatient department visits
  with asthma as the primary diagnosis.

- The 2012 NHAMCS reported 10.5 million physician office visits
  with asthma as the primary diagnosis.

- The NHAMCS: 2014 emergency department summary tables
  showed that asthma was the primary diagnosis for more than
  2.0 million emergency department visits.

- The 2011 to 2012 *National Survey for Children's Health* (NSCH)
  reported that children who have asthma (3.4%) are more likely
  to use a hospital emergency department as their usual place for
  medical care than children without asthma (2.1%).

Asthma is a common chronic disease in children.

- In 2016, the prevalence of asthma in children was 8.3 percent,
  meaning about 1 in 12 children had asthma.

- In 2013, approximately 13.8 million missed school days were
  reported due to asthma.

Non-Hispanic Blacks have a higher asthma mortality rate than
people of other races or ethnicities.

- According to the CDC's 2015 summary of *Asthma Mortality Data*, Black Americans have a higher asthma death rate, at 23.9 deaths per million persons, than non-Hispanic whites (8.4 deaths per million persons), Hispanics (7.3 deaths per million persons), and other non-Hispanics (10.0 deaths per million persons).

The economic costs of asthma are high.

- The annual economic cost of asthma in 2007, including medical costs and lost school and work days, amounted to more than $56 billion.

- In 2012, the median annual medical cost of asthma was $983 per child, with a range of $833 in Arizona to $1,121 in Michigan.

Reducing exposure to environmental factors, such as indoor asthma triggers, is important for asthma management. On average, Americans spend about 90 percent of their time indoors. Indoor environmental factors called "asthma triggers," such as dust mites, mold, cockroaches, pet dander, and secondhand smoke, can exacerbate asthma symptoms.

With an asthma action plan that includes medical treatment and control of environmental triggers, people with asthma can lead healthy, active lives.

Section 8.3

Chronic Obstructive Pulmonary Disease Stats

This section includes text excerpted from "Chronic Obstructive Pulmonary Disease (COPD) Includes: Chronic Bronchitis and Emphysema," Centers for Disease Control and Prevention (CDC), May 3, 2017.

This section provides statistics on chronic obstructive pulmonary disease (COPD), including chronic bronchitis and emphysema.

Morbidity

- Number of adults with diagnosed chronic bronchitis in the past year: 8.6 million

- Percent of adults with diagnosed chronic bronchitis in the past year: 3.5 percent

- Number of adults who have ever been diagnosed with emphysema: 3.4 million

- Percent of adults who have ever been diagnosed with emphysema: 1.4 percent

Physician Office Visits

- Percent of visits to office-based physicians with COPD indicated on the medical record: 3.6 percent

Emergency Department Visits

- Percent of visits to emergency departments with COPD indicated on the medical record: 5.6 percent

Mortality

- Number of deaths from chronic lower respiratory diseases (including asthma): 154,596

- Chronic lower respiratory diseases (including asthma) deaths per 100,000 population: 47.8

- Cause of death rank: 4

- Number of bronchitis (chronic and unspecified) deaths: 518

- Bronchitis (chronic and unspecified) deaths per 100,000 population: 0.2

- Number of emphysema deaths: 6,977

- Emphysema deaths per 100,000 population: 2.2

- Number of deaths from other chronic lower respiratory diseases (excluding asthma): 143,583

- Other chronic lower respiratory diseases (excluding asthma) deaths per 100,000 population: 44.4

Section 8.4

Lung and Bronchus Cancer

This section includes text excerpted from "Cancer Stat Facts: Lung and Bronchus Cancer," Surveillance, Epidemiology, and End Results Program (SEER), National Cancer Institute (NCI), April 16, 2019.

Statistics at a Glance

Table 8.1. Lung and Bronchus Cancer Statistics

Estimated New Cases in 2019	228,150
Percent of All New Cancer Cases	12.9 percent
Estimated Deaths in 2019	142,670
Percent of All Cancer Deaths	23.5 percent
Percent Surviving 5 Years (2009 to 2015)	19.4 percent

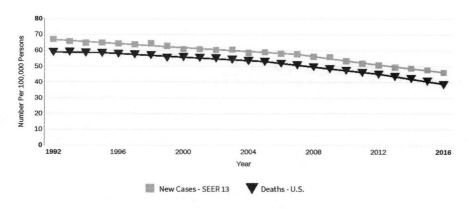

Figure 8.1. *Lung and Bronchus Cancer Statistics*

Number of New Cases and Deaths per 100,000

The number of new cases of lung and bronchus cancer was 54.9 per 100,000 men and women per year. The number of deaths was 41.9 per 100,000 men and women per year. These rates are age-adjusted and based on 2012 to 2016 cases and deaths.

83

Lifetime Risk of Developing Lung and Bronchus Cancer

Approximately 6.3 percent of men and women will be diagnosed with lung and bronchus cancer at some point during their lifetime, based on 2014 to 2016 data.

Prevalence of Lung and Bronchus Cancer

In 2016, there were an estimated 538,243 people living with lung and bronchus cancer in the United States.

Survival Statistics
How Many People Survive Five Years or More after Being Diagnosed with Lung and Bronchus Cancer?

Relative survival statistics compare the survival of patients diagnosed with cancer with the survival of people in the general population who are the same age, race, and sex and who have not been diagnosed with cancer. Because survival statistics are based on large groups of people, they cannot be used to predict exactly what will happen to an individual patient. No two patients are exactly alike, and treatment and responses to treatment can vary greatly.

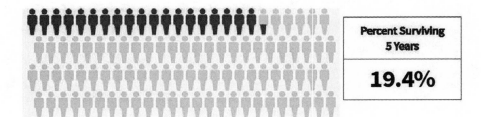

Figure 8.2. *Percent Surviving Being Diagnosed with Lung and Bronchus Cancer*

Based on data from Surveillance, Epidemiology, and End Results Program (SEER) 18 2009 to 2015. Gray figures represent those who have died from lung and bronchus cancer.

Survival by Stage

Cancer stage at diagnosis, which refers to the extent of a cancer in the body, determines treatment options and has a strong influence on the length of survival. In general, if the cancer is found only in the part of the body where it started it is localized (sometimes referred to as "stage 1") If it has spread to a different part of the body, the stage is regional or distant. The earlier lung and bronchus cancer is caught, the better chance a person has of surviving five years after being diagnosed. For lung and bronchus cancer, 16.4 percent are diagnosed at the local stage. The 5-year survival for localized lung and bronchus cancer is 57.4 percent.

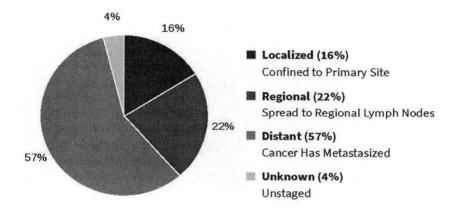

Figure 8.3. *Percent of Cases by Stage*

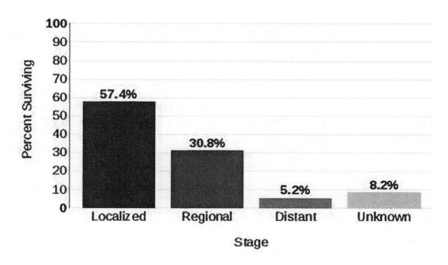

Figure 8.4. *Five-Year Relative Survival*

Surveillance, Epidemiology, and End Results Program (SEER) 2009 to 2015, All Races, Both Sexes by SEER Summary Stage 2000.

Number of New Cases and Deaths
How Common Is Lung and Bronchus Cancer?

Compared to other cancers, lung and bronchus cancer is fairly common.

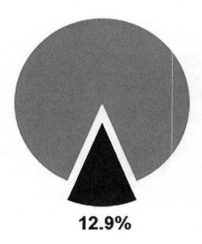

12.9%

Figure 8.5. *Percentage of New Lung and Bronchus Cancer Cases in the United States*

Lung and bronchus cancer represents 12.9 percent of all new cancer cases in the United States.

Table 8.2. How Common Lung and Bronchus Cancer Is

Rank	Common Types of Cancer	Estimated New Cases 2019	Estimated Deaths 2019
1	Breast Cancer (Female)	268,600	41,760
2	Lung and Bronchus Cancer	228,150	142,670
3	Prostate Cancer	174,650	31,620
4	Colorectal Cancer	145,600	51,020
5	Melanoma of the Skin	96,480	7,230
6	Bladder Cancer	80,470	17,670
7	Non-Hodgkin Lymphoma	74,200	19,970
8	Kidney and Renal Pelvis Cancer	73,820	14,770
9	Uterine Cancer	61,880	12,160
10	Leukemia	61,780	22,840

Who Gets Lung and Bronchus Cancer

Lung cancer is more common in women than men, particularly African American men. Smoking is widely recognized as the leading cause of lung cancer. The number of new cases of lung and bronchus cancer was 54.9 per 100,000 women and men per year based on 2012 to 2016 cases.

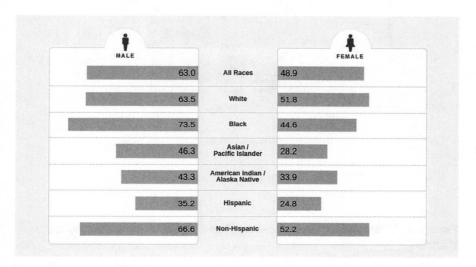

Figure 8.6. *Number of New Cases per 100,000 Persons by Race/Ethnicity and Sex: Lung and Bronchus Cancer*

Surveillance, Epidemiology, and End Results Program (SEER) 2012 to 2016, Age-Adjusted

Who Dies from Lung and Bronchus Cancer

Death rates for lung cancer are higher among the middle-aged and older populations. Lung and bronchus cancer is the leading cause of cancer death in the United States. The number of deaths was 41.9 per 100,000 women and men per year based on 2012 to 2016 deaths.

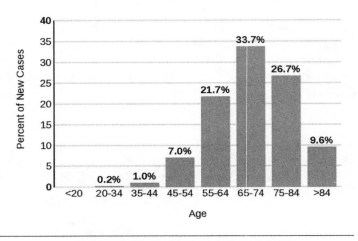

Lung and bronchus cancer is most frequently diagnosed among people aged 65-74.

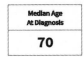

Figure 8.7. *Percent of New Cases by Age Group: Lung and Bronchus Cancer*

Surveillance, Epidemiology, and End Results Program (SEER) 2012 to 2016, All Races, Both Sexes

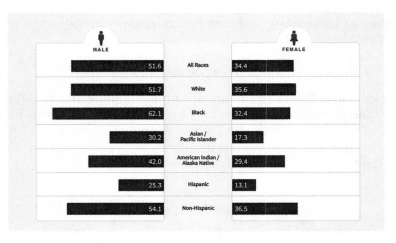

Figure 8.8. *Number of Deaths*

U.S. 2012 to 2016, Age-Adjusted

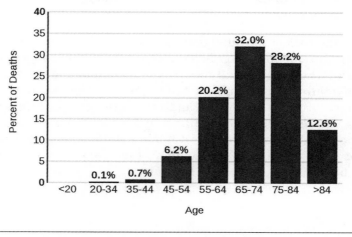

The percent of lung and bronchus cancer deaths is highest among people aged 65-74.

Median Age At Death
72

Figure 8.9. *Percent of Deaths by Age Group: Lung and Bronchus Cancer*
U.S. 2012 to 2016, All Races, Both Sexes

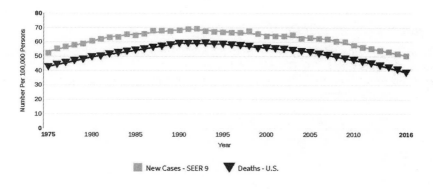

Figure 8.10. *New Cases and Deaths*

New cases come from Surveillance, Epidemiology, and End Results Program (SEER) Incidence. Deaths come from U.S. Mortality. 1975 to 2016. All races, both sexes. Rates are age-adjusted.
Modeled trend lines were calculated from the underlying rates using the Joinpoint Trend Analysis Software.

Trends in Rates
Changes over Time

Keeping track of the number of new cases, deaths, and survival over time (trends) can help scientists understand whether progress is being made and where additional research is needed to address challenges, such as improving screening or finding better treatments.

Using statistical models for analysis, rates for new lung and bronchus cancer cases have been falling on average 2.3 percent each year over the last 10 years. Death rates have been falling on average 2.9 percent each year over 2007 to 2016. Five-year survival trends are shown below.

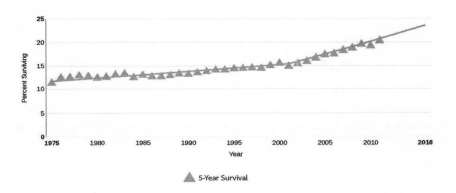

Figure 8.11. *Five-Year Relative Survival*

Surveillance, Epidemiology, and End Results Program (SEER) 5-Year Relative Survival percent from 1975 to 2011, All races, both sexes.
Modeled trend lines were calculated from the underlying rates using the Joinpoint Survival Model Software.

Section 8.5

Tuberculosis—United States, 2018

This section includes text excerpted from
"Tuberculosis—United States, 2018," Centers for
Disease Control and Prevention (CDC), March 21, 2019.

In 2018, a total of 9,029 new tuberculosis (TB) cases were reported in the United States, representing a 0.7 percent decrease from 2017. The U.S. TB incidence in 2018 (2.8 per 100,000 persons) represented a 1.3 percent decrease from 2017; the rate among non-U.S.-born persons was greater than 14 times of that in U.S.-born persons. Although the total number of cases and incidence are the lowest ever reported in the United States, it has been predicted that the U.S. TB elimination goal (annual incidence of less than one case per one million persons) will not be attained in the 21st century without greatly increased investment in detection and treatment of latent TB infection (LTBI) programs to identify, test, and treat populations at high risk for TB remain important to eliminating TB in the United States.

The health departments in the 50 states and in the District of Columbia (DC) electronically report provisional case data that meet the national TB surveillance case definition to the Centers for Disease Control and Prevention (CDC). Data reported include demographic information (e.g., birth date, sex, self-reported race/ethnicity, and country of birth), clinical information (e.g., reason for TB evaluation, anatomic site of disease, test results, and therapy administered), and information on TB risk factors (e.g., human immunodeficiency virus (HIV) infection status, history of homelessness, and residence in a congregate setting). According to U.S. Census Bureau definitions, a "U.S.-born" person is classified as one born in the United States, or a U.S. territory, or born abroad to a U.S. citizen parent. Race/ethnicity data are collected and reported using federal classification standards; Hispanics/ Latinx can be of any race, and all other reported race categories are non-Hispanic/Latinx. The CDC derived the denominators used to calculate national and state TB incidence from July 2018 U.S. Census Bureau population estimates and the denominators used to calculate TB incidence by national origin and race/ethnicity from July 2018 Current Population Survey data. The number of reported TB cases and TB incidence (cases per 100,000 persons) for 2017 and 2018, as well as the percent changes from 2017 to 2018, were calculated for the 50 states and DC and for each U.S.

91

Census Bureau division. The numbers of TB cases and TB incidence per 100,000 persons were calculated by national origin and race/ethnicity for 2015 to 2018.

Tuberculosis incidence declined 1.3 percent from 2017 to 2018 and an average of 1.6 percent per year between 2014 and 2018, a slower pace of decline than the 4.7 percent annual decline during 2010 to 2014. State-specific TB incidence for 2018 ranged from 0.2 per 100,000 in Wyoming to 8.5 in Alaska, with a median rate of 1.9. Ten states (Alaska, California, Florida, Hawaii, Maryland, Massachusetts, Minnesota, New Jersey, New York, and Texas) and DC reported TB incidence above the national rate. As has been the case for over two decades, four states (California, Florida, New York, and Texas) accounted for approximately half of the reported cases of TB in the United States.

Among the 9,029 TB cases reported in the United States in 2018, approximately two thirds (6,276 (69.5%)) occurred in non-U.S.-born persons, whereas 2,662 (29.5%) occurred in U.S.-born persons; 91 (1.0%) cases occurred in persons for whom no national origin was documented. This distribution is similar to that in 2017, when 6,392 (70.3%) cases occurred in non-U.S.-born persons, 2,693 (29.6%) occurred in U.S.-born persons, and 9 (0.1%) occurred in persons for whom no national origin was documented. TB incidence among non-U.S.-born persons (14.2 cases per 100,000) decreased by 3.8 percent from 2017 to 2018, and the incidence among U.S.-born persons (1.0 cases per 100,000) decreased by 1.8 percent.

Among non-U.S.-born persons with TB, incidence in 2018 was highest among Asians, followed by Native Hawaiians/Pacific Islanders, non-Hispanic Blacks (Blacks), Hispanics, and American Indian/Alaska Natives, and was lowest among non-Hispanic Whites (Whites). Among TB cases in non-U.S.-born persons, incidence decreased from 2017 to 2018 among Asians, Blacks, and Whites, but increased in Hispanics. The top five countries of birth of non-U.S.-born persons with TB were Mexico (1,195 cases; 19.0% of all non-U.S.-born cases), Philippines (781; 12.4%), India (616; 9.8%), Vietnam (503; 8.0%), and China (374; 6.0%). Among TB cases in non-U.S.-born persons, 2,905 (46.3%) were diagnosed greater than or equal to 10 years after the patient first arrived in the United States.

The highest TB incidence for U.S.-born persons occurred among Native Hawaiians/Pacific Islanders, followed by American Indians/Alaska Natives, Blacks, Asians, and Hispanics, and was lowest in Whites. Among U.S.-born persons, TB incidence decreased from 2017 to 2018 among Blacks, but remained stable among Asians, Hispanics, and Whites.

During 2018, 4.1 percent of TB cases were reported among persons who experienced homelessness within the year preceding diagnosis, 3.3 percent among residents of a correctional facility at the time of diagnosis, and 1.6 percent among residents of a long-term care facility at the time of diagnosis. Among cases diagnosed in persons who experienced homelessness and among residents of long-term care facilities, 60.8 percent and 56.8 percent, respectively, were in persons who were U.S.-born, whereas among residents of a correctional facility, only 33.6 percent were U.S.-born. HIV status was known for 85.3 percent of TB cases reported in 2018. Overall, 5.3 percent of TB patients with known HIV status were coinfected with HIV, including 8.6 percent among persons aged 25 to 44 years.

Initial drug-susceptibility testing for at least isoniazid and rifampin was performed for 73.5 percent of all TB cases (and 93.8% of culture-confirmed cases) in 2017, the most recent year for which complete data are available. Among the 6,684 TB cases reported in 2017 with available drug-susceptibility testing results, 128 (1.9%) were multidrug-resistant TB. Of these multidrug-resistant TB cases, 110 (85.9%) were in non-U.S.-born persons; 26 (20.3%) multidrug-resistant TB patients reported a previous episode of TB. Three cases of extensively drug-resistant TB were reported, all of which occurred in non-U.S.-born persons.

Discussion

In 2018, the provisional TB case count and incidence for the United States declined slightly, compared with those in 2017. Lower counts and incidences were seen in U.S.-born persons as well as in non-U.S.-born persons, who continue to represent a large majority of TB cases and have an incidence greater than 14 times that of U.S.-born persons.

In 2018, approximately half (46.3%) of TB cases in non-U.S.-born persons received a TB diagnosis greater than or equal to 10 years after first arriving in the United States, consistent with a published estimate that reactivation of remotely acquired LTBI has been responsible for greater than 80 percent of domestic TB cases. Therefore, TB elimination will require a concerted effort to enhance surveillance, detection, and treatment for LTBI among populations at increased risk.

Between 3.1 percent and 5.0 percent of the U.S. population has LTBI. Without treatment, 5 to 10 percent of persons with LTBI will develop TB disease in their lifetime. The CDC and the U.S. Preventive Services Task Force (USPSTF) recommend testing populations that are at increased risk for TB, including persons born in or who frequently travel to countries where TB is prevalent and persons who currently live, or previously lived, in congregate settings. The CDC also recommends testing for TB in healthcare workers and others who work in places where there is a high risk of TB transmission, persons who are contacts of a person with infectious TB disease, and immunocompromised persons, who have a higher risk for developing TB disease once infected. According to one model, increased uptake of LTBI screening and treatment among populations at higher risk for TB would result in an incidence of 26 new infections per million by 2050. Detection of LTBI can be improved by the preferential use of interferon-γ release assays over the tuberculin skin test, especially in persons with a history of Bacillus Calmette-Guérin vaccination or who are unlikely to return to have their tuberculin skin test read. In addition, the adoption of shorter, safer, and more convenient LTBI treatment regimens continues to be critical in improving treatment initiation and completion. Therefore, the CDC recommends either three months of once-weekly rifapentine plus isoniazid or four months of daily rifampin for treatment of LTBI; these regimens may be used instead of longer courses of isoniazid alone. Given that the estimated prevalence of LTBI is higher among non-U.S.-born persons and that rates of TB disease are much higher in this group, the detection and treatment of LTBI among non-U.S.-born persons should be prioritized. The CDC is working with its state and local partners to develop an LTBI surveillance system to track the effectiveness of public health measures to address LTBI.

There are two limitations to the findings. First, this analysis is limited to the reported provisional number of TB cases and incidence for 2018. Second, incidences are calculated using estimated population numbers as denominators.

TB case counts and incidence in the United States in 2018 are the lowest ever reported, but this progress has slowed recently. To achieve TB elimination, the United States must expand the detection and treatment of LTBI and TB disease. TB is a global problem, and its elimination will depend on cooperative measures to detect and treat LTBI and TB disease around the world.

Chapter 9

Research on Respiratory Disorders

Chapter Contents

Section 9.1

Inhaled Corticosteroids and Its Effect on Patients with Mild Persistent Asthma and Low Sputum Eosinophils

This section includes text excerpted from "Large Portion of Patients with Mild Persistent Asthma and Low Sputum Eosinophils Respond Equally Well to Inhaled Corticosteroids as Placebo," National Institutes of Health (NIH), May 19, 2019.

A study of nearly 300 patients with mild persistent asthma found that inhaled steroids—long considered the gold standard for asthma treatment—were no more effective than placebo in nearly three-fourths of the study patients, all over age 12. Inhaled steroids were better than placebo for a subset of the patients who had high levels of a particular type of inflammatory cells, called "eosinophils," in their sputum, but they represented about a fourth of patients enrolled in the trial.

The study was funded by the National Heart, Lung, and Blood Institute (NHLBI), part of the National Institutes of Health (NIH), and appeared online on May 19 in the *New England Journal of Medicine* (NEJM). The publication coincides with the study's presentation at the international conference of the American Thoracic Society, which takes place in Dallas.

The research highlights the need for developing more effective treatments for asthma and suggests that it may be possible to target particular therapies to subsets of patients, such as those with high or low eosinophils. New approaches to treating the "low eosinophil" group could be especially helpful for improving the overall effectiveness of treatments for mild asthma, the most common type of this respiratory condition.

"We are intrigued by the results of this study and believe it raises questions about the way doctors manage mild persistent asthma," said Stephen Lazarus, M.D., lead study author and a professor of medicine at the University of California, San Francisco. "We are not saying that steroids are unimportant for mild asthma, but our study does suggest that treatment guidelines should be re-evaluated for patients with mild persistent asthma who have low sputum eosinophils."

James Kiley, Ph.D., director of the Division of Lung Diseases at NHLBI, said the research underscored the value of customizing treatments to help people with asthma. "This study adds to a growing body of evidence that different patients with mild asthma should be treated differently, perhaps using biomarkers like sputum eosinophils to select which drugs should be used—a precision medicine approach," he said.

Asthma affects nearly 25 million Americans, according to the Centers for Disease Control and Prevention (CDC). Despite significant research strides, increasing numbers of people continue to have poorly controlled asthma. Mild persistent asthma is characterized by symptoms, such as coughing, wheezing, and chest tightness, symptoms that occur less frequently than in people with severe asthma and are generally easier to control with steroids. However, daily steroid use can have adverse side effects over time, including weight gain and diabetes, and, at $200 to $400 per inhaler, can be expensive. A growing number of studies suggest that it may be possible to manage mild persistent asthma safely without daily steroid use.

In the quest to improve treatments for this type of asthma, researchers in the current study focused on sputum eosinophils, white blood cells (WBCs) found in the lung that can serve as biomarkers of airway inflammation. Biomarkers are generally used to guide treatment only in the most severe forms of asthma. Past studies have estimated that about half of the population with mild persistent asthma have less than two percent sputum eosinophils and that most people with low eosinophils do not respond well to steroid treatment. But laboratory tests to measure sputum eosinophils are relatively complex and not routinely used in most clinics.

The multicenter study included 295 people over the age of 12 with mild persistent asthma. The researchers further divided the group based on low or high sputum eosinophil levels (low equals to less than 2%; high equal to greater than or equal to 2%). The researchers assigned the participants in random sequence to three treatment groups for 12-week periods: inhaled steroids; long-acting muscarinic antagonists (LAMA), a nonsteroidal treatment for uncontrolled asthma; or placebo. By the end of the study, every participant had received each treatment. The inhaled steroid used in this study was mometasone and the LAMA drug was tiotropium.

The researchers were surprised to find that nearly 73 percent of the participants, or 221 people, were classified as having low sputum eosinophils, a much higher frequency than expected. Among those participants who were classified as "Eos-low," the number who responded better to active treatment with steroids was no different than the number who responded better to placebo. By contrast, those who were classified as "Eos-high" were nearly three times as likely to respond to inhaled steroids than placebo.

Among those who were 'Eos-low' and had a better response to one of the treatments, 60 percent had superior results on LAMA, versus 40 percent who had better symptom control on placebo. While Lazarus cautioned that this difference is not large enough to conclude that patients are more likely to do better on LAMA drugs, he said it does highlight the need to study alternatives to inhaled steroids in mild asthma.

Section 9.2

Long-Term Oxygen Treatment Does Not Benefit Some COPD Patients

This section includes text excerpted from "Long-Term Oxygen Treatment Does Not Benefit Some COPD Patients," National Institutes of Health (NIH), October 27, 2016.

The data from the Long-Term Oxygen Treatment Trial (LOTT) show that oxygen use is not beneficial for most people with chronic obstructive pulmonary disease (COPD) and moderately low levels of blood oxygen. It neither boosted their survival nor reduced hospital admissions for study participants. Previous research showed that long-term oxygen treatment improves survival in those with COPD and severely low levels of blood oxygen. However, a long-standing question remained whether a different group of COPD patients—those with moderately low levels of blood oxygen—also benefit. The study was funded by the National Heart, Lung, and Blood Institute (NHLBI)—a part of the National Institutes of Health (NIH)—and the Centers for Medicare & Medicaid Services (CMS).

The study, the largest of its kind to evaluate the effectiveness of home oxygen in this group of patients, was published in the online issue of the *New England Journal of Medicine*. The 738 patients enrolled in this study had COPD and moderately low levels of blood oxygen (in contrast to severely low blood oxygen levels) at rest or during exercise.

In the current study, patients with moderately low levels of blood oxygen are defined as those with a blood oxygen saturation (SpO2) between 89 and 93 percent at rest (moderate resting hypoxemia), or a

SpO2 below 90 percent during the 6-minute walk test. Patients with severely low blood oxygen levels are defined as those with a SpO2 equal to or less than 88 percent at rest. This latter group was excluded from the LOTT study because prior studies showed that they benefit from long-term oxygen treatment. Blood oxygen saturation or SpO2 refers to the percentage of oxygen-saturated hemoglobin relative to total hemoglobin in the blood and is measured through a pulse oximeter. A pulse oximeter is a special probe that indirectly measures oxygen levels in the blood, often by attachment to the finger.

"These results provide insight into a long-standing question about oxygen use in patients with COPD and moderately low levels of blood oxygen. For the most part, this treatment did not improve or prolong life in study participants," said James P. Kiley, Ph.D., director of NHL-BI's Division of Lung Diseases. "The findings also underscore the need for new treatments for COPD."

Researchers say patients with any form of COPD should check with their doctors before making changes in their treatment plans. "We want to make it clear that LOTT was not designed to assess individual responses to oxygen treatment and that individual responses can vary. Each COPD patient should discuss their own personal situation with their healthcare provider," said William C. Bailey, M.D., Professor Emeritus at the University of Alabama at Birmingham School of Medicine, and study Chair.

Chronic obstructive pulmonary disease, the third leading cause of death in the United States, is a progressive lung disease triggered primarily by cigarette smoking, although up to 20 percent of patients with COPD never smoked. Symptoms include shortness of breath, chronic coughing, and wheezing. The disease also causes low oxygen levels in the blood. About 15 million people have been diagnosed with COPD in the United States and another 10 million may be undiagnosed.

For decades, oxygen has been one of the main treatment tools for patients with COPD and low oxygen levels. It involves the use of metal tank cylinders containing oxygen or concentrators that extract oxygen from air; both systems deliver the gas through a nasal tube or mask.

The LOTT study is a randomized clinical trial to determine whether oxygen use could help COPD patients with moderately low levels of blood oxygen. The 7-year study, which included patients from 42 medical centers throughout the United States, began in 2009 and was completed in 2015.

In the study, half of the patients received long-term oxygen and the other half did not. The researchers found no significant differences between the two groups based on how long patients survived, and the amount of time leading to their first hospitalization. They also found no differences in other important benchmarks, such as the rate at which the patients were hospitalized or experienced worsening of COPD symptoms. Nor did researchers find statistically significant differences between the groups in quality of life, levels of depression or anxiety, lung function, or ability to walk for short periods.

Although no cure for COPD exists, there are a number of treatment options, including the use of bronchodilators and steroids, as well as pulmonary rehabilitation, surgery, and lung transplantation. Researchers worldwide are also studying new medications and exploring other approaches such as gene therapy. They continue to emphasize the importance of not smoking tobacco in preventing or slowing the progression of COPD.

Section 9.3

New Study Offers Insights on Genetic Indicators of COPD Risk

This section includes text excerpted from "New Study Offers Insights on Genetic Indicators of COPD Risk," National Institutes of Health (NIH), January 16, 2018.

Researchers have discovered that genetic variations in the anatomy of the lungs could serve as indicators to help identify people who have low, but stable, lung function early in life, and those who are particularly at risk for chronic obstructive pulmonary disease (COPD) because of a smoke-induced decline in lung function. The results of the study, which was funded by the National Heart, Lung and Blood Institute (NHLBI), part of the National Institutes of Health (NIH), appeared in the journal *Proceedings of the National Academy of Sciences* (PNAS).

Cigarette smoking has long been the most common cause of COPD, but not all smokers develop the condition, and many nonsmokers do. Why that is so has never been fully understood, but a team of researchers now have a clue after discovering that genetically programmed airway tree variation is linked to a higher prevalence of COPD among older adults.

"This work raises many interesting questions for researchers. Understanding precisely why these genes influence the development of COPD may lead to entirely new and more effective ways of preventing or treating this disease," said James Kiley, M.D., Director of the NHLBI's Division of Lung Diseases. "This novel study suggests that a computed tomography (CT) scan, which is widely available, can be used to measure airway structure and predict who is at higher risk for smoke-induced lung injury."

Chronic obstructive pulmonary disease, a progressive disease that makes it hard to breathe, is the fourth leading cause of death in the United States. An estimated 16 million people are currently diagnosed with COPD, and millions more are believed to have the condition.

Until recently, researchers believed that COPD developed later in life as a result of prolonged exposure to cigarette smoke or air pollution, which accelerated the decline in lung function. However, recent studies have shown that many older adults with COPD had low lung function early in life and experienced the normal lung function decline associated with aging, not an accelerated decline.

"In the current study, we found that central airway branches of the lungs, which are believed to form early in life, do not follow the textbook pattern in one quarter of the adult population and these nontextbook variations in airway branches are associated with higher COPD prevalence among older adults," said the study's first author Benjamin M. Smith, M.D. M.S., assistant professor at Columbia University Medical Center. "Interestingly, one of the airway branch variants was associated with COPD among smokers and nonsmokers. The other was associated with COPD, but only among smokers."

These airway tree variations are identifiable on low-dose screening lung CT scans, which are currently indicated clinically for lung cancer screening in older patients with a history of heavy smoking in the prior 15 years. Before CT scans are used outside of this group for the identification of airway variants in clinical practice, the study authors say more research will be needed to confirm that preventive or therapeutic interventions based on the presence of airway tree variations can improve patients' outcomes.

In the meantime, the researchers say they will be investigating another important finding—this one around family history. Their study identified a common airway branch variation that occurs within families and is associated with COPD among nonsmokers. Smith said while other developmental events that occur within families may be involved, his research team is looking into whether there is a genetic basis for this variant. "If proven," he said, "this would represent a novel mechanism of COPD among nonsmokers."

Section 9.4

Genetics and Pollution Drive Severity of Asthma Symptoms

This section includes text excerpted from "Genetics and Pollution Drive Severity of Asthma Symptoms," National Institutes of Health (NIH), August 31, 2018.

Asthma patients, with a specific genetic profile, exhibit more intense symptoms following exposure to traffic pollution, according to researchers at the National Institutes of Health (NIH) and collaborators. The study appeared online in *Scientific Reports*.

The research team, made up of scientists from the National Institute of Environmental Health Sciences (NIEHS), part of NIH, and Rice University, Houston, also found that asthma patients that lack this genetic profile do not have the same sensitivity to traffic pollution and do not experience worse asthma symptoms. The work brings scientists closer to being able to use precision medicine, an emerging field that intends to prevent and treat disease based on factors specific to an individual.

The co-lead author Shepherd Schurman, M.D., associate medical director of the NIEHS Clinical Research Unit, stated the results are based on genetic variation, the subtle differences in deoxyribonucleic acid (DNA) that make each person unique. He further added that to understand the concept, one should think of human genes, which are made up of DNA base pairs A, C, G, and T, as written instructions for making proteins.

"All humans have the same genes, in other words the same basic instructions, but in some people one DNA base pair has been changed," Schurman said. "This common type of genetic variation is called a "single nucleotide polymorphism" or SNP, and it can alter the way proteins are made and make individuals more or less prone to illness."

Schurman is also head of the Environmental Polymorphisms Registry (EPR), the DNA bank in North Carolina that provided volunteers for the study. The EPR studies how SNPs impact disease risk in combination with environmental exposures.

Together with NIEHS colleague and lung disease expert Stavros Garantziotis, M.D., medical director of the NIEHS Clinical Research Unit, the two scientists examined four SNPs that are involved in a biochemical pathway that leads to inflammatory responses in the body. They explained that SNPs are usually studied one at a time, but they wanted to learn if different combinations of these SNPs, along with pollution exposure, could worsen symptoms in a person with an inflammatory disease such as asthma.

Schurman and Garantziotis gathered information about the SNPs, severity of asthma symptoms, and residential addresses of 2,704 EPR participants with asthma. Using the SNPs data, they divided the participants into three groups: hyperresponders, or those who are very sensitive to air pollution and likely to develop inflammation; hyporesponders, or those insensitive to air pollution and less likely to develop inflammation; and those in between. With the help of collaborators at Rice University, the team used the participants' addresses to calculate their distance from a major road. Participants were categorized depending on whether they lived more or less than 275 yards from a major roadway. Data suggest that air pollution levels are elevated closer to major roads.

The researchers found that asthma sufferers who were hyper-responders and lived closer to heavily traveled roads had the worst asthma symptoms, such as difficulty breathing, chest pain, cough, and wheezing, compared to the other groups. In contrast, asthma patients who were hypo-responders and lived further away from busy roads had milder symptoms. Garantziotis concluded the work could greatly enhance the quality of life (QOL) for people with asthma.

"Based on this research, we could propose that hyperresponders, who are exposed to traffic pollution, receive air purification intervention, such as high-efficiency particulate air (HEPA) filters, for their home," Garantziotis said.

The NIEHS Clinical Director Janet Hall, M.D., said the results emphasize the importance of gene-environment interactions in the progression of disease.

"This research is a great example of how we can approach disease prevention on a personal level, and tailor our treatments to suit individual patients," she said. "That way we can be more efficient with our treatments and preventative measures, while at the same time cutting healthcare costs."

Section 9.5

NIH Research Improves Health for People with Asthma

This section includes text excerpted from "NIH Research Improves Health for People with Asthma," National Institutes of Health (NIH), May 1, 2017.

May is Asthma Awareness Month, and the National Institutes of Health is finding solutions to improve the health of the nearly 25 million people in the United States who currently have asthma. In recent decades, the prevalence of asthma has been increasing, resulting in millions of urgent medical visits and missed days of work and school each year.

Asthma is a chronic, and sometimes fatal, disease in which the airways become inflamed from a variety of triggers in the air, like indoor allergens from dust mites, mold, and cockroaches, and outdoor air pollution. Once the airways become swollen and inflamed, they become narrower, causing symptoms, such as wheezing, coughing, chest tightness, and difficulty breathing.

Together, three institutes lead asthma research at the National Institutes of Health (NIH): the National Institute of Environmental Health Sciences (NIEHS), the National Heart, Lung, and Blood Institute (NHLBI), and the National Institute of Allergy and Infectious Diseases (NIAID). These three institutes support different aspects of asthma research but are united in a commitment to reduce the burden of this debilitating disease, as highlighted here through recent studies funded collaboratively by all three institutes.

For example, research funded by NIEHS, NHLBI, and NIAID has demonstrated the importance of healthy school environments. A study of students from inner-city schools linked airborne mouse allergens at schools to increased symptoms and decreased lung function in asthmatic children. This suggests there are steps schools can take to improve air quality and potentially benefit children with asthma.

In fact, a preliminary study tested high-efficiency particulate air filters, commonly known as "high-efficiency particulate air (HEPA) filters," in three urban elementary schools, which yielded two indoor air quality improvements: about a 40 percent reduction in fine dust particles, along with about a 55 percent reduction in traffic-related black carbon levels. Both pollutants can irritate the lungs of people with asthma.

The NIH—supported researchers also are evaluating how much outdoor air pollution may come inside school buildings. One study found that levels of traffic-related black carbon were lower inside than outside, but when outdoor levels increased, so did the indoor levels. Fine dust particles inside schools came from both indoor and outdoor sources.

In addition to studying school environments, research funded by NIEHS, NHLBI, and NIAID has explored the complex role of the immune system in asthma. A study published in 2016 showed that children exposed to a wide range of bacteria and microbes, as found in dust on traditional Amish farms that use animals rather than machines, may be protected against asthma through the stimulation and shaping of nonspecific, or innate, immune responses.

The study also took genetic factors into account by comparing genetically similar Amish and Hutterite children who live in communities with different agricultural practices. The researchers further strengthened the findings by reproducing the observed protective effect in mouse studies. The difference in triggering of the innate immune response may help explain why asthma remains rare among the Amish but affects nearly 1 in 10 U.S. children, who typically do not live in a rich microbial environment.

While bacteria and microbes can benefit the immune system, exposure to mold may make asthma worse. Scientists funded by NIEHS, NHLBI, and NIAID showed that children with high exposure to molds and fungi were more likely to have asthma at age seven. For children with allergies, the association was especially strong.

Part Two

Infectious
Respiratory Disorders

Chapter 10

Preventing Infectious Diseases

Chapter Contents

Section 10.1

Tips to Prevent Seasonal Flu

This section includes text excerpted from "CDC Says "Take 3"
Actions to Fight the Flu," Centers for Disease Control
and Prevention (CDC), December 10, 2018.

Flu is a serious contagious disease that can lead to hospitalization and even death.

Take Time to Get a Flu Vaccine

The Centers for Disease Control and Prevention (CDC) recommends a yearly flu vaccine as the first and most important step in protecting against flu viruses. While there are many different flu viruses, a flu vaccine protects against the viruses that research suggests will be most common.

Flu vaccination can reduce flu illnesses, doctors' visits, and missed work and school due to flu, as well as prevent flu-related hospitalizations. Everyone 6 months of age and older should get a flu vaccine every year before flu activity begins in their community.

Vaccination of high risk persons is especially important to decrease their risk of severe flu illness. People at high risk of serious flu complications include young children, pregnant women, people with certain chronic health conditions like asthma, diabetes or heart and lung disease and people 65 years and older. Vaccination is also important for healthcare workers, and other people who live with or care for high risk people to keep from spreading flu to them.

Children younger than 6 months are at high risk of serious flu illness, but are too young to be vaccinated. People who care for infants should be vaccinated instead.

Take Everyday Preventive Actions to Stop the Spread of Germs

You can do the following to stop spreading of germs.

- Try to avoid close contact with sick people.
- While sick, limit contact with others as much as possible to keep from infecting them.
- If you are sick with flu symptoms, the CDC recommends that you stay home for at least 24 hours after your fever is gone

except to get medical care or for other necessities. (Your fever should be gone for 24 hours without the use of a fever-reducing medicine.)

- Cover your nose and mouth with a tissue when you cough or sneeze. Throw the tissue in the trash after you use it.

- Wash your hands often with soap and water. If soap and water are not available, use an alcohol-based hand rub.

- Avoid touching your eyes, nose, and mouth. Germs spread this way.

- Clean and disinfect surfaces and objects that may be contaminated with germs like the flu.

Take Flu Antiviral Drugs If Your Doctor Prescribes Them

Follow the directions given by the doctor. Take flu antiviral drugs if she or he prescribes them for you.

- If you get the flu, antiviral drugs can be used to treat your illness.

- Antiviral drugs are different from antibiotics. They are prescription medicines (pills, liquid or an inhaled powder) and are not available over-the-counter (OTC).

- Antiviral drugs can make illness milder and shorten the time you are sick. They may also prevent serious flu complications. For people with high-risk factors treatment with an antiviral drug can mean the difference between having a milder illness versus a very serious illness that could result in a hospital stay.

- Studies show that flu antiviral drugs work best for treatment when they are started within two days of getting sick, but starting them later can still be helpful, especially if the sick person has a high-risk factor or is very sick from the flu. Follow your doctor's instructions for taking this drug.

- Flu symptoms include fever, cough, sore throat, runny or stuffy nose, body aches, headache, chills and fatigue. Some people also may have vomiting and diarrhea. People may be infected with the flu, and have respiratory symptoms without a fever.

Section 10.2

Handwashing Prevents Infectious Diseases

This section includes text excerpted from "Show Me the Science—Why Wash Your Hands?" Actions to Fight the Flu," Centers for Disease Control and Prevention (CDC), September 17, 2018.

How Germs Get onto Hands and Make People Sick

Feces (poop) from people or animals is an important source of germs like *Salmonella*, *E. coli O157*, and norovirus that cause diarrhea, and it can spread some respiratory infections such as adenovirus and hand-foot-mouth disease. These kinds of germs can get onto hands after people use the toilet or change a diaper, but also in less obvious ways, such as after handling raw meats that have invisible amounts of animal poop on them. A single gram of human feces—which is about the weight of a paper clip—can contain one trillion germs. Germs can also get onto hands if people touch any object that has germs on it because someone coughed or sneezed on it or was touched by some other contaminated object. When these germs get onto hands and are not washed off, they can be passed from person to person and make people sick.

Washing Hands Prevents Illnesses and Spread of Infections to Others

Handwashing with soap removes germs from hands. This helps prevent infections because:

- People frequently touch their eyes, nose, and mouth without even realizing it. Germs can get into the body through the eyes, nose and mouth and make us sick.

- Germs from unwashed hands can get into foods and drinks while people prepare or consume them. Germs can multiply in some types of foods or drinks, under certain conditions, and make people sick.

- Germs from unwashed hands can be transferred to other objects, like handrails, table tops, or toys, and then transferred to another person's hands.

- Removing germs through handwashing, therefore, helps prevent diarrhea and respiratory infections and may even help prevent skin and eye infections.

Teaching people about handwashing helps them and their communities stay healthy.

Handwashing education in the community:

- Reduces the number of people who get sick with diarrhea by 23 to 40 percent

- Reduces diarrheal illness in people with weakened immune systems by 58 percent

- Reduces respiratory illnesses, like colds, in the general population by 16 to 21 percent

- Reduces absenteeism due to gastrointestinal illness in schoolchildren by 29 to 57 percent

Not Washing Hands Harms Children around the World

About 1.8 million children under the age of 5 die each year from diarrheal diseases and pneumonia, the top two killers of young children around the world.

- Handwashing with soap could protect about 1 out of every 3 young children who get sick with diarrhea and almost 1 out of 5 young children with respiratory infections like pneumonia.

- Although people around the world clean their hands with water, very few use soap to wash their hands. Washing hands with soap removes germs much more effectively.

- Handwashing education and access to soap in schools can help improve attendance.

- Good handwashing early in life may help improve child development in some settings.

- Estimated global rates of handwashing after using the toilet are only 19 percent.

Handwashing Helps Battle the Rise in Antibiotic Resistance

Preventing sickness reduces the amount of antibiotics people use and the likelihood that antibiotic resistance will develop. Handwashing can prevent about 30 percent of diarrhea-related sicknesses and about 20 percent of respiratory infections (e.g., colds). Antibiotics often are prescribed unnecessarily for these health issues. Reducing the number of these infections by washing hands frequently helps prevent the overuse of antibiotics—the single most important factor leading to antibiotic resistance around the world. Handwashing can also prevent people from getting sick with germs that are already resistant to antibiotics and that can be difficult to treat.

Section 10.3

Influenza Vaccination

This section includes text excerpted from "Key Facts about Seasonal Flu Vaccine," Centers for Disease Control and Prevention (CDC), September 6, 2018.

Why Should People Get Vaccinated against the Flu?

Influenza is a potentially serious disease that can lead to hospitalization and sometimes even death. Every flu season is different, and influenza infection can affect people differently, but millions of people get the flu every year, hundreds of thousands of people are hospitalized and thousands or tens of thousands of people die from flu-related causes every year. An annual seasonal flu vaccine is the best way to help protect against flu. Vaccination has been shown to have many benefits including reducing the risk of flu illnesses, hospitalizations and even the risk of flu-related death in children.

How Do Flu Vaccines Work?

Flu vaccines cause antibodies to develop in the body about two weeks after vaccination. These antibodies provide protection against infection with the viruses that are in the vaccine.

The seasonal flu vaccine protects against the influenza viruses that research indicates will be most common during the upcoming season. Traditional flu vaccines (called "trivalent" vaccines) are made to protect against three flu viruses; an influenza A (H1N1) virus, an influenza A (H3N2) virus, and an influenza B virus. There are also flu vaccines made to protect against four flu viruses (called "quadrivalent" vaccines). These vaccines protect against the same viruses as the trivalent vaccine and an additional B virus.

What Kinds of Flu Vaccines Are Available?

The Centers for Disease Control and Prevention (CDC) recommends the use of any licensed, age-appropriate influenza vaccine during the 2018 to 2019 influenza season, including inactivated influenza vaccine (IIV), recombinant influenza vaccine (RIV), or live attenuated influenza vaccine (LAIV). No preference is expressed for any influenza vaccine over another. Both trivalent (three-component) and quadrivalent (four-component) flu vaccines will be available.

Trivalent flu vaccines include:

- One standard-dose trivalent flu shot (IIV3) manufactured using virus grown in eggs. This shot (Afluria) can be given either with a needle (for people aged 5 years and older) or with a jet injector (or people aged 18 through 64 years only).

- A high-dose trivalent flu shot (Fluzone High-dose), approved for people 65 years and older.

- A trivalent flu shot made with adjuvant (Fluad), approved for people 65 years and older.

Quadrivalent flu vaccines include:

- Standard-dose quadrivalent flu shots that are manufactured using virus grown in eggs. These include Afluria Quadrivalent, Fluarix Quadrivalent, FluLaval Quadrivalent, and Fluzone Quadrivalent. Different flu shots are approved for different age groups. Some are approved for children as young as 6 months of age. Most flu shots are given in the arm (muscle) with a needle. One quadrivalent flu shot (Afluria Quadrivalent) can be given either with a needle (for people aged 5 years and older) or with a jet injector (for people aged 18 through 64 years only).

- A quadrivalent cell-based flu shot (Flucelvax Quadrivalent) containing virus grown in cell culture (that is egg-free), which is approved for people 4 years and older.

- A recombinant quadrivalent flu shot (Flublok Quadrivalent) approved for people 18 years and older.

Who Should Get Vaccinated This Season?

Everyone six months of age and older should get a flu vaccine every season. Vaccination to prevent influenza is particularly important for people who are at high risk of serious complications from influenza.

Who Should Not Be Vaccinated?

Different flu vaccines are approved for use in different age groups. In addition, some vaccines are not recommended for certain groups. Factors that can determine a person's suitability for vaccination, or vaccination with a particular vaccine, include a person's age, health (current and past), and any allergies to flu vaccine or its components.

- People who cannot get a flu shot
- People who should talk to their doctor before getting the flu shot

When Should You Get Vaccinated?

You should get a flu vaccine before flu begins spreading in your community. It takes about two weeks after vaccination for antibodies that protect against flu to develop in the body. The CDC recommends that people get a flu vaccine by the end of October. Getting vaccinated later, however, can still be beneficial and vaccination should continue to be offered throughout the flu season, even into January or later.

Children who need two doses of vaccine to be protected should start the vaccination process sooner, because the two doses must be given at least four weeks apart.

Where Can You Get a Flu Vaccine?

Flu vaccines are offered in many doctor's offices, clinics, health departments, pharmacies and college health centers, as well as by many employers, and even in some schools. Even if you do not have a regular doctor or nurse, you can get a flu vaccine somewhere else, such as a health department, pharmacy, urgent care clinic, and often your school, college health center, or workplace.

Why Do You Need a Flu Vaccine Every Year?

A flu vaccine is needed every season for two reasons. First, the body's immune response from vaccination declines over time, so an annual vaccine is needed for optimal protection. Second, because flu viruses are constantly changing, the formulation of the flu vaccine is reviewed each year and updated as needed to keep up with changing flu viruses. For the best protection, everyone six months and older should get vaccinated annually.

Does Flu Vaccine Work Right Away?

No. It takes about two weeks after vaccination for antibodies to develop in the body and provide protection against influenza virus infection. That is why it is better to get vaccinated by the end of October, before the flu season really gets under way.

Can You Get Seasonal Flu Even Though You Got a Flu Vaccine This Year?

Yes. It is possible to get sick with flu even if you have been vaccinated (although you will not know for sure unless you get a flu test). This is possible for the following reasons:

- You may be exposed to a flu virus shortly before getting vaccinated or during the period that it takes the body to gain protection after getting vaccinated. This exposure may result in you becoming ill with the flu before the vaccine begins to protect you. (Antibodies that provide protection develop in the body about two weeks after vaccination.)

- You may be exposed to a flu virus that is not included in the seasonal flu vaccine. There are many different flu viruses that circulate every year. A flu vaccine is made to protect against the three or four flu viruses that research suggests will be most common.

- Unfortunately, some people can become infected with a flu virus a flu vaccine is designed to protect against, despite getting vaccinated. Protection provided by flu vaccination can vary widely, based in part on health and age factors of the person getting vaccinated. In general, a flu vaccine works best among healthy younger adults and older children. Some older people and people with certain chronic illnesses may develop less immunity after vaccination. Flu vaccination is not a perfect tool, but it is the best way to protect against flu infection.

Section 10.4

Pneumococcal Vaccination

This section includes text excerpted from "Pneumococcal Vaccination," Centers for Disease Control and Prevention (CDC), December 6, 2017.

Vaccines help prevent pneumococcal disease, which is any type of infection caused by *Streptococcus pneumoniae* bacteria. There are two kinds of pneumococcal vaccines available in the United States:

- Pneumococcal conjugate vaccine

- Pneumococcal polysaccharide vaccine

The Centers for Disease Control and Prevention (CDC) recommends pneumococcal conjugate vaccine for all children younger than 2 years old, all adults 65 years or older, and people 2 through 64 years old with certain medical conditions. The CDC recommends pneumococcal polysaccharide vaccine for all adults 65 years or older, people 2 through 64 years old with certain medical conditions, and adults 19 through 64 years old who smoke cigarettes.

Talk with your or your child's healthcare professional if you have questions about pneumococcal vaccines.

Who Should Get Pneumococcal Vaccines?

The CDC recommends pneumococcal vaccination for all children younger than 2 years old and all adults 65 years or older. In certain situations, other children and adults should also get pneumococcal vaccines.

Who Should Not Get Pneumococcal Vaccines?

Because of age or health conditions, some people should not get certain vaccines or should wait before getting them.

What Types of Pneumococcal Vaccines Are There?

There are two pneumococcal vaccines licensed for use in the United States by the U.S. Food and Drug Administration (FDA):

- Pneumococcal conjugate vaccine (PCV13 or Prevnar 13®)

- Pneumococcal polysaccharide vaccine (PPSV23 or Pneumovax23®)

What Are the Possible Side Effects of Pneumococcal Vaccines?

Most people who get a pneumococcal vaccine do not have any serious problems with it. With any medicine, including vaccines, there is a chance of side effects. These are usually mild and go away on their own within a few days, but serious reactions are possible.

Mild Problems
Pneumococcal Conjugate Vaccine

Mild problems following pneumococcal conjugate vaccination can include:
- Reactions where the shot was given:
  - Redness
  - Swelling
  - Pain or tenderness
- Fever
- Loss of appetite
- Fussiness (irritability)
- Feeling tired
- Headache
- Chills

Young children who get pneumococcal conjugate vaccine at the same time as inactivated flu vaccine may be at increased risk for seizures caused by fever.

Pneumococcal Polysaccharide Vaccine

Mild problems following pneumococcal polysaccharide vaccination can include:
- Reactions where the shot was given:
  - Redness
  - Pain

- Fever

- Muscle aches

If these problems occur, they usually go away within about two days.

Chapter 11

Colds

Chapter Contents

Section 11.1

Common Cold

This section includes text excerpted from "Common Colds:
Protect Yourself and Others," Centers for Disease
Control and Prevention (CDC), February 11, 2019.

Sore throat and runny nose are usually the first signs of a cold, followed by coughing and sneezing. Most people recover in about 7 to 10 days. You can help reduce your risk of getting a cold: wash your hands often, avoid close contact with sick people, and do not touch your face with unwashed hands.

Common colds are the main reason that children miss school and adults miss work. Each year in the United States, there are millions of cases of the common cold. Adults have an average of 2 to 3 colds per year, and children have even more.

Most people get colds in the winter and spring, but it is possible to get a cold any time of the year. Symptoms usually include:

- Sore throat

- Runny nose

- Coughing

- Sneezing

- Headaches

- Body aches

Most people recover within about 7 to 10 days. However, people with weakened immune systems, asthma, or respiratory conditions may develop serious illness, such as bronchitis or pneumonia.

How to Protect Yourself

Viruses that cause colds can spread from infected people to others through the air and close personal contact. You can also get infected through contact with stool (poop) or respiratory secretions from an infected person. This can happen when you shake hands with someone who has a cold, or touch a surface, such as a doorknob, that has respiratory viruses on it, then touch your eyes, mouth, or nose.

You can help reduce your risk of getting a cold:

- Wash your hands often with soap and water. Wash them for 20 seconds, and help young children do the same. If soap and water are not available, use an alcohol-based hand sanitizer. Viruses that cause colds can live on your hands, and regular handwashing can help protect you from getting sick.

- Avoid touching your eyes, nose, and mouth with unwashed hands. Viruses that cause colds can enter your body this way and make you sick

- Stay away from people who are sick. Sick people can spread viruses that cause the common cold through close contact with others.

How to Protect Others

If you have a cold, you should follow these tips to help prevent spreading it to other people:

- Stay at home while you are sick and keep children out of school or day care while they are sick.

- Avoid close contact with others, such as hugging, kissing, or shaking hands.

- Move away from people before coughing or sneezing.

- Cough and sneeze into a tissue then throw it away, or cough and sneeze into your upper shirt sleeve, completely covering your mouth and nose.

- Wash your hands after coughing, sneezing, or blowing your nose.

- Disinfect frequently touched surfaces and objects, such as toys and doorknobs.

There is no vaccine to protect you against the common cold.

How to Feel Better

There is no cure for a cold. To feel better, you should get lots of rest and drink plenty of fluids. Over-the-counter (OTC) medicines may help ease symptoms but will not make your cold go away any faster. Always read the label and use medications as directed. Talk to your doctor before giving your child nonprescription cold medicines, since some medicines contain ingredients that are not recommended for children.

Antibiotics will not help you recover from a cold caused by a respiratory virus. They do not work against viruses, and they may make it harder for your body to fight future bacterial infections if you take them unnecessarily.

When to See a Doctor

You should call your doctor if you or your child has one or more of these conditions:

- Symptoms that last more than 10 days

- Symptoms that are severe or unusual

- If your child is younger than 3 months of age and has a fever or is lethargic

You should also call your doctor right away if you are at high risk for serious flu complications and get flu symptoms, such as fever, chills, and muscle or body aches. People at high risk for flu complications include young children (younger than 5 years old), adults 65 years and older, pregnant women, and people with certain medical conditions, such as asthma, diabetes, and heart disease.

Your doctor can determine if you or your child has a cold or the flu and can recommend treatment to help with symptoms.

Causes of the Common Cold

Many different respiratory viruses can cause the common cold, but rhinoviruses are the most common. *Rhinoviruses* can also trigger asthma attacks and have been linked to sinus and ear infections. Other viruses that can cause colds include a respiratory syncytial virus, human parainfluenza viruses, adenovirus, human coronaviruses, and human metapneumovirus (hMPV).

Know the Difference between Common Cold and Flu

The flu, which is caused by influenza viruses, also spreads and causes illness around the same time as the common cold. Because these two illnesses have similar symptoms, it can be difficult (or even impossible) to tell the difference between them based on symptoms alone. In general, flu symptoms are worse than the common cold and can include fever or feeling feverish/chills, cough, sore throat, runny or stuffy nose, muscle or body aches, headaches and fatigue (tiredness). Flu can also have very serious complications.

Section 11.2

Bronchitis

This section includes text excerpted from "Bronchitis,"
Centers for Disease Control and Prevention (CDC), April 7, 2017.

Bronchitis occurs when the airways of the lungs swell and produce mucus. That is what makes you cough. Acute bronchitis, often called a "chest cold," is the most common type of bronchitis. The symptoms last less than three weeks. Antibiotics are not indicated to treat acute bronchitis. Using antibiotics when not needed could do more harm than good.

If you are a healthy person without underlying heart or lung problems or a weakened immune system, this information is for you.

Symptoms of Bronchitis

Symptoms of acute bronchitis include:

• Coughing with or without mucus production

You may also experience:

• Soreness in the chest

• Fatigue (feeling tired)

• Mild headache

• Mild body aches

• Watery eyes

Causes of Bronchitis

Acute bronchitis is usually caused by a virus and often occurs after an upper respiratory infection. Bacteria can sometimes cause acute bronchitis, but even in these cases antibiotics are NOT recommended and will not help you get better.

When to Seek Medical Care

See a healthcare professional if you or your child have any of the following:

• Temperature higher than 100.4°F

- Cough with bloody mucus

- Shortness of breath or trouble breathing

- Symptoms that last more than 3 weeks

- Repeated episodes of bronchitis

Recommended Treatment

Acute bronchitis almost always gets better on its own—without antibiotics. Using antibiotics when they are not needed can do more harm than good. Unintended consequences of antibiotics include side effects, such as rash and diarrhea, as well as more serious consequences, such as an increased risk for an antibiotic-resistant infection or *Clostridium difficile* infection, sometimes deadly diarrhea.

To feel better:

- Get plenty of rest.

- Drink plenty of fluids.

- Use a clean humidifier or cool mist vaporizer.

- Breathe in steam from a bowl of hot water or shower.

- Use lozenges. (Do not give lozenges to children younger than four years of age).

- Ask your healthcare professional or pharmacist about over-the-counter (OTC) medicines that can help you feel better.

Remember, always use OTC medicines as directed. Do not use cough and cold medicines in children younger than four years of age unless specifically told to do so by a healthcare professional.

Your healthcare professional will most likely prescribe antibiotics for a diagnosis of whooping cough (pertussis) or pneumonia.

Prevention of Bronchitis

In order to prevent bronchitis you should:

- Practice good hand hygiene.

- Keep you and your child up to date with recommended vaccines.

- Avoid smoking.

- Avoid secondhand smoke, chemicals, dust, or air pollution.

- Always cover your mouth and nose when coughing or sneezing.
- Make sure you and your child are to up-to-date with all recommended vaccines.

Remember, antibiotics will not treat acute bronchitis. Using antibiotics when not needed could do more harm than good.

Chapter 12

Influenza

Chapter Contents

Section 12.1

Types of Influenza Viruses

This section includes text excerpted from "About Flu," Centers for
Disease Control and Prevention (CDC), August 23, 2018.

What Is Influenza Virus?

Influenza (flu) is a contagious respiratory illness caused by influenza viruses. It can cause mild to severe illness. Serious outcomes of
flu infection can result in hospitalization or death. Some people, such
as older people, young children, and people with certain health conditions, are at high risk of serious flu complications.

How Many Types of Influenza Viruses Are There?

There are four types of influenza viruses: A, B, C, and D. Human
influenza A and B viruses cause seasonal epidemics of disease almost
every winter in the United States. The emergence of a new and very
different influenza A virus to infect people can cause an influenza pandemic. Influenza type C infections generally cause a mild respiratory
illness and are not thought to cause epidemics. Influenza D viruses
primarily affect cattle and are not known to infect or cause illness in
people.

Influenza A viruses are divided into subtypes based on two proteins on the surface of the virus: the hemagglutinin (H) and the neuraminidase (N). There are 18 different hemagglutinin subtypes and 11
different neuraminidase subtypes. (H1 through H18 and N1 through
N11, respectively.)

Influenza A viruses can be further broken down into different
strains. Current subtypes of influenza A viruses found in people are
influenza A (H1N1) and influenza A (H3N2) viruses. In the spring
of 2009, a new influenza A (H1N1) virus emerged to cause illness in
people. This virus was very different from the human influenza A
(H1N1) viruses circulating at that time. The new virus caused the first
influenza pandemic in more than 40 years. That virus (often called
"2009 H1N1") has now replaced the H1N1 virus that was previously
circulating in humans.

Influenza B viruses are not divided into subtypes, but can be further
broken down into lineages and strains. Currently circulating influenza
B viruses belong to one of two lineages: B/Yamagata and B/Victoria.

Naming Influenza Viruses

The Centers for Disease Control and Prevention (CDC) follows an internationally accepted naming convention for influenza viruses. This convention was accepted by World Health Organization (WHO) in 1979 and published in February 1980 in *The Bulletin of the World Health Organization*. The approach uses the following components:

- The antigenic type (e.g., A, B, C)
- The host of origin (e.g., swine, equine, chicken, etc. For human-origin viruses, no host of origin designation is given.)
- Geographical origin (e.g., Denver, Taiwan, etc.)
- Strain number (e.g., 15, 7, etc.)
- Year of isolation (e.g., 57, 2009, etc.)
- For influenza A viruses, the hemagglutinin and neuraminidase antigen (e.g., H1N1, H5N1)

For example:

- A/duck/Alberta/35/76 (H1N1) for a virus from duck origin
- A/Perth/16/2009 (H3N2) for a virus from human origin

Influenza Vaccine Viruses

Influenza A (H1N1), A (H3N2), and one or two influenza B viruses (depending on the vaccine) are included in each year's influenza vaccine. Getting a flu vaccine can protect against flu viruses that are the same or related to the viruses in the vaccine. The seasonal flu vaccine does not protect against influenza C viruses. Additionally, flu vaccines will NOT protect against infection and illness caused by other viruses that also can cause influenza-like symptoms. There are many other nonflu viruses that can result in influenza-like illness (ILI) that spread during flu season.

Section 12.2

Key Facts about Seasonal Influenza

This section includes text excerpted from "Key Facts about
Influenza (Flu)," Centers for Disease Control and
Prevention (CDC), August 27, 2018.

What Is Influenza (Flu)?

Flu is a contagious respiratory illness caused by influenza viruses
that infect the nose, throat, and sometimes the lungs. It can cause
mild to severe illness, and at times can lead to death. The best way to
prevent flu is by getting a flu vaccine each year.

Flu Symptoms

Flu is different from a cold. As it usually comes on suddenly. People
who are sick with flu often feel some or all of these symptoms:

- Fever* or feeling feverish/chills

- Cough

- Sore throat

- Runny or stuffy nose

- Muscle or body aches

- Headaches

- Fatigue (tiredness)

It is important to note that not everyone with flu will have a fever.

Some people may have vomiting and diarrhea, though this is more
common in children than adults.

How Flu Spreads

Most experts believe that flu viruses spread mainly by tiny droplets made when people with flu cough, sneeze or talk. These droplets can land in the mouths or noses of people who are nearby. Less
often, a person might get flu by touching a surface or object that has

flu virus on it and then touching their own mouth, nose or possibly their eyes.

How Many People Get Sick with Flu Every Year?

The Centers for Disease Control and Prevention (CDC) study published in *Clinical Infectious Diseases* in 2018, looked at the percentage of the U.S. population who were sickened by the flu using two different methods and compared the findings. Both methods had similar findings, which suggested that on average, about 8 percent of the U.S. population gets sick from flu each season, with a range of between 3 percent and 11 percent, depending on the season.

Why Is the 3 to 11 Percent Estimate Different from the Previously Cited 5 to 20 Percent Range?

The commonly cited 5 to 20 percent estimate was based on a study that examined both symptomatic and asymptomatic influenza illness, which means it also looked at people who may have had the flu but never knew it because they did not have any symptoms. The 3 to 11 percent range is an estimate of the proportion of people who have symptomatic flu illness.

Who Is Most Likely to Be Infected with Influenza?

The same CID study found that children are most likely to get sick from the flu and that people 65 and older are least likely to get sick from influenza. Median incidence values (or attack rate) by age group were 9.3 percent for children 0 to 17 years, 8.8 percent for adults 18 to 64 years, and 3.9 percent for adults 65 years and older. This means that children younger than 18 are more than twice as likely to develop a symptomatic flu infection than adults 65 and older.

How Is Seasonal Incidence of Influenza Estimated?

Influenza virus infection is so common that the number of people infected each season can only be estimated. These statistical estimations are based on CDC-measured flu hospitalization rates that are adjusted to produce an estimate of the total number of influenza infections in the United States for a given flu season.

The estimates for the number of infections are then divided by the census population to estimate the seasonal incidence (or attack rate) of influenza.

Does Seasonal Incidence of Influenza Change Based on the Severity of Flu Season?

Yes. The proportion of people who get sick from the flu varies. A paper published in CID found that between 3 percent and 11 percent of the U.S. population gets infected and develops flu symptoms each year. The 3 percent estimate is from the 2011 to 2012 season, which was an H1N1-predominant season classified as being of low severity. The estimated incidence of flu illness during two seasons was around 11 percent; 2012 to 2013 was an H3N2-predominant season classified as being of moderate severity, while 2014 to 2015 was an H3N2 predominant season classified as being of high severity.

Period of Contagiousness

You may be able to pass on flu to someone else before you know you are sick, as well as while you are sick.

- People with flu are most contagious in the first three to four days after their illness begins.
- Some otherwise healthy adults may be able to infect others beginning one day before symptoms develop and up to five to seven days after becoming sick.
- Some people, especially young children and people with weakened immune systems, might be able to infect others with flu viruses for an even longer time.

Onset of Symptoms

The time from when a person is exposed and infected with flu to when symptoms begin is about two days, but can range from about one to four days.

Complications of Flu

Complications of flu can include bacterial pneumonia, ear infections, sinus infections and worsening of chronic medical conditions, such as congestive heart failure, asthma, or diabetes.

Table 12.1. Estimates of the Incidence of Symptomatic Influenza by Season and Age-Group, United States, 2010 to 2016

Season	Predominant Virus(es)	Season Severity	Incidence and Percent by Age Group						
			0 to 4 yrs	5 to 17 yrs	18 to 49 yrs	50 to 64 yrs	≥65 yrs	All Ages
2010–11	A/H3N2, A/H1N1pdm09	Moderate	14.1	8.4	5.3	8.1	4.3	6.8
2011–12	A/H3N2	Low	4.8	3.6	2.5	3.1	2.3	3
2012–13	A/H3N2	Moderate	18.6	12.7	8.9	14.3	9.9	11.3
2013–14	A/H1N1pdm09	Moderate	12.4	7.2	9.2	13	3.4	9
2014–15	A/H3N2	High	150	12.7	7.8	12.9	12.4	10.8
2015–16	A/H1N1pdm09	Moderate	11.1	7.4	7.1	11	3.5	7.6
Median			13.2	7.9	7.4	12	3.9	8.3

People at High Risk from Flu

Anyone can get flu (even healthy people), and serious problems related to flu can happen at any age, but some people are at high risk of developing serious flu-related complications if they get sick. This includes people 65 years and older, people of any age with certain chronic medical conditions (such as asthma, diabetes, or heart disease), pregnant women, and children younger than 5 years.

Preventing Seasonal Flu

The first and most important step in preventing flu is to get a flu vaccine each year. Flu vaccine has been shown to reduce flu related illnesses and the risk of serious flu complications that can result in hospitalization or even death. The CDC also recommends everyday preventive actions (such as staying away from people who are sick, covering coughs and sneezes and frequent handwashing) to help slow the spread of germs that cause respiratory (nose, throat, and lungs) illnesses, such as flu.

Diagnosing Flu

It is very difficult to distinguish flu from other viral or bacterial respiratory illnesses based on symptoms alone. There are tests available to diagnose flu.

Treating Flu

There are influenza antiviral drugs that can be used to treat flu illness.

Section 12.3

Avian Influenza

This section includes text excerpted from "Avian Influenza A Virus Infections in Humans," Centers for Disease Control and Prevention (CDC), April 18, 2017.

Although avian influenza A viruses usually do not infect people, rare cases of human infection with these viruses have been reported. Infected birds shed avian influenza virus in their saliva, mucus and feces. Human infections with bird flu viruses can happen when enough virus gets into a person's eyes, nose or mouth, or is inhaled. This can happen when virus is in the air (in droplets or possibly dust) and a person breathes it in, or when a person touches something that has virus on it then touches their mouth, eyes or nose. Rare human infections with some avian viruses have occurred most often after unprotected contact with infected birds or surfaces contaminated with avian influenza viruses. However, some infections have been identified where direct contact was not known to have occurred. Illness in people has ranged from mild to severe.

The spread of avian influenza A viruses from one ill person to another has been reported very rarely, and when it has been reported it has been limited, inefficient and not sustained. However, because of the possibility that avian influenza A viruses could change and gain the ability to spread easily between people, monitoring for human infection and person-to-person spread is extremely important for public health.

Signs and Symptoms of Avian Influenza a Virus Infections in Humans

The reported signs and symptoms of avian influenza A virus infections in humans have ranged from mild to severe and included conjunctivitis, influenza-like illness (e.g., fever, cough, sore throat, muscle aches) sometimes accompanied by nausea, abdominal pain, diarrhea, and vomiting, severe respiratory illness (e.g., shortness of breath, difficulty breathing, pneumonia, acute respiratory distress, viral pneumonia, respiratory failure), neurologic changes (altered mental status, seizures), and the involvement of other organ systems. Asian lineage H7N9 and HPAI Asian lineage H5N1 viruses have been responsible for most human illness worldwide to date, including most serious illnesses and highest mortality.

Detecting Avian Influenza A Virus Infection in Humans

Avian influenza A virus infection in people cannot be diagnosed by clinical signs and symptoms alone; laboratory testing is needed. Avian influenza A virus infection is usually diagnosed by collecting a swab from the upper respiratory tract (nose or throat) of the sick person. (Testing is more accurate when the swab is collected during the first few days of illness.) This specimen is sent to a laboratory; the laboratory looks for avian influenza A virus either by using a molecular test, by trying to grow the virus, or both. (Growing avian influenza A viruses should only be done in laboratories with high levels of biosafety.)

For critically ill patients, collection and testing of lower respiratory tract specimens also may lead to diagnosis of avian influenza virus infection. However for some patients who are no longer very sick or who have fully recovered, it may be difficult to detect the avian influenza A virus in the specimen. Sometimes it may still be possible to diagnose avian influenza A virus infection by looking for evidence of antibodies the body has produced in response to the virus. This is not always an option because it requires two blood specimens (one taken during the first week of illness and another taken three to four weeks later). Also, it can take several weeks to verify the results, and testing must be performed in a special laboratory, such as at the CDC.

Treating Avian Influenza A Virus Infections in Humans

The Centers for Disease Control and Prevention (CDC) recommends a neuraminidase inhibitor for treatment of human infection with avian influenza A viruses. Analyses of available avian influenza viruses circulating worldwide suggest that most viruses are susceptible to oseltamivir, peramivir, and zanamivir. However, some evidence of antiviral resistance has been reported in Asian H5N1 and Asian H7N9 viruses isolated from some human cases. Monitoring for antiviral resistance among avian influenza A viruses is crucial and ongoing.

Preventing Human Infection with Avian Influenza A Viruses

The best way to prevent infection with avian influenza A viruses is to avoid sources of exposure. Most human infections with avian influenza A viruses have occurred following direct or close contact with infected poultry.

People who have had contact with infected birds may be given influenza antiviral drugs preventatively. While antiviral drugs are most often used to treat influenza, they also can be used to prevent infection in someone who has been exposed to influenza viruses. When used to prevent seasonal influenza, antiviral drugs are 70 to 90 percent effective.

Seasonal influenza vaccination will not prevent infection with avian influenza A viruses, but can reduce the risk of co-infection with human and avian influenza A viruses. It is also possible to make a vaccine that can protect people against avian influenza viruses. For example, the United States government maintains a stockpile of vaccines to protect against some Asian avian influenza A H5N1 viruses. The stockpiled vaccine could be used if similar H5N1 viruses were to begin transmitting easily from person to person. Creating a candidate vaccine virus is the first step in producing a vaccine.

Chapter 13

Otitis Media

What Is Otitis Media?

Otitis media is an infection or inflammation of the middle ear. This inflammation often begins when infections that cause sore throats, colds, or other respiratory or breathing problems spread to the middle ear. These can be viral or bacterial infections. 75 percent of children experience at least one episode of otitis media by their third birthday. Almost half of these children will have three or more ear infections during their first three years.

It is estimated that medical costs and lost wages because of otitis media amount to $5 billion a year in the United States. Although otitis media is primarily a disease of infants and young children, it can also affect adults.

How Do We Hear?

The ear consists of three major parts: the outer ear, the middle ear, and the inner ear. The outer ear includes the pinna—the visible part of the ear—and the ear canal. The outer ear extends to the tympanic membrane or eardrum, which separates the outer ear from the middle ear. The middle ear is an air-filled space that is located behind the eardrum. The middle ear contains three tiny bones, the malleus, incus,

This chapter includes text excerpted from "Otitis Media," National Institute on Deafness and Other Communication Disorders (NIDCD), October 2000. Reviewed August 2019.

and stapes, which transmit sound from the eardrum to the inner ear. The inner ear contains the hearing and balance organs. The cochlea contains the hearing organ which converts sound into electrical signals which are associated with the origin of impulses carried by nerves to the brain where their meanings are appreciated.

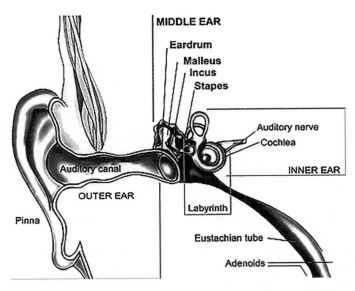

Figure 13.1. *Parts of Ear* (Source: "Ear Infections in Children," National Institute on Deafness and Other Communication Disorders (NIDCD).)

Why Are More Children Affected by Otitis Media Than Adults?

There are many reasons why children are more likely to suffer from otitis media than adults. First, children have more trouble fighting infections. This is because their immune systems are still developing. Another reason has to do with the child's eustachian tube. The eustachian tube is a small passageway that connects the upper part of the throat to the middle ear. It is shorter and straighter in the child than in the adult. It can contribute to otitis media in several ways.

The eustachian tube is usually closed but opens regularly to ventilate or replenish the air in the middle ear. This tube also equalizes middle ear air pressure in response to air pressure changes in the environment. However, a eustachian tube that is blocked by swelling of its lining or plugged with mucus from a cold or for some other reason cannot open to ventilate the middle ear. The lack of ventilation may allow fluid from the tissue that lines the middle ear to accumulate. If the eustachian tube remains plugged, the fluid cannot drain and begins to collect in the normally air-filled middle ear.

One more factor that makes children more susceptible to otitis media is that adenoids in children are larger than they are in adults. Adenoids are composed largely of cells (lymphocytes) that help fight infections. They are positioned in the back of the upper part of the throat near the eustachian tubes. Enlarged adenoids can, because of their size, interfere with the eustachian tube opening. In addition, adenoids may themselves become infected, and the infection may spread into the eustachian tubes.

Bacteria reach the middle ear through the lining or the passageway of the eustachian tube and can then produce infection, which causes swelling of the lining of the middle ear, blocking of the eustachian tube, and migration of white cells from the bloodstream to help fight the infection. In this process the white cells accumulate, often killing bacteria and dying themselves, leading to the formation of pus, a thick yellowish-white fluid in the middle ear. As the fluid increases, the child may have trouble hearing because the eardrum and middle ear bones are unable to move as freely as they should. As the infection worsens, many children also experience severe ear pain. Too much fluid in the ear can put pressure on the eardrum and eventually tear it.

What Are the Effects of Otitis Media?

Otitis media not only causes severe pain but may result in serious complications if it is not treated. An untreated infection can travel from the middle ear to the nearby parts of the head, including the brain. Although the hearing loss caused by otitis media is usually temporary, untreated otitis media may lead to permanent hearing impairment. Persistent fluid in the middle ear and chronic otitis media can reduce a child's hearing at a time that is critical for speech and language development. Children who have early hearing impairment from frequent ear infections are likely to have speech and language disabilities.

Can Anything Be Done to Prevent Otitis Media?

Specific prevention strategies applicable to all infants and children, such as immunization against viral respiratory infections or specifically against the bacteria that cause otitis media are not available. Nevertheless, it is known that children who are cared for in group settings, as well as children who live with adults who smoke cigarettes, have more ear infections. Therefore, a child who is prone to otitis media should avoid contact with sick playmates and environmental tobacco smoke.

Infants who nurse from a bottle while lying down also appear to develop otitis media more frequently. Children who have been breastfed often have fewer episodes of otitis media. Research has shown that cold and allergy medications, such as antihistamines and decongestants are not helpful in preventing ear infections. The best hope for avoiding ear infections is the development of vaccines against the bacteria that most often cause otitis media. Scientists are nowadays, developing vaccines that show promise in preventing otitis media. Additional clinical research must be completed to ensure their effectiveness and safety.

How Does a Child's Physician Diagnose Otitis Media?

The simplest way to detect an active infection in the middle ear is to look in the child's ear with an otoscope, a light instrument that allows the physician to examine the outer ear and the eardrum. Inflammation of the eardrum indicates an infection. There are several ways that a physician checks for middle ear fluid. The use of a special type of otoscope called a "pneumatic otoscope" allows the physician to blow a puff of air onto the eardrum to test eardrum movement. (An eardrum with fluid behind it does not move as well as an eardrum with air behind it.)

A useful test of middle ear function is called "tympanometry." This test requires insertion of a small soft plug into the opening of the child's ear canal. The plug contains a speaker, a microphone, and a device that is able to change the air pressure in the ear canal, allowing for several measures of the middle ear. The child feels air pressure changes in the ear or hears a few brief tones. While this test provides information on the condition of the middle ear, it does not determine how well the child hears. A physician may suggest a hearing test for a child who has frequent ear infections to determine the extent of hearing loss. The hearing test is usually performed by an audiologist, a person who is specially trained to measure hearing.

How Is Otitis Media Treated?

Many physicians recommend the use of an antibiotic (a drug that kills bacteria) when there is an active middle ear infection. If a child is experiencing pain, the physician may also recommend a pain reliever.

Following the physician's instructions is very important. Once started, the antibiotic should be taken until it is finished. Most physicians will have the child return for a followup examination to see if the infection has cleared. Unfortunately, there are many bacteria that can cause otitis media, and some have become resistant to some antibiotics. This happens when antibiotics are given for coughs, colds, flu, or viral infections where antibiotic treatment is not useful. When bacteria become resistant to antibiotics, those treatments are then less effective against infections. This means that several different antibiotics may have to be tried before an ear infection clears. Antibiotics may also produce unwanted side effects, such as nausea, diarrhea, and rashes.

Once the infection clears, fluid may remain in the middle ear for several months. Middle ear fluid that is not infected often disappears after 3 to 6 weeks. Neither antihistamines nor decongestants are recommended as helpful in the treatment of otitis media at any stage in the disease process. Sometimes physicians will treat the child with an antibiotic to hasten the elimination of the fluid. If the fluid persists for more than 3 months and is associated with a loss of hearing, many physicians suggest the insertion of "tubes" in the affected ears. This operation, called a "myringotomy," can usually be done on an outpatient basis by a surgeon, who is usually an otolaryngologist (a physician who specializes in the ears, nose, and throat). While the child is asleep under general anesthesia, the surgeon makes a small opening in the child's eardrum. A small metal or plastic tube is placed into the opening in the eardrum. The tube ventilates the middle ear and helps keep the air pressure in the middle ear equal to the air pressure in the environment. The tube normally stays in the eardrum for 6 to 12 months, after which time it usually comes out spontaneously. If a child has enlarged or infected adenoids, the surgeon may recommend removal of the adenoids at the same time the ear tubes are inserted. Removal of the adenoids has been shown to reduce episodes of otitis media in some children, but not those who are under 4 years of age. Research, however, has shown that removal of a child's tonsils does not reduce occurrences of otitis media. Tonsillotomy and adenoidectomy may be appropriate for reasons other than middle ear fluid.

Hearing should be fully restored once the fluid is removed. Some children may need to have the operation again if the otitis media returns after the tubes come out. While the tubes are in place, water should be kept out of the ears. Many physicians recommend that a child with tubes wear special earplugs while swimming or bathing so that water does not enter the middle ear.

Chapter 14

Pertussis

Pertussis, also known as "whooping cough," is a highly contagious respiratory disease. It is caused by the bacterium *Bordetella pertussis*.

Pertussis is known for uncontrollable, violent coughing which often makes it hard to breathe. After cough fits, someone with pertussis often needs to take deep breaths, which result in a "whooping" sound. Pertussis can affect people of all ages, but can be very serious, even deadly, for babies less than a year old.

The best way to protect against pertussis is by getting vaccinated.

Causes of Pertussis

Bordetella pertussis bacteria attach to the cilia (tiny, hair-like extensions) that line part of the upper respiratory system. The bacteria release toxins (poisons), which damage the cilia and cause airways to swell.

Transmission of Pertussis

Pertussis is a very contagious disease only found in humans. Pertussis spreads from person to person. People with pertussis usually spread the disease to another person by coughing or sneezing or when spending a lot of time near one another where you share breathing

---

This chapter includes text excerpted from "Pertussis (Whooping Cough)," Centers for Disease Control and Prevention (CDC), August 7, 2017.

space. Many babies who get pertussis are infected by older siblings, parents, or caregivers who might not even know they have the disease.

Infected people are most contagious up to about two weeks after the cough begins. Antibiotics may shorten the amount of time someone is contagious.

While pertussis vaccines are the most effective tool to prevent this disease, no vaccine is 100 percent effective. When pertussis circulates in the community, there is a chance that a fully vaccinated person, of any age, can catch this disease. If you have gotten the pertussis vaccine but still get sick, the infection is usually not as bad.

Signs and Symptoms of Pertussis

Pertussis (whooping cough) can cause serious illness in babies, children, teens, and adults. Symptoms of pertussis usually develop within 5 to 10 days after you are exposed. Sometimes pertussis symptoms do not develop for as long as 3 weeks.

Early Symptoms

The disease usually starts with cold-like symptoms and maybe a mild cough or fever. In babies, the cough can be minimal or not even there. Babies may have a symptom known as "apnea." Apnea is a pause in the child's breathing pattern. Pertussis is most dangerous for babies. About half of babies younger than one year who get the disease need care in the hospital.

Early symptoms can last for one to two weeks and usually include:

- Runny nose

- Low-grade fever (generally minimal throughout the course of the disease)

- Mild, occasional cough

- Apnea—a pause in breathing (in babies)

Pertussis in its early stages appears to be nothing more than the common cold. Therefore, healthcare professionals often do not suspect or diagnose it until more severe symptoms appear.

Later-Stage Symptoms

After one to two weeks and as the disease progresses, the traditional symptoms of pertussis may appear and include:

- Paroxysms (fits) of many, rapid coughs followed by a high-pitched "whoop" sound

- Vomiting (throwing up) during or after coughing fits

- Exhaustion (very tired) after coughing fits

Pertussis can cause violent and rapid coughing, over and over, until the air is gone from your lungs. When there is no more air in the lungs, you are forced to inhale with a loud "whooping" sound. This extreme coughing can cause you to throw up and be very tired. Although you are often exhausted after a coughing fit, you usually appear fairly well in-between. Coughing fits generally become more common and bad as the illness continues, and can occur more often at night. The coughing fits can go on for up to 10 weeks or more. In China, pertussis is known as the "100 day cough."

The "whoop" is often not there if you have milder (less serious) disease. The infection is generally milder in teens and adults, especially those who have gotten the pertussis vaccine.

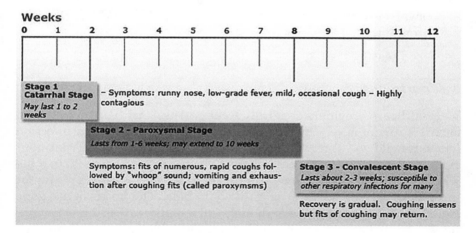

Figure 14.1. *Disease Progression*

Symptoms among Those Who Got Pertussis Vaccine

In those who have gotten the pertussis vaccine:

- In most cases, the cough will not last as many days

- Coughing fits, whooping, and vomiting after coughing fits occur less often

- The percentage of children with apnea (long pause in breathing), cyanosis (blue/purplish skin coloration due to lack of oxygen) and vomiting is less

Recovery

Recovery from pertussis can happen slowly. The cough becomes milder and less common. However, coughing fits can return with other respiratory infections for many months after the pertussis infection started.

Diagnosis and Treatment of Pertussis
Diagnosis

Healthcare providers diagnose pertussis (whooping cough) by considering if you have been exposed to pertussis and by doing a:

- History of typical signs and symptoms

- Physical examination

- Laboratory test which involves taking a sample of mucus (with a swab or syringe filled with saline) from the back of the throat through the nose

- Blood test

Treatment

Healthcare providers generally treat pertussis with antibiotics and early treatment is very important. Treatment may make your infection less serious if you start it early, before coughing fits begin. Treatment can also help prevent spreading the disease to close contacts (people who have spent a lot of time around the infected person). Treatment after three weeks of illness is unlikely to help. The bacteria are gone from your body by then, even though you usually will still have symptoms. This is because the bacteria have already done damage to your body.

There are several antibiotics (medications that can help treat diseases caused by bacteria) available to treat pertussis. If a healthcare professional diagnoses you or your child with pertussis, they will explain how to treat the infection.

Pertussis can sometimes be very serious, requiring treatment in the hospital. Babies are at greatest risk for serious complications from pertussis. View photos of a baby getting treatment for pertussis in the hospital.

If Your Child Gets Treatment for Pertussis at Home

Do not give your child cough medications unless instructed to do so by your doctor. Giving cough medicine probably will not help and is often not recommended for kids younger than four years old.

Manage pertussis and reduce the risk of spreading it to others by:

- Following the schedule for giving antibiotics exactly as your child's doctor prescribed.

- Keeping your home free from irritants—as much as possible—that can trigger coughing, such as smoke, dust, and chemical fumes.

- Using a clean, cool mist vaporizer to help loosen mucus and soothe the cough.

- Practicing good handwashing.

- Encouraging your child to drink plenty of fluids, including water, juices, and soups, and eating fruits to prevent dehydration (lack of fluids). Report any signs of dehydration to your doctor immediately. These include dry, sticky mouth, sleepiness or tiredness, or thirst. They also include decreased urination or fewer wet diapers, few or no tears when crying, muscle weakness, headache, dizziness or lightheadedness.

- Encouraging your child to eat small meals every few hours to help prevent vomiting (throwing up) from occurring.

If Your Child Gets Treatment for Pertussis in the Hospital

Your child may need help keeping breathing passages clear, which may require suctioning (drawing out) of mucus. Doctors monitor breathing and give oxygen, if needed. Children might need intravenous (IV, through the vein) fluids if they show signs of dehydration or have difficulty eating. You should take precautions, such as practicing good hand hygiene and keeping surfaces clean.

Prevention of Pertussis
Vaccines

The best way to prevent pertussis (whooping cough) among babies, children, teens, and adults is to get vaccinated. Also, keep babies and other people at high risk for pertussis complications away from infected people.

In the United States, the recommended pertussis vaccine for babies and children is called "DTaP." This is a combination vaccine that helps protect against three diseases: diphtheria, tetanus, and pertussis.

Vaccine protection for these three diseases fades with time. Before 2005, the only booster (called "Tetanus-Diphtheria" (Td)) available contained protection against tetanus and diphtheria. This vaccine was recommended for teens and adults every 10 years. Nowadays there is a booster (called "tetanus-diphtheria-acellular pertussis" or "Tdap") for preteens, teens, and adults that contains protection against tetanus, diphtheria, and pertussis.

Being up-to-date with pertussis vaccines is especially important for families with and caregivers of new babies.

Infection

If your doctor confirms that you have pertussis, your body will have a natural defense (immunity) to future pertussis infections. Some observational studies suggest that pertussis infection can provide immunity for 4 to 20 years. Since this immunity fades and does not offer lifelong protection, the Centers for Disease Control and Prevention (CDC) still recommends pertussis vaccination.

Antibiotics

If you or a member of your household has been diagnosed with pertussis, your doctor or local health department may recommend preventive antibiotics (medications that can help prevent diseases caused by bacteria) to other members of the household to help prevent the spread of disease. Additionally, they may recommend preventive antibiotics to some other people outside the household who have been exposed to a person with pertussis, including:

- People at risk for serious disease

- People who have routine contact with someone that is considered at high risk of serious disease

Babies younger than one-year-old are most at risk for serious complications from pertussis. Pregnant women are not at increased risk for serious disease. However, experts consider those in their third trimester to be at increased risk since they could, in turn, expose their newborn to pertussis. You should discuss whether or not you need preventive antibiotics with your doctor. This is especially important if there is a baby or pregnant woman in your household. It is also important if you plan to have contact with a baby or pregnant woman.

Hygiene

Like many respiratory illnesses, pertussis spreads by coughing and sneezing while in close contact with others, who then breathe in the bacteria. The CDC recommends practicing good hygiene to prevent the spread of respiratory illnesses. To practice good hygiene you should:

- Cover your mouth and nose with a tissue when you cough or sneeze.

- Put your used tissue in the wastebasket.

- Cough or sneeze into your upper sleeve or elbow, not your hands, if you do not have a tissue.

- Wash your hands often with soap and water for at least 20 seconds.

- Use an alcohol-based hand rub if soap and water are not available.

Chapter 15

Pneumonia

Pneumonia is a bacterial, viral, or fungal infection of one or both sides of the lungs that causes the air sacs, or alveoli, of the lungs to fill up with fluid or pus. Symptoms can be mild or severe and may include a cough with phlegm (a slimy substance), fever, chills, and trouble breathing. Many factors affect how serious pneumonia is, such as the type of germ causing the lung infection, your age, and your overall health. Pneumonia tends to be more serious for children under the age of five, adults over the age of 65, people with certain conditions, such as heart failure, diabetes, or chronic obstructive pulmonary disease (COPD), or people who have weak immune systems due to human immunodeficiency virus (HIV) and acquired immunodeficiency syndrome (AIDS), chemotherapy (a treatment for cancer), or organ or blood and marrow stem cell transplant procedures.

To diagnose pneumonia, your doctor will review your medical history, perform a physical exam, and order diagnostic tests. This information can help your doctor determine what type of pneumonia you have. If your doctor suspects you got your infection while in a hospital, you may be diagnosed with hospital-acquired pneumonia. If you have been on a ventilator to help you breathe, you may have ventilator-associated pneumonia. The most common form of pneumonia is community-acquired pneumonia, which is when you get an infection outside of a hospital.

This chapter includes text excerpted from "Pneumonia," National Heart, Lung, and Blood Institute (NHLBI), September 27, 2016.

Treatment depends on whether bacteria, viruses, or fungi are causing your pneumonia. If bacteria are causing your pneumonia, you usually are treated at home with oral antibiotics. Most people respond quickly to treatment. If your symptoms worsen you should see a doctor right away. If you have severe symptoms or underlying health problems, you may need to be treated in a hospital. It may take several weeks to recover from pneumonia.

Causes of Pneumonia

Bacteria, viruses, and fungi infections can cause pneumonia. These infections cause inflammation in the air sacs, or alveoli, of the lungs. This inflammation causes the air sacs to fill with fluid and pus.

Bacteria

Bacteria are the most common cause of pneumonia in adults. Many types of bacteria can cause bacterial pneumonia. *Streptococcus pneumoniae* or pneumococcus bacteria are the most common cause of bacterial pneumonia in the United States.

If your pneumonia is caused by one of the following types of bacteria, it is called "atypical pneumonia."

- *Legionella pneumophila.* This type of pneumonia sometimes is called "Legionnaire disease," and it has caused serious outbreaks. Outbreaks have been linked to exposure to cooling towers, whirlpool spas, and decorative fountains.

- *Mycoplasma pneumoniae.* This is a common type of pneumonia that usually affects people younger than 40 years old. People who live or work in crowded places, such as schools, homeless shelters, and prisons are at higher risk for this type of pneumonia. It is usually mild and responds well to treatment with antibiotics. However, *Mycoplasma pneumoniae* can be very serious. It may be associated with a skin rash and hemolysis. This type of bacteria is a common cause of "walking pneumonia."

- *Chlamydia pneumoniae.* This type of pneumonia can occur all year and often is mild. The infection is most common in people 65 to 79 years old.

Bacterial pneumonia can occur on its own or develop after you have had a viral cold or the flu. Bacterial pneumonia often affects just one lobe, or area, of a lung. When this happens, the condition is called "lobar pneumonia."

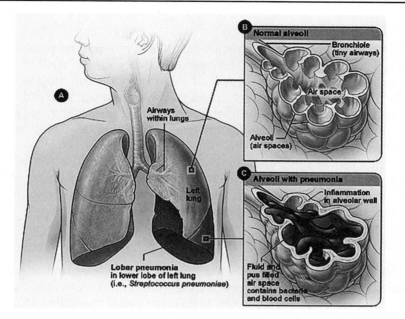

Figure 15.1. *Location of Lungs and Airways, Normal Alveoli, and Alveoli with Pneumonia*

This figure shows pneumonia affecting the single lower lobe of the left lung. Figure A shows the location of the lungs and airways in the body. Figure B shows normal alveoli. Figure C shows infected alveoli or air sacs.

Most of the time, the body filters bacteria out of the air that we breathe to protect the lungs from infection. Your immune system, the shape of your nose and throat, your ability to cough, and fine, hair-like structures called "cilia" help stop the germs from reaching your lungs.

Sometimes bacteria manage to enter the lungs and cause infections. This is more likely to occur if:

- Your immune system is weak

- A germ is very strong

- Your body fails to filter out the bacteria from the air that you breathe. For example, if you cannot cough because you have had a stroke or are sedated, bacteria may remain in your airways.

When bacteria reach your lungs, your immune system goes into action. It sends many kinds of cells to attack the bacteria. These cells cause inflammation in alveoli (air sacs) and can cause these spaces to fill up with fluid and pus. This causes the symptoms of pneumonia.

Virus

Viruses that infect the respiratory tract may cause pneumonia. The influenza or flu virus is the most common cause of viral pneumonia in adults. Respiratory syncytial virus (RSV) is the most common cause of viral pneumonia in children younger than one year old. Other viruses can cause pneumonia, such as the common cold virus known as "rhinovirus," "human parainfluenza virus (HPIV)," and "human metapneumovirus (HMPV)."

Most cases of viral pneumonia are mild. They get better in about one to three weeks without treatment. Some cases are more serious and may require treatment in a hospital. If you have viral pneumonia, you run the risk of getting bacterial pneumonia.

Fungi

Pneumocystis pneumonia is a serious fungal infection caused by *Pneumocystis jirovecii*. It occurs in people who have weak immune systems due to HIV/AIDS or the long-term use of medicines that suppress their immune systems such as those used to treat cancer or as part of organ or blood and marrow stem cell transplant procedures.

Other fungal infections also can lead to pneumonia. The following are three fungi that occur in the soil in some parts of the United States and can cause some people to get pneumonia.

- **Coccidioidomycosis.** This fungus is found in Southern California and the desert Southwest. It is the cause of valley fever.

- **Histoplasmosis.** This fungus is found in the Ohio and Mississippi River Valleys.

- *Cryptococcus.* This fungus is found throughout the United States in bird droppings and soil contaminated with bird droppings.

Risk Factors for Pneumonia
Age

Pneumonia can affect people of all ages. However, two age groups are at greater risk of developing pneumonia and having more severe pneumonia:

- **Infants who are two years old or younger** because their immune systems are still developing during the first few years of life.

- **People who are 65 years old or older** because their immune systems begin to change as a normal part of aging.

Environment

Your risk for pneumonia may increase if you have been exposed to certain chemicals, pollutants, or toxic fumes.

Lifestyle Habits

Smoking cigarettes, excessive use of alcohol, or being undernourished also increases your risk for pneumonia.

Other Medical Conditions

Other conditions and factors also increase your risk for pneumonia. Your risk also goes up if you:

- Have trouble coughing because of a stroke or other condition, or have problems swallowing

- Cannot move around much or are sedated

- Recently had a cold or the flu

- Have a lung disease or other serious diseases including cystic fibrosis (CF), asthma, chronic obstructive pulmonary disease (COPD), bronchiectasis, diabetes, heart failure, or sickle cell disease (SCD)

- Are in a hospital intensive-care unit, especially if you are using a ventilator to help you breathe

- Have a weak or suppressed immune system due to HIV/AIDS, organ transplant or blood and marrow stem cell transplant, chemotherapy (a treatment for cancer), or long-term steroid use

Screening and Prevention of Pneumonia

Pneumonia can be very serious and even life-threatening. Vaccines can help prevent certain types of pneumonia. Good hygiene, quitting smoking, and keeping your immune system strong by exercising and healthy eating are other ways to prevent pneumonia.

Vaccines

Vaccines are available to prevent pneumonia caused by pneumococcal bacteria or the flu virus, or influenza. Vaccines cannot prevent all cases of infection. However, compared to people who do not get vaccinated, those who are vaccinated and still get pneumonia tend to have:

- Milder infections

- Pneumonia that does not last as long

- Fewer serious complications

Pneumococcal Pneumonia Vaccines

Two vaccines are available to prevent pneumococcal pneumonia and potentially fatal complications, such as bacteremia and meningitis. Pneumococcal vaccines are particularly important for:

- Adults who are 65 years old or older

- People who have chronic (ongoing) diseases, serious long-term health problems, or weak immune systems. For example, this may include people who have cancer, HIV/AIDS, asthma, SCD, or damaged or removed spleens

- People who smoke

- Children who are younger than five years old

- Children older than five years of age with certain medical conditions, such as heart or lung diseases or cancer

The Centers for Disease Control and Prevention (CDC) recommends that adults who are 65 and older should have two pneumococcal vaccinations.

Influenza (Flu) Vaccine

Because many people get pneumonia after having influenza or the flu, your yearly flu vaccine can help you and your family not get pneumonia. The flu vaccine is usually given in September through November before the months when influenza or the flu is most frequently spread.

Haemophilus Influenzae Type B *Vaccine*

Haemophilus influenzae type b (Hib) is a type of bacteria that can cause pneumonia and meningitis. The Hib vaccine is given to children to help prevent these infections. The vaccine is recommended for all children in the United States who are younger than five years old. The vaccine often is given to infants starting at two months of age.

Other Ways to Help Prevent Pneumonia

You also can take the following steps to help prevent pneumonia:

- **Wash your hands** with soap and water or alcohol-based rubs to kill germs.
- **Do not smoke.** Smoking damages your lungs' ability to filter out and defend against germs.
- **Keep your immune system strong.** Get plenty of rest and physical activity and follow a healthy diet.

Signs, Symptoms, and Complications of Pneumonia

The signs and symptoms of pneumonia vary from mild to severe. But, some people are at risk for developing more severe pneumonia or potentially fatal complications.

Signs and Symptoms

See your doctor promptly if you have the following signs and symptoms:

- Have a high fever
- Have shaking chills
- Have a cough with phlegm (a slimy substance), which does not improve or worsens
- Develop shortness of breath with normal daily activities
- Have chest pain when you breathe or cough
- Feel suddenly worse after a cold or the flu

If you have pneumonia, you also may have other symptoms, including nausea (feeling sick to the stomach), vomiting, and diarrhea.

Symptoms may vary in certain populations. Newborns and infants may not show any signs of the infection. Or, they may vomit, have a fever and cough, or appear restless, sick, or tired and without energy.

Older adults and people who have serious illnesses or weak immune systems may have fewer and milder symptoms. They may even have a lower than normal temperature. If they already have a lung disease, it may get worse. Older adults who have pneumonia sometimes have sudden changes in mental awareness.

Complications

Often, people who have pneumonia can be successfully treated and do not have complications. Possible complications of pneumonia may include:

- **Bacteremia and septic shock.** Bacteremia is a serious complication in which bacteria from the initial site of infection spread into the blood. It may lead to septic shock, a potentially fatal complication.

- **Lung abscesses.** Lung abscesses usually are treated with antibiotics. Sometimes surgery or drainage with a needle is needed to remove the pus.

- **Pleural effusions, empyema, and pleurisy.** These painful or even potentially fatal complications can occur if pneumonia is not treated. The pleura is a membrane that consists of two large, thin layers of tissue. One layer wraps around the outside of your lungs and the other layer lines the inside of your chest cavity. Pleurisy is when the two layers of the pleura become irritated and inflamed, causing sharp pain each time you breathe in. The pleural space is a very thin space between the two pleura. Pleural effusions are the buildup of fluid in the pleural space. If the fluid becomes infected, it is called "empyema." If this happens, you may need to have the fluid drained through a chest tube or removed with surgery.

- **Renal failure**

- **Respiratory failure**

Diagnosis of Pneumonia

Sometimes pneumonia is hard to diagnose because it may cause symptoms commonly seen in people with colds or the flu. You may not realize it is more serious until it lasts longer than these other conditions. Your doctor will diagnose pneumonia based on your medical history, a physical exam, and test results. Your doctor may be able to diagnose you with a certain type of pneumonia based on how you got your infection and the type of germ causing your infection.

Medical History

Your doctor will ask about your signs and symptoms and how and when they began. To find out whether you have bacterial, viral, or fungal pneumonia, your doctor also may ask about:

- Any recent traveling you have done
- Your hobbies
- Your exposure to animals
- Your exposure to sick people at home, school, or work
- Your past and current medical conditions, and whether any have gotten worse recently
- Any medicines you take
- Whether you smoke
- Whether you have had flu or pneumonia vaccinations

Physical Exam

Your doctor will listen to your lungs with a stethoscope. If you have pneumonia, your lungs may make crackling, bubbling, and rumbling sounds when you inhale. Your doctor also may hear wheezing. Your doctor may find it hard to hear sounds of breathing in some areas of your chest.

Diagnostic Tests

If your doctor thinks you have pneumonia, she or he may recommend one or more of the following tests.

- **Chest x-ray** to look for inflammation in your lungs. A chest x-ray is the best test for diagnosing pneumonia. However, this test will not tell your doctor what kind of germ is causing pneumonia.
- **Blood tests** such as a complete blood count (CBC) to see if your immune system is actively fighting an infection.

- **Blood culture** to find out whether you have a bacterial infection that has spread to your bloodstream. If so, your doctor can decide how to treat the infection.

Your doctor may recommend other tests if you are in the hospital, have serious symptoms, are older, or have other health problems.

- **Sputum test.** Your doctor may collect a sample of sputum (spit) or phlegm (slimy substance from deep in your lungs) that was produced from one of your deep coughs and send the sample to the lab for testing. This may help your doctor find out if bacteria are causing your pneumonia. Then, she or he can plan your treatment.

- **Chest computed tomography (CT) scan** to see how much of your lungs is affected by your condition or to see if you have complications, such as lung abscesses or pleural effusions. A CT scan shows more detail than a chest x-ray.

- **Pleural fluid culture.** For this test, a fluid sample is taken from the pleural space (a thin space between two layers of tissue that line the lungs and chest cavity). Doctors use a procedure called "thoracentesis" to collect the fluid sample. The fluid is studied for bacteria that may cause pneumonia.

- **Pulse oximetry.** For this test, a small sensor is attached to your finger or ear. The sensor uses light to estimate how much oxygen is in your blood. Pneumonia can keep your lungs from moving enough oxygen into your bloodstream. If you are very sick, your doctor may need to measure the level of oxygen in your blood using a blood sample. The sample is taken from an artery, usually in your wrist. This test is called an "arterial blood gas test."

- **Bronchoscopy** is a procedure used to look inside the lungs' airways. If you are in the hospital and treatment with antibiotics is not working well, your doctor may use this procedure. Your doctor passes a thin, flexible tube through your nose or mouth, down your throat, and into the airways. The tube has a light and small camera that allow your doctor to see your windpipe and airways and take pictures. Your doctor can see whether something is blocking your airways or whether another factor is contributing to your pneumonia. Your doctor may use this procedure to collect samples of fluid from the site of pneumonia (called "bronchoalveolar lavage" or BAL) or to take small biopsies of lung tissue to help find the cause of your pneumonia.

Types of Pneumonia

Your doctor may also diagnose you with a certain type of pneumonia. Pneumonia is named for the way in which a person gets the infection or for the germ that causes the infection.

- **Community-acquired pneumonia (CAP).** CAP is the most common type of pneumonia and is usually caused by pneumococcus bacteria. Most cases occur during the winter. CAP occurs outside of hospitals and other healthcare settings. Most people get CAP by breathing in germs (especially while sleeping) that live in the mouth, nose, or throat.

- **Hospital-acquired pneumonia (HAP).** HAP is when people catch pneumonia during a hospital stay for another illness. HAP tends to be more serious than CAP because you are already sick. Also, hospitals tend to have more germs that are resistant to antibiotics that are used to treat bacterial pneumonia.

- **Ventilator-associated pneumonia (VAP).** VAP is when people who are on a ventilator machine to help them breathe get pneumonia.

- **Atypical pneumonia.** Atypical pneumonia is a type of CAP. It is caused by lung infections with less common bacteria than the pneumococcus bacteria that cause CAP. Atypical bacteria include *Legionella pneumophila, Mycoplasma pneumoniae,* or *Chlamydia pneumoniae.*

- **Aspiration pneumonia.** This type of pneumonia can occur if you inhale food, drink, vomit, or saliva from your mouth into your lungs. This may happen if something disturbs your normal gag reflex, such as a brain injury, swallowing problems, or excessive use of alcohol or drugs. Aspiration pneumonia can cause lung abscesses.

Treatment of Pneumonia

Treatment for pneumonia depends on the type of pneumonia you have, the germ causing your infection, and how severe your pneumonia is. Most people who have community-acquired pneumonia—the most common type of pneumonia—are treated at home. The goals of treatment are to cure the infection and prevent complications.

Bacterial Pneumonia

Bacterial pneumonia is treated with medicines called "antibiotics." You should take antibiotics as your doctor prescribes. You may start to feel better before you finish the medicine, but you should continue taking it as prescribed. If you stop too soon, pneumonia may come back.

Most people begin to improve after one to three days of antibiotic treatment. This means that they should feel better and have fewer symptoms such as cough and fever.

Viral Pneumonia

Antibiotics do not work when the cause of pneumonia is a virus. If you have viral pneumonia, your doctor may prescribe an antiviral medicine to treat it. Viral pneumonia usually improves in one to three weeks.

Treating Severe Symptoms

You may need to be treated in a hospital if:

• Your symptoms are severe

• You are at risk for complications because of other health problems

If the level of oxygen in your bloodstream is low, you may receive oxygen therapy. If you have bacterial pneumonia, your doctor may give you antibiotics through an intravenous (IV) line inserted into a vein.

General Treatment Advice and Follow-Up Care

If you have pneumonia, follow your treatment plan, take all medicines as prescribed, and get follow-up medical care.

Living with Pneumonia

If you have pneumonia, you can take steps to recover from the infection and prevent complications.

• Get plenty of rest.

- Follow your treatment plan as your doctor advises.

- Take all medicines as your doctor prescribes. If you are using antibiotics, continue to take the medicine until it is all gone. You may start to feel better before you finish the medicine, but you should continue to take it. If you stop too soon, the bacterial infection and your pneumonia may come back.

- Ask your doctor when you should schedule follow-up care. Your doctor may recommend a chest x-ray to make sure the infection is gone.

It may take time to recover from pneumonia. Some people feel better and are able to return to their normal routines within a week. For other people, it can take a month or more. Most people continue to feel tired for about a month. Talk to your doctor about when you can go back to your normal routine.

If you have pneumonia, limit contact with family and friends. Cover your nose and mouth while coughing or sneezing, get rid of used tissues right away, and wash your hands. These actions help keep the infection from spreading to other people.

Chapter 16

Sinusitis

A sinus infection (sinusitis) does not typically need to be treated with antibiotics in order to get better. If you or your child is diagnosed with a sinus infection, your healthcare professional can decide if antibiotics are needed.

Causes of Sinusitis

Sinus infections occur when fluid is trapped or blocked in the sinuses, allowing germs to grow. Sinus infections are usually (9 out of 10 cases in adults; 5 to 7 out of 10 cases in children) caused by a virus. They are less commonly (1 out of 10 cases in adults; 3 to 5 out of 10 cases in children) caused by bacteria.

Other conditions can cause symptoms similar to a sinus infection, including:

- Allergies
- Pollutants (airborne chemicals or irritants)
- Fungal infections

Risk Factors of Sinusitis

Several conditions can increase your risk of getting a sinus infection:

- A previous respiratory tract infection (RTI), such as the common cold

This chapter includes text excerpted from "Sinus Infection (Sinusitis)," Centers for Disease Control and Prevention (CDC), September 25, 2017.

- Structural problems within the sinuses

- A weak immune system or taking drugs that weaken the immune system

- Nasal polyps

- Allergies

In children, the following are also risk factors for a sinus infection:

- Going to day care

- Using a pacifier

- Drinking a bottle while laying down

- Being exposed to secondhand smoke

Signs and Symptoms of Sinusitis

Common signs and symptoms of a sinus infection include:

- Headache

- Stuffy or runny nose

- Loss of the sense of smell

- Facial pain or pressure

- Postnasal drip (mucus drips down the throat from the nose)

- Sore throat

- Fever

- Coughing

- Fatigue (being tired)

- Bad breath

When to Seek Medical Care

See a healthcare professional if you or your child has any of the following:

- Temperature higher than 100.4°F

- Symptoms that are getting worse or lasting more than 10 days

- Multiple sinus infections in the past year

- Symptoms that are not relieved with over-the-counter (OTC) medicines

If your child is younger than three months of age and has a fever, it is important to call your healthcare professional right away.

You may have chronic sinusitis if your sinus infection lasts more than 8 weeks or if you have more than 4 sinus infections each year. If you are diagnosed with chronic sinusitis, or believe you may have chronic sinusitis, you should visit your healthcare professional for evaluation. Chronic sinusitis can be caused by nasal growths, allergies, or respiratory tract infections (RTI) (viral, bacterial, or fungal).

Diagnosis and Treatment of Sinusitis

Your healthcare professional will determine if you or your child has a sinus infection by asking about symptoms and doing a physical examination. Sometimes they will also swab the inside of your nose.

Antibiotics may be needed if the sinus infection is likely to be caused by bacteria. Antibiotics will not help a sinus infection caused by a virus or an irritation in the air (such as secondhand smoke). These infections will almost always get better on their own. Antibiotic treatment in these cases may even cause harm in both children and adults.

If symptoms continue for more than 10 days, schedule a follow-up appointment with your healthcare professional for re-evaluation.

Sinusitis Symptom Relief

Rest, OTC medicines, and other self-care methods may help you or your child feel better. Always use OTC products as directed since many OTC products are not recommended for children of certain ages.

Prevention of Sinusitis

There are several steps you can take to help prevent a sinus infection, including:

- Practice good hand hygiene

- Keep you and your child up to date with recommended immunizations

- Avoid close contact with people who have colds or other upper respiratory infections

- Avoid smoking and exposure to secondhand smoke

- Use a clean humidifier to moisten the air at home

Chapter 17

Streptococcal Pharyngitis (Strep Throat) and Tonsillitis

Chapter Contents

Section 17.1

Strep Throat

This section includes text excerpted from "Strep Throat:
All You Need to Know," Centers for Disease Control
and Prevention (CDC), November 1, 2018.

Viruses are the most common cause of a sore throat. However, strep throat is an infection in the throat and tonsils caused by bacteria called "group A streptococcus (group A strep)."

How You Get Strep Throat

Group A strep live in the nose and throat and can easily spread to other people. It is important to know that all infected people do not have symptoms or seem sick. People who are infected spread the bacteria by coughing or sneezing, which creates small respiratory droplets that contain the bacteria.

People can get sick if they:

- Breathe in those droplets

- Touch something with droplets on it and then touch their mouth or nose

- Drink from the same glass or eat from the same plate as a sick person

- Touch sores on the skin caused by group A strep (impetigo)

Rarely, people can spread group A strep through food that is not handled properly. Experts do not believe pets or household items, such as toys, spread these bacteria.

Common Signs and Symptoms of Strep Throat

In general, strep throat is a mild infection, but it can be very painful. The most common symptoms of strep throat include:

- Sore throat that can start very quickly

- Pain when swallowing

- Fever

- Red and swollen tonsils, sometimes with white patches or streaks of pus

- Tiny, red spots (petechiae) on the roof of the mouth (the soft or hard palate)

- Swollen lymph nodes in the front of the neck

Other symptoms may include headache, stomach pain, nausea, or vomiting—especially in children. Someone with strep throat may also have a rash known as "scarlet fever" (also called "scarlatina").

The following symptoms suggest a virus is the cause of the illness instead of strep throat:

- Cough

- Runny nose

- Hoarseness (changes in your voice that makes it sound breathy, raspy, or strained)

- Conjunctivitis (also called "pink eye")

It usually takes two to five days for someone exposed to group A strep to become ill.

Who Are at Risk of Getting Strep Throat?

Anyone can get strep throat, but there are some factors that can increase the risk of getting this common infection.

Strep throat is more common in children than adults. It is most common in children 5 through 15 years old. It is rare in children younger than 3 years old. Adults who are at increased risk for strep throat include:

- Parents of school-aged children

- Adults who are often in contact with children

Close contact with another person with strep throat is the most common risk factor for illness. For example, if someone has strep throat, it often spreads to other people in their household.

Infectious illnesses tend to spread wherever large groups of people gather together. Crowded conditions can increase the risk of getting a group A strep infection. These settings include:

- Schools

- Day care centers

- Military training facilities

Diagnosis of Strep Throat

Only a rapid strep test or throat culture can determine if group A strep is the cause. A doctor cannot tell if someone has strep throat just by looking at his or her throat.

A rapid strep test involves swabbing the throat and running a test on the swab. The test quickly shows if group A strep is causing the illness. If the test is positive, doctors can prescribe antibiotics. If the test is negative, but a doctor still suspects strep throat, then the doctor can take a throat culture swab. A throat culture takes time to see if group A strep bacteria grow from the swab. While it takes more time, a throat culture sometimes finds infections that the rapid strep test misses. Culture is important to use in children and teens since they can get rheumatic fever from an untreated strep throat infection. For adults, it is usually not necessary to do a throat culture following a negative rapid strep test. Adults are generally not at risk of getting rheumatic fever following a strep throat infection.

How Is Strep Throat Treated?

Doctors treat strep throat with antibiotics. Either penicillin or amoxicillin are recommended as a first choice for people who are not allergic to penicillin. Doctors can use other antibiotics to treat strep throat in people who are allergic to penicillin.

Benefits of antibiotics include:

- Decreasing how long someone is sick

- Decreasing symptoms (feeling better)

- Preventing the bacteria from spreading to others

- Preventing serious complications, such as rheumatic fever

Someone who tests positive for strep throat but has no symptoms (called a "carrier") usually does not need antibiotics. They are less likely to spread the bacteria to others and very unlikely to get complications. If a carrier gets a sore throat illness caused by a virus, the rapid strep test can be positive. In these cases it can be hard to know what is causing the sore throat. If someone keeps getting a sore throat after taking the right antibiotics, they may be a strep carrier and have a viral throat infection. Talk to a doctor if you think you or your child may be a strep carrier.

What Complications Are Associated with Strep Throat?

Complications can occur after a strep throat infection. This can happen if the bacteria spread to other parts of the body. Complications can include:

- Abscesses (pockets of pus) around the tonsils
- Swollen lymph nodes in the neck
- Sinus infections
- Ear infections
- Rheumatic fever (a heart disease)
- Poststreptococcal glomerulonephritis (a kidney disease)

What Can Be Done to Prevent Strep Throat?

People can get strep throat more than once. Having strep throat does not protect someone from getting it again in the future. While there is no vaccine to prevent strep throat, there are things people can do to protect themselves and others.

Good Hygiene Helps Prevent Group A Strep Infections

The best way to keep from getting or spreading group A strep is to wash your hands often. This is especially important after coughing or sneezing and before preparing foods or eating. To practice good hygiene you should:

- Cover your mouth and nose with a tissue when you cough or sneeze
- Put your used tissue in the wastebasket
- Cough or sneeze into your upper sleeve or elbow, not your hands, if you do not have a tissue
- Wash your hands often with soap and water for at least 20 seconds
- Use an alcohol-based hand rub if soap and water are not available

You should also wash glasses, utensils, and plates after someone who is sick uses them. These items are safe for others to use once washed.

Antibiotics Help Prevent Spreading the Infection to Others

People with strep throat should stay home from work, school, or day care until they:

- No longer have a fever

- Have taken antibiotics for at least 24 hours

Take the prescription exactly as the doctor says to. Do not stop taking the medicine, even if you or your child feel better, unless the doctor says to stop. Wash your hands often to help prevent germs from spreading.

Section 17.2

Tonsillitis

This section includes text excerpted from "Tonsillitis," MedlinePlus, National Institutes of Health (NIH), April 11, 2017.

What Are Tonsils?

Tonsils are lumps of tissue at the back of the throat. There are two of them, one on each side. Along with the adenoids, tonsils are part of the lymphatic system. The lymphatic system clears away infection and keeps body fluids in balance. Tonsils and adenoids work by trapping the germs coming in through the mouth and nose.

What Is Tonsillitis?

Tonsillitis is an inflammation (swelling) of the tonsils. Sometimes along with tonsillitis, the adenoids are also swollen.

What Causes Tonsillitis

The cause of tonsillitis is usually a viral infection. Bacterial infections, such as strep throat can also cause tonsillitis.

Who Is at Risk for Tonsillitis?

Tonsillitis is most common in children over age two. Almost every child in the United States gets it at least once. Tonsillitis caused by bacteria is more common in kids who are 5 to 15-years old. Tonsillitis caused by a virus is more common in younger children. Adults can get tonsillitis, but it is not very common.

Is Tonsillitis Contagious?

Although tonsillitis is not contagious, the viruses and bacteria that cause it are contagious. Frequent handwashing can help prevent spreading or catching the infections.

What Are the Symptoms of Tonsillitis?

The symptoms of tonsillitis include:

- A sore throat, which may be severe
- Red, swollen tonsils
- Trouble swallowing
- A white or yellow coating on the tonsils
- Swollen glands in the neck
- Fever
- Bad breath

How Is Tonsillitis Diagnosed?

To diagnose tonsillitis, your child's healthcare provider will first ask you about your child's symptoms and medical history. The provider will look at your child's throat and neck, checking for things, such as redness or white spots on the tonsils and swollen lymph nodes.

Your child will probably also have one or more tests to check for strep throat, since it can cause tonsillitis and it requires treatment. It could be a rapid strep test, a throat culture, or both. For both tests, the provider uses a cotton swab to collect a sample of fluids from your child's tonsils and the back of the throat. With the rapid strep test, testing is done in the office, and you get the results within minutes. The throat culture is done in a lab, and it usually takes a few days to get the results. The throat culture is a more reliable test. So sometimes if the rapid strep test is negative (meaning that it does not show any strep bacteria), the provider will also do a throat culture just to make sure that your child does not have strep.

What Are the Treatments for Tonsillitis?

Treatment for tonsillitis depends on the cause. If the cause is a virus, there is no medicine to treat it. If the cause is a bacterial infection, such as strep throat, your child will need to take antibiotics. It is important for your child to finish the antibiotics even if he or she feels better. If treatment stops too soon, some bacteria may survive and reinfect your child.

No matter what is causing the tonsillitis, there are some things you can do to help your child feel better. Make sure that your child:

- Gets a lot of rest
- Drinks plenty of fluids
- Tries eating soft foods if it hurts to swallow
- Tries eating warm liquids or cold foods, such as popsicles to soothe the throat
- Is not around cigarette smoke or do anything else that could irritate the throat
- Sleeps in a room with a humidifier
- Gargles with saltwater
- Sucks on a lozenge (but do not give them to children under four; they can choke on them)
- Takes an over-the-counter (OTC) pain reliever, such as acetaminophen. Children and teenagers should not take aspirin.

Chapter 18

Tuberculosis

Tuberculosis (TB) is caused by a bacterium called *"Mycobacterium tuberculosis."* The bacteria usually attack the lungs, but TB bacteria can attack any part of the body, such as the kidney, spine, and brain. Not everyone infected with TB bacteria becomes sick. As a result, two TB-related conditions exist: latent TB infection (LTBI) and TB disease. If not treated properly, TB disease can be fatal.

How Tuberculosis Spreads

Tuberculosis bacteria are spread through the air from one person to another. The TB bacteria are put into the air when a person with TB disease of the lungs or throat coughs, speaks, or sings. People nearby may breathe in these bacteria and become infected.

Tuberculosis is NOT spread by:

- Shaking someone's hand
- Sharing food or drink
- Touching bed linens or toilet seats
- Sharing toothbrushes
- Kissing

This chapter includes text excerpted from "Basic TB Facts," Centers for Disease Control and Prevention (CDC), March 20, 2016.

When a person breathes in TB bacteria, the bacteria can settle in the lungs and begin to grow. From there, they can move through the blood to other parts of the body, such as the kidney, spine, and brain.

Tuberculosis disease in the lungs or throat can be infectious. This means that the bacteria can be spread to other people. TB in other parts of the body, such as the kidney or spine, is usually not infectious.

People with TB disease are most likely to spread it to people they spend time with every day. This includes family members, friends, and coworkers or schoolmates.

Latent Tuberculosis Infection and Tuberculosis Disease

Not everyone infected with TB bacteria becomes sick. As a result, two TB-related conditions exist: latent TB infection and TB disease.

Latent Tuberculosis Infection

Tuberculosis bacteria can live in the body without making you sick. This is called "latent TB infection." In most people who breathe in TB bacteria and become infected, the body is able to fight the bacteria to stop them from growing.

People with latent TB infection:

- Have no symptoms

- Do not feel sick

- Cannot spread TB bacteria to others

- Usually, have a positive TB skin test reaction or positive TB blood test

- May develop TB disease if they do not receive treatment for latent TB infection

Many people who have latent TB infection never develop TB disease. In these people, the TB bacteria remain inactive for a lifetime without causing disease. But in other people, especially people who have a weak immune system, the bacteria become active, multiply, and cause TB disease.

Tuberculosis Disease

Tuberculosis bacteria become active if the immune system cannot stop them from growing. When TB bacteria are active (multiplying in your body), this is called "TB disease." People with TB disease are sick. They may also be able to spread the bacteria to people they spend time with every day.

Many people who have latent TB infection never develop TB disease. Some people develop TB disease soon after becoming infected (within weeks) before their immune system can fight the TB bacteria. Other people may get sick years later when their immune system becomes weak for another reason.

For people whose immune systems are weak, especially those with human immunodeficiency virus (HIV) infection, the risk of developing TB disease is much higher than for people with normal immune systems.

Table 18.1. Differences between Latent Tuberculosis Infection and Tuberculosis Disease

A Person with Latent Tuberculosis Infection	A Person with Tuberculosis Disease
Has no symptoms	Has symptoms that may include: • A bad cough that lasts three weeks or longer • Pain in the chest • Coughing up blood or sputum • Weakness or fatigue • Weight loss • No appetite • Chills • Fever • Sweating at night
Does not feel sick	Usually feels sick
Cannot spread TB bacteria to others	May spread TB bacteria to others
Usually has a skin test or blood test result indicating TB infection	Usually has a skin test or blood test result indicating TB infection
Has a normal chest x-ray and a negative sputum smear	May have an abnormal chest x-ray, or positive sputum smear or culture
Needs treatment for latent TB infection to prevent TB disease	Needs treatment to treat TB disease

Signs and Symptoms of Tuberculosis

Symptoms of TB disease depend on where in the body the TB bacteria are growing. TB bacteria usually grow in the lungs (pulmonary TB).

TB disease in the lungs may cause symptoms, such as:

- A bad cough that lasts three weeks or longer
- Pain in the chest
- Coughing up blood or sputum (phlegm from deep inside the lungs)

Other symptoms of TB disease are:

- Weakness or fatigue
- Weight loss
- No appetite
- Chills
- Fever
- Sweating at night

Symptoms of TB disease in other parts of the body depend on the area affected.

People who have latent TB infection do not feel sick, do not have any symptoms, and cannot spread TB to others.

Risk Factors of Tuberculosis

Some people develop TB disease soon after becoming infected (within weeks) before their immune system can fight the TB bacteria. Other people may get sick years later, when their immune system becomes weak for another reason.

Overall, about 5 to 10 percent of infected persons who do not receive treatment for latent TB infection will develop TB disease at some time in their lives. For persons whose immune systems are weak, especially those with HIV infection, the risk of developing TB disease is much higher than for persons with normal immune systems.

Generally, persons at high risk for developing TB disease fall into two categories:

- Persons who have been recently infected with TB bacteria
- Persons with medical conditions that weaken the immune system

Persons Who Have Been Recently Infected with Tuberculosis Bacteria

This includes:

- Close contacts of a person with infectious TB disease

- Persons who have immigrated from areas of the world with high rates of TB

- Children less than five years of age who have a positive TB test

- Groups with high rates of TB transmission, such as homeless persons, injection drug users, and persons with HIV infection

- Persons who work or reside with people who are at high risk for TB in facilities or institutions, such as hospitals, homeless shelters, correctional facilities, nursing homes, and residential homes for those with HIV

Persons with Medical Conditions That Weaken the Immune System

Babies and young children often have weak immune systems. Other people can have weak immune systems, too, especially people with any of these conditions:

- HIV infection (the virus that causes acquired immunodeficiency syndrome (AIDS))

- Substance abuse

- Silicosis

- Diabetes mellitus

- Severe kidney disease

- Low body weight

- Organ transplants

- Head and neck cancer

- Medical treatments, such as corticosteroids or organ transplant

- Specialized treatment for rheumatoid arthritis (RA) or Crohn disease

Exposure to Tuberculosis
What to Do If You Have Been Exposed to Tuberculosis

You may have been exposed to TB bacteria if you spent time near someone with TB disease. The TB bacteria are put into the air when a person with active TB disease of the lungs or throat coughs, sneezes, speaks, or sings. You cannot get TB from:

- Clothes
- Drinking glass
- Eating utensils
- Handshake
- Toilet
- Other surfaces

If you think you have been exposed to someone with TB disease, you should contact your doctor or local health department about getting a TB skin test or a special TB blood test. Be sure to tell the doctor or nurse when you spent time with the person who has TB disease.

It is important to know that a person who is exposed to TB bacteria is not able to spread the bacteria to other people right away. Only persons with active TB disease can spread TB bacteria to others. Before you would be able to spread TB to others, you would have to breathe in TB bacteria and become infected. Then the active bacteria would have to multiply in your body and cause active TB disease. At this point, you could possibly spread TB bacteria to others. People with TB disease are most likely to spread the bacteria to people they spend time with every day, such as family members, friends, coworkers, or schoolmates.

Some people develop TB disease soon (within weeks) after becoming infected, before their immune system can fight the TB bacteria. Other people may get sick years later, when their immune system becomes weak for another reason. Many people with TB infection never develop TB disease.

Prevention of Tuberculosis
Preventing Latent Tuberculosis Infection from Progressing to Tuberculosis Disease

Many people who have latent TB infection never develop TB disease. But some people who have latent TB infection are more likely to develop TB disease than others. Those at high risk for developing TB disease include:

- People with HIV infection
- People who became infected with TB bacteria in the last two years

- Babies and young children
- People who inject illegal drugs
- People who are sick with other diseases that weaken the immune system
- Elderly people

People who were not treated correctly for TB in the past

If you have latent TB infection and you are in one of these high-risk groups, you should take medicine to keep from developing TB disease. There are several treatment options for latent TB infection. You and your healthcare provider must decide which treatment is best for you. If you take your medicine as instructed, it can keep you from developing TB disease. Because there are less bacteria, treatment for latent TB infection is much easier than treatment for TB disease. A person with TB disease has a large amount of TB bacteria in the body. Several drugs are needed to treat TB disease.

Preventing Exposure to Tuberculosis Disease While Traveling Abroad

In many countries, TB is much more common than in the United States. Travelers should avoid close contact or prolonged time with known TB patients in crowded, enclosed environments (for example, clinics, hospitals, prisons, or homeless shelters).

Although multidrug-resistant (MDR) and extensively drug-resistant (XDR) TB are occurring globally, they are still rare. HIV-infected travelers are at greatest risk if they come in contact with a person with MDR or XDR TB.

Air travel itself carries a relatively low risk of infection with TB of any kind. Travelers who will be working in clinics, hospitals, or other healthcare settings where TB patients are likely to be encountered should consult infection control or occupational health experts. They should ask about administrative and environmental procedures for preventing exposure to TB. Once those procedures are implemented, additional measures could include using personal respiratory protective devices.

Travelers who anticipate possible prolonged exposure to people with TB (for example, those who expect to come in contact routinely with clinic, hospital, prison, or homeless shelter populations) should have a TB skin test or a TB blood test before leaving the United States. If the test reaction is negative, they should have a repeat test 8 to 10 weeks after returning to the United States. Additionally, annual testing may be recommended for those who anticipate repeated or prolonged exposure or an extended stay over a period of years. Because people with HIV infection are more likely to have an impaired response to TB tests, travelers who are HIV positive should tell their physicians about their HIV infection status.

Chapter 19

Other Viral Respiratory Infections

Chapter Contents

Section 19.1

Adenovirus

This section includes text excerpted from "Adenoviruses," Centers for Disease Control and Prevention (CDC), April 26, 2018.

Adenoviruses are common viruses that cause a range of illness. They can cause cold-like symptoms, sore throat, bronchitis, pneumonia, diarrhea, and pink eye (conjunctivitis). You can get an adenovirus infection at any age. People with weakened immune systems or existing respiratory or cardiac disease are more likely than others to get very sick from an adenovirus infection.

Symptoms

Adenoviruses can cause a wide range of illnesses, such as:

- Common cold
- Sore throat
- Bronchitis (a condition that occurs when the airways in the lungs become filled with mucus and may spasm, which causes a person to cough and have shortness of breath)
- Pneumonia (infection of the lungs)
- Diarrhea
- Pink eye (conjunctivitis)
- Fever
- Bladder inflammation or infection
- Inflammation of stomach and intestines
- Neurologic disease (conditions that affect the brain and spinal cord)

Adenoviruses can cause mild to severe illness, though serious illness is less common. People with weakened immune systems, or existing respiratory or cardiac disease, are at higher risk of developing severe illness from an adenovirus infection.

Transmission of Adenoviruses

Adenoviruses are usually spread from an infected person to others through:

- Close personal contact, such as touching or shaking hands
- The air by coughing and sneezing
- Touching an object or surface with adenoviruses on it, then touching your mouth, nose, or eyes before washing your hands

Some adenoviruses can spread through an infected person's stool, for example, during diaper changing. Adenovirus can also spread through the water, such as swimming pools, but this is less common.

Sometimes the virus can be shed (released from the body) for a long time after a person recovers from an adenovirus infection, especially among people who have weakened immune systems. This "virus shedding" usually occurs without any symptoms, even though the person can still spread adenovirus to other people.

Prevention

Adenovirus Vaccine Is for U.S. Military Only

There is currently no adenovirus vaccine available to the general public.

A vaccine specific for adenovirus types 4 and 7 was approved by the U.S. Food and Drug Administration (FDA) in March 2011, for use only in U.S. military personnel who may be at higher risk for infection from these two adenovirus types.

Follow Simple Steps to Protect Yourself and Others

You can protect yourself and others from adenoviruses and other respiratory illnesses by following a few simple steps:

- Wash your hands often with soap and water.
- Avoid touching your eyes, nose, or mouth with unwashed hands.
- Avoid close contact with people who are sick.

If you are sick you can help protect others:

- Stay home when you are sick.
- Cover your mouth and nose when coughing or sneezing.
- Avoid sharing cups and eating utensils with others.
- Refrain from kissing others.

- Wash your hands often with soap and water, especially after using the bathroom.

- Frequent handwashing is especially important in child care settings and healthcare facilities.

Maintain Proper Chlorine Levels to Prevent Outbreaks

Adenoviruses are resistant to many common disinfectant products and can remain infectious for long periods on surfaces and objects. It is important to keep adequate levels of chlorine in swimming pools to prevent outbreaks of conjunctivitis caused by adenoviruses.

Treatment

There is no specific treatment for people with adenovirus infection. Most adenovirus infections are mild and may require only care to help

Section 19.2

Bronchiolitis Obliterans Organizing Pneumonia

This section includes text excerpted from "Bronchiolitis Obliterans Organizing Pneumonia," Genetic and Rare Diseases Information Center (GARD), National Center for Advancing Translational Sciences (NCATS), February 16, 2016.

Bronchiolitis obliterans organizing pneumonia (BOOP) is a lung disease that causes inflammation in the small air tubes (bronchioles) and air sacs (alveoli). BOOP typically develops in individuals between 40 to 60 years old; however, the disorder may affect individuals of any age. The signs and symptoms of BOOP vary but often include shortness of breath, a dry cough, and fever. BOOP can be caused by viral infections, various drugs, and other medical conditions. If the cause is known, the condition is called "secondary BOOP." In many cases, the underlying cause of BOOP is unknown. These cases are called "idiopathic BOOP" or "cryptogenic organizing pneumonia." Treatment often includes corticosteroid medications

Symptoms of Bronchiolitis Obliterans Organizing Pneumonia

Signs and symptoms of BOOP vary. Some individuals with BOOP may have no apparent symptoms, while others may have severe respiratory distress as in acute, rapidly-progressive BOOP. The most common signs and symptoms of BOOP include shortness of breath (dyspnea), dry cough, and fever. Some people with BOOP develop a flu-like illness with cough, fever, fatigue, and weight loss.

Cause of Bronchiolitis Obliterans Organizing Pneumonia

Bronchiolitis obliterans organizing pneumonia may be caused by a variety of factors, including viral infections, inhalation of toxic gases, drugs, connective tissue disorders, radiation therapy, cocaine, inflammatory bowel disease, and HIV infection. In many cases, the underlying cause of BOOP is unknown. These cases are called "idiopathic BOOP" or "cryptogenic organizing pneumonia (COP)."

Diagnosis of Bronchiolitis Obliterans Organizing Pneumonia

Bronchiolitis obliterans organizing pneumonia is typically diagnosed by lung biopsy, although imaging tests and pulmonary function tests can also provide information for diagnosis.

Treatment of Bronchiolitis Obliterans Organizing Pneumonia

Most cases of BOOP respond well to treatment with corticosteroids. If the condition is caused by a particular drug, stopping the drug can also improve a patient's condition.

Other medications reported in the medical literature to be beneficial for individuals on a case-by-case basis include: cyclophosphamide, erythromycin in the form of azithromycin, and Mycophenolate Mofetil (CellCept). In rare cases, lung transplantation may be necessary for individuals with BOOP who do not respond to standard treatment options.

Section 19.3

Hantavirus Pulmonary Syndrome

This section includes text excerpted from "Hantavirus Pulmonary Syndrome (HPS)," Centers for Disease Control and Prevention (CDC), February 6, 2013. Reviewed August 2019.

Hantavirus pulmonary syndrome (HPS) is a severe, sometimes fatal, respiratory disease in humans caused by infection with *Hantaviruses*.

Anyone who comes into contact with rodents that carry *Hantaviruses* is at risk of HPS. Rodent infestation in and around the home remains the primary risk for *Hantavirus* exposure. Even healthy individuals are at risk for HPS infection if exposed to the virus.

To date, no cases of HPS have been reported in the United States in which the virus was transmitted from one person to another. In fact, in a study of healthcare workers who were exposed to either patients or specimens infected with related types of *Hantaviruses* (which cause a different disease in humans), none of the workers showed evidence of infection or illness.

In Chile and Argentina, rare cases of person-to-person transmission have occurred among close contacts of a person who was ill with a type of *Hantavirus* called "Andes virus."

Transmission of Hantavirus Pulmonary Syndrome
How People Get Hantavirus Infection
Where Hantavirus Is Found

Cases of human *Hantavirus* infection occur sporadically, usually in rural areas where forests, fields, and farms offer suitable habitat for the virus's rodent hosts. Areas around the home or work where rodents may live (for example, houses, barns, outbuildings, and sheds) are potential sites where people may be exposed to the virus. In the United States and Canada, the Sin Nombre *Hantavirus* is responsible for the majority of cases of *Hantavirus* infection. The host of the Sin Nombre virus is the deer mouse (Peromyscus maniculatus), present throughout the western and central United States and Canada.

Several other *hantaviruses* are capable of causing hantavirus infection in the United States. The New York *Hantavirus*, carried by the white-footed mouse, is associated with HPS cases in the northeastern U.S. The Black Creek *Hantavirus*, carried by the cotton rat, is found in the southeastern U.S. Cases of HPS have been confirmed elsewhere in the Americas, including Canada, Argentina, Bolivia, Brazil, Chile, Panama, Paraguay, and Uruguay.

How People Become Infected with Hantaviruses

In the United States, deer mice (along with cotton rats and rice rats in the southeastern states and the white-footed mouse in the Northeast) are reservoirs of the *Hantaviruses*. The rodents shed the virus in their urine, droppings, and saliva. The virus is mainly transmitted to people when they breathe in air contaminated with the virus.

When fresh rodent urine, droppings, or nesting materials are stirred up, tiny droplets containing the virus get into the air. This process is known as "airborne transmission."

There are several other ways rodents may spread *Hantavirus* to people:

- If a rodent with the virus bites someone, the virus may be spread to that person, but this type of transmission is rare.

- Scientists believe that people may be able to get the virus if they touch something that has been contaminated with rodent urine, droppings, or saliva, and then touch their nose or mouth.

- Scientists also suspect people can become sick if they eat food contaminated by urine, droppings, or saliva from an infected rodent.

The *Hantaviruses* that cause human illness in the United States cannot be transmitted from one person to another. For example, you cannot get these viruses from touching or kissing a person who has HPS or from a healthcare worker who has treated someone with the disease.

In Chile and Argentina, rare cases of person-to-person transmission have occurred among close contacts of a person who was ill with a type of *Hantavirus* called "Andes virus."

People at Risk for Hantavirus Infection

Anyone who comes into contact with rodents that carry *Hantavirus* is at risk of HPS. Rodent infestation in and around the home remains the primary risk for *Hantavirus* exposure. Even healthy individuals are at risk for HPS infection if exposed to the virus.

Any activity that puts you in contact with rodent droppings, urine, saliva, or nesting materials can place you at risk for infection.

Hantavirus is spread when virus-containing particles from rodent urine, droppings, or saliva are stirred into the air. It is important to avoid actions that raise dust, such as sweeping or vacuuming. Infection occurs when you breathe in virus particles.

Potential Risk Activities for Hantavirus Infection
Opening and Cleaning Previously Unused Buildings

Opening or cleaning cabins, sheds, and outbuildings, including barns, garages, and storage facilities, that have been closed during the winter are potential risks for *Hantavirus* infections, especially in rural settings.

House Cleaning Activities

Cleaning in and around your own home can put you at risk if rodents have made it their home too. Many homes can expect to shelter rodents, especially as the weather turns cold.

Work-Related Exposure

Construction, utility and pest control workers can be exposed when they work in crawl spaces, under houses, or in vacant buildings that may have a rodent population.

Campers and Hikers

Campers and hikers can also be exposed when they use infested trail shelters or camp in other rodent habitats. The chance of being exposed to *Hantavirus* is greatest when people work, play, or live in closed spaces where rodents are actively living. However, research results show that many people who have become ill with HPS were infected with the disease after continued contact with rodents and/or their droppings. In addition, many people who have contracted HPS reported that they had not seen rodents or their droppings before becoming ill. Therefore, if you live in an area where the carrier rodents, such as the deer mouse, are known to live, take sensible precautions-even if you do not see rodents or their droppings.

Signs and Symptoms of Hantavirus Pulmonary Syndrome

Due to the small number of HPS cases, the "incubation time" is not positively known. However, on the basis of limited information, it appears that symptoms may develop between one and eight weeks after exposure to fresh urine, droppings, or saliva of infected rodents.

Early Symptoms

Early symptoms include fatigue, fever and muscle aches, especially in the large muscle groups—thighs, hips, back, and sometimes shoulders. These symptoms are universal.

There may also be headaches, dizziness, chills, and abdominal problems, such as nausea, vomiting, diarrhea, and abdominal pain. About half of all HPS patients experience these symptoms.

Late Symptoms

4 to 10 days after the initial phase of illness, the late symptoms of HPS appear. These include coughing and shortness of breath, with the sensation of, as one survivor put it, a "tight band around my chest and a pillow over my face" as the lungs fill with fluid.

Is the Disease Fatal?

Yes. HPS can be fatal. It has a mortality rate of 38 percent.

Diagnosis of Hantavirus Pulmonary Syndrome

Diagnosing HPS in an individual who has only been infected a few days is difficult because early symptoms, such as fever, muscle aches, and fatigue are easily confused with influenza. However, if the individual is experiencing fever and fatigue and has a history of potential rural rodent exposure, together with shortness of breath, would be strongly suggestive of HPS. If the individual is experiencing these symptoms they should see their physician immediately and mention their potential rodent exposure.

Are There Any Complications?

Previous observations of patients that develop HPS from New World *Hantaviruses* recover completely. No chronic infection has been detected in humans. Some patients have experienced longer than expected recovery times, but the virus has not been shown to leave lasting effects on the patient.

Treatment of Hantavirus Pulmonary Syndrome
Treating Hantavirus Pulmonary Syndrome

There is no specific treatment, cure, or vaccine for *Hantavirus* infection. However, it is known that if infected individuals are recognized early and receive medical care in an intensive care unit, they may do better. In intensive care, patients are intubated and given oxygen therapy to help them through the period of severe respiratory distress.

The earlier the patient is brought in to intensive care, the better. If a patient is experiencing full distress, it is less likely the treatment will be effective.

Therefore, if you have been around rodents and have symptoms of fever, deep muscle aches, and severe shortness of breath, see your doctor immediately. Be sure to tell your doctor that you have been around rodents—this will alert your physician to look closely for any rodent-carried disease, such as HPS.

Prevention of Hantavirus Pulmonary Syndrome

Eliminate or minimize contact with rodents in your home, workplace, or campsite. If rodents do not find that where you are is a good place for them to be, then you are less likely to come into contact with them. Seal up holes and gaps in your home or garage. Place traps in and around your home to decrease rodent infestation. Clean up any easy-to-get-to food.

Research results show that many people who became ill with HPS developed the disease after having been in frequent contact with rodents and/or their droppings around a home or a workplace. On the other hand, many people who became ill reported that they had not seen rodents or rodent droppings at all. Therefore, if you live in an area where the carrier rodents are known to live, try to keep your home, vacation place, workplace, or campsite clean.

Got Mice?

- Seal up holes inside and outside the home to keep rodents out.

- Trap rodents around the home to help reduce the population.

- Avoid illness: Take precautions before and while cleaning rodent-infested areas.

Section 19.4

Legionella *(Legionnaires Disease)*

This section includes text excerpted from "*Legionella* (Legionnaires'
Disease and Pontiac Fever)," Centers for Disease
Control and Prevention (CDC), April 30, 2018.

Legionella bacteria can cause a serious type of pneumonia (lung
infection) called "Legionnaires' disease." The bacteria can also cause
a less serious illness called "Pontiac fever."

Causes and Common Sources of Legionella *Infection*

Legionella is a type of bacterium found naturally in freshwater
environments, such as lakes and streams. It can become a health
concern when it grows and spreads in human-made building water
systems, such as:

- Showerheads and sink faucets

- Cooling towers (structures that contain water and a fan as part
  of centralized air-cooling systems for building or industrial
  processes)

- Hot tubs that are not drained after each use

- Decorative fountains and water features

- Hot water tanks and heaters

- Large plumbing systems

Home and car air-conditioning units do not use water to cool the
air, so they are not a risk for *Legionella* growth.

How Legionella *Infection Spreads*

After *Legionella* grows and multiplies in a building water system,
water containing *Legionella* then has to spread in droplets small
enough for people to breathe in. People can get Legionnaires' disease
or Pontiac fever when they breathe in small droplets of water in the
air that contain the bacteria.

Less commonly, people can get sick by aspiration of drinking water
containing *Legionella*. This happens when water accidentally goes into

the lungs while drinking. People at increased risk of aspiration include those with swallowing difficulties.

In general, people do not spread Legionnaires' disease and Pontiac fever to other people. However, this may be possible under rare circumstances.

Talk to your doctor or local health department if:

- You believe you were exposed to *Legionella*

- You develop symptoms, such as fever, cough, chills, or muscle aches

Your local health department can determine whether to investigate. Be sure to mention if you spent any nights away from home in the last 10 days.

People at Increased Risk of Legionella Infection

Most healthy people exposed to *Legionella* do not get sick. People at increased risk of getting sick are:

- People 50 years or older

- Current or former smokers

- People with a chronic lung disease (such as chronic obstructive pulmonary disease or emphysema)

- People with weak immune systems or who take drugs that weaken the immune system, (such as after a transplant operation or chemotherapy)

- People with cancer

- People with underlying illnesses, such as diabetes, kidney failure, or liver failure

Signs and Symptoms of Legionella Infection
Legionnaires' Disease

Legionnaires' disease is very similar to other types of pneumonia (lung infection), with symptoms that include:

- Cough

- Shortness of breath

- Fever

- Muscle aches

- Headaches

Legionnaires' disease can also be associated with other, such as diarrhea, nausea, and confusion. Symptoms usually begin 2 to 10 days after being exposed to the bacteria, but it can take longer so people should watch for symptoms for about 2 weeks after exposure.

If you develop pneumonia symptoms, see a doctor right away. Be sure to mention if you may have been exposed to *Legionella*, have used a hot tub, spent any nights away from home, or stayed in a hospital in the last two weeks.

Pontiac Fever

Pontiac fever symptoms are primarily fever and muscle aches; it is a milder infection than Legionnaires' disease. Symptoms begin between a few hours to three days after being exposed to the bacteria and usually last less than a week. Pontiac fever is different from Legionnaires' disease because someone with Pontiac fever does not have pneumonia.

Diagnosis, Treatment, and Complications of Legionella *Infection*

Legionellosis can present as two types of illness: Legionnaires' disease and Pontiac fever. The two illnesses can be diagnosed with similar tests, but are treated differently.

Legionnaires' Disease
Diagnosis

People with Legionnaires' disease have pneumonia (lung infection), which can be confirmed by chest x-ray. Clinicians typically use two preferred types of tests to see if a patient's pneumonia is caused by *Legionella*:

- Urine test

- Laboratory test that involves taking a sample of sputum (phlegm) or washing from the lung

Treatment and Complications

Legionnaires' disease requires treatment with antibiotics (medicines that kill bacteria in the body), and most cases of this illness can be treated successfully. Healthy people usually get better after being sick with Legionnaires' disease, but they often need care in the hospital.

Possible complications of Legionnaires' disease include:

- Lung failure

- Death

About 1 out of every 10 people who gets sick with Legionnaires' disease will die due to complications from their illness. For those who get Legionnaires' disease during a stay in a healthcare facility, about 1 out of every 4 will die.

Pontiac Fever
Diagnosis

Clinicians can use a urine or blood test to see if someone has Pontiac fever. However, a negative test does not rule out that someone may have it (this is called a "false negative"). Clinicians most often diagnose Pontiac fever when there are other known laboratory-confirmed legionellosis cases (either Legionnaires' disease or Pontiac fever) who may have been exposed to *Legionella* at the same time or place.

Treatment and Complications

Pontiac fever goes away without specific treatment.

Prevention of Legionella *Infection*
Water Management Programs

There are no vaccines that can prevent Legionnaires' disease.

Instead, the key to preventing Legionnaires' disease is to make sure that building owners and managers maintain building water systems in order to reduce the risk of *Legionella* growth and spread. Examples of building water systems that might grow and spread *Legionella* include:

- Hot tubs

- Hot water tanks and heaters

- Large plumbing systems

- Cooling towers (structures that contain water and a fan as part of centralized air-cooling systems for building or industrial processes)

- Decorative fountains

The Centers for Disease Control and Prevention (CDC) developed a toolkit to help building owners and managers develop and implement a water management program to reduce their building's risk for growing and spreading *Legionella*.

Legionella *and Hot Tubs*

Legionella grows best in warm water, such as the water temperatures used in hot tubs. However, warm temperatures also make it hard to keep disinfectants, such as chlorine, at the levels needed to kill germs, such as *Legionella*. Disinfectant and other chemical levels in hot tubs should be checked regularly and hot tubs should be cleaned as recommended by the manufacturer.

Section 19.5

Psittacosis

This section includes text excerpted from "Psittacosis," Centers for Disease Control and Prevention (CDC), February 11, 2019.

Chlamydia psittaci is a type of bacteria that often infects birds. Less commonly, these bacteria can infect people and cause a disease called "psittacosis." Psittacosis causes a wide range of symptoms, including fever, headache, and a dry cough. This illness can also cause pneumonia (a lung infection) that may require treatment or care in a hospital. Rarely, psittacosis can be deadly.

Causes of Psittacosis, How It Spreads, and People at Increased Risk
Causes

Chlamydia psittaci is a type of bacteria that often infects birds. Less commonly, these bacteria can infect people and cause a disease called "psittacosis." Psittacosis in people is most commonly associated with pet birds, such as parrots and cockatiels, and poultry, such as turkeys or ducks.

How It Spreads

The bacteria can infect people exposed to infected birds. It is important to know that infected birds do not always have symptoms or seem sick. Both sick birds and birds without symptoms shed the bacteria in their droppings and respiratory secretions. When the droppings and secretions dry, small dust particles (including the bacteria) can get into the air. The most common way someone gets infected is by breathing in the dust from these dried secretions. Less commonly, birds infect people through bites and beak-to-mouth contact.

In general, people do not spread psittacosis to other people. However, this is possible in rare cases. There is no evidence that the bacteria spread by preparing or eating chicken meat.

People at Increased Risk

People of all ages can get psittacosis, but it is more commonly reported among adults. Those who have contact with pet birds and poultry, including people who work in bird-related occupations, are at increased risk:

- Bird owners

- Aviary and pet shop employees

- Poultry workers

- Veterinarians

Signs and Symptoms of Psittacosis
In People

In general, psittacosis causes mild illness. The most common symptoms include:

- Fever and chills

- Headache

- Muscle aches

- Dry cough

Psittacosis can also cause pneumonia (a lung infection) that may require treatment or care in a hospital. Rarely, psittacosis can result in death.

Most people begin developing signs and symptoms within 5 to 14 days after exposure to the bacteria (*Chlamydia psittaci*). Less commonly, people report symptoms starting after 14 days.

In Birds

The signs of *C. psittaci* infection in birds are nonspecific and include:

- Poor appetite

- Inflamed eyes

- Breathing difficulty

- Diarrhea

Infected birds may not have symptoms or seem sick. When birds have symptoms caused by *C. psittaci* infection, veterinarians call the disease "avian chlamydiosis."

Diagnosis, Treatment, and Complications of Psittacosis
Diagnosis

Symptoms of psittacosis are similar to many other respiratory illnesses. In addition, tests to detect the bacteria directly may not be readily available. For these reasons, healthcare professionals may not suspect it, making psittacosis difficult to diagnose. The Centers for Disease Control and Prevention (CDC) rarely receives reports of psittacosis. Tell your healthcare professional if you get sick after buying or handling a pet bird or poultry.

There are a number of tests healthcare professionals can use to determine if someone has psittacosis. These tests include collecting sputum (phlegm) or swabs from the nose and/or throat to detect the bacteria.

Treatment

People diagnosed with psittacosis usually take antibiotics to treat the infection. Most people improve quickly if they start antibiotics soon after they first get sick.

If your healthcare professional prescribes antibiotics for you, take it exactly as your healthcare professional tells you.

Complications

Most people who get treatment for psittacosis make a full recovery. However, some people have serious complications and need care or treatment in a hospital. Complications include:

- Lung infection (pneumonia)

- Inflammation of the heart valves (endocarditis)

- Inflammation of the liver (hepatitis)

- Inflammation of the nerves or the brain, leading to neurologic problems

With appropriate antibiotic treatment, psittacosis rarely (less than 1 in 100 cases) results in death.

Prevention of Psittacosis

While there is no vaccine to prevent psittacosis, there are things you can do to protect yourself and others. Buy pet birds only from a well-known pet store. If you own pet birds or poultry, follow good precautions when handling and cleaning birds and cages.

Previous Infections

Getting psittacosis will not prevent you from future illness. If you get psittacosis, you may still get sick from it again in the future.

Safe Bird and Cage Care

One important aspect of preventing psittacosis is to control infection among birds.

- Keep cages clean; clean cages and food and water bowls daily.

- Position cages so that food, feathers, and feces cannot spread between them (i.e., do not stack cages, use solid-sided cases or barriers if cages are next to each other).

- Avoid overcrowding.

- Isolate and treat infected birds.

Use water or disinfectant to wet surfaces before cleaning bird cages or surfaces contaminated with bird droppings. Avoid dry sweeping or vacuuming to minimize circulation of feathers and dust. Also, remember to thoroughly wash your hands with running water and soap after contact with birds or their droppings.

Use personal protective equipment (PPE), such as gloves and appropriate masks, when handling infected birds or cleaning their cages.

Chapter 20

Fungal Infections That Cause Respiratory Complications

Chapter Contents

Section 20.1

Aspergillosis

This section includes text excerpted from "Aspergillosis," Centers for Disease Control and Prevention (CDC), January 2, 2019.

Aspergillosis is an infection caused by *Aspergillus*, a common mold (a type of fungus) that lives indoors and outdoors. Most people breathe in *Aspergillus* spores every day without getting sick. However, people with weakened immune systems or lung diseases are at a higher risk of developing health problems due to *Aspergillus*. The types of health problems caused by *Aspergillus* include allergic reactions, lung infections, and infections in other organs.

Symptoms of Aspergillosis

The different types of aspergillosis can cause different symptoms. The symptoms of allergic bronchopulmonary aspergillosis (ABPA) are similar to asthma symptoms, including:

- Wheezing
- Shortness of breath
- Cough
- Fever (in rare cases)

Symptoms of allergic *Aspergillus sinusitis* include:

- Stuffiness
- Runny nose
- Headache
- Reduced ability to smell

Symptoms of an aspergilloma ("fungus ball") include:

- Cough
- Coughing up blood
- Shortness of breath

Symptoms of chronic pulmonary aspergillosis include:

- Weight loss

- Cough
- Coughing up blood
- Fatigue
- Shortness of breath

Invasive aspergillosis usually occurs in people who are already sick from other medical conditions, so it can be difficult to know which symptoms are related to an *Aspergillus* infection. However, the symptoms of invasive aspergillosis in the lungs include:

- Fever
- Chest pain
- Cough
- Coughing up blood
- Shortness of breath
- Other symptoms can develop if the infection spreads from the lungs to other parts of the body.

Contact your healthcare provider if you have symptoms that you think are related to any form of aspergillosis.

Aspergillosis Risk and Prevention
Who Gets Aspergillosis

The different types of aspergillosis affect different groups of people.

- **Allergic bronchopulmonary aspergillosis (ABPA)** most often occurs in people who have cystic fibrosis or asthma.

- **Aspergillomas** usually affect people who have other lung diseases like tuberculosis. Also called a "fungus ball."

- **Chronic pulmonary aspergillosis** typically occurs in people who have other lung diseases, including tuberculosis, chronic obstructive pulmonary disease (COPD), or sarcoidosis.

- **Invasive aspergillosis** affects people who have weakened immune systems, such as people who have had a stem cell transplant or organ transplant, are getting chemotherapy for cancer, or are taking high doses of corticosteroids. Invasive aspergillosis has been described among hospitalized patients with severe influenza.

211

How Does Someone Get Aspergillosis?

People can get aspergillosis by breathing in microscopic *Aspergillus* spores from the environment. Most people breathe in *Aspergillus* spores every day without getting sick. However, people with weakened immune systems or lung diseases are at a higher risk of developing health problems due to *Aspergillus*.

How Can I Prevent Aspergillosis?

It is difficult to avoid breathing in *Aspergillus* spores because the fungus is common in the environment. For people who have weakened immune systems, there may be some ways to lower the chances of developing a severe *Aspergillus* infection.

- **Protect yourself from the environment.** It is important to note that although these actions are recommended, they have not been proven to prevent aspergillosis.

  - Try to avoid areas with a lot of dust such as construction or excavation sites. If you cannot avoid these areas, wear an N95 respirator (a type of face mask) while you are there.

- Avoid activities that involve close contact to soil or dust, such as yard work or gardening. If this is not possible,

  - Wear shoes, long pants, and a long-sleeved shirt when doing outdoor activities such as gardening, yard work, or visiting wooded areas.

  - Wear gloves when handling materials such as soil, moss, or manure.

- To reduce the chances of developing a skin infection, clean skin injuries well with soap and water, especially if they have been exposed to soil or dust.

- **Antifungal medication.** If you are at high risk for developing invasive aspergillosis (for example, if you have had an organ transplant or a stem cell transplant), your healthcare provider may prescribe medication to prevent aspergillosis. Scientists are still learning about which transplant patients are at highest risk and how to best prevent fungal infections.

- **Testing for early infection.** Some high-risk patients may benefit from blood tests to detect invasive aspergillosis. Talk to your doctor to determine if this type of test is right for you.

How Is Aspergillosis Diagnosed?

Healthcare providers consider your medical history, risk factors, symptoms, physical examinations, and lab tests when diagnosing aspergillosis. You may need imaging tests such as a chest x-ray or a computed tomography (CT) scan of your lungs or other parts of your body depending on the location of the suspected infection. If your healthcare provider suspects that you have an *Aspergillus* infection in your lungs, she or he might collect a sample of fluid from your respiratory system to send to a laboratory. Healthcare providers may also perform a tissue biopsy, in which a small sample of affected tissue is analyzed in a laboratory for evidence of *Aspergillus* under a microscope or in a fungal culture. A blood test can help diagnose invasive aspergillosis early in people who have severely weakened immune systems.

Treatment of Aspergillosis
Allergic Forms of Aspergillosis

For allergic forms of aspergillosis such as allergic bronchopulmonary aspergillosis (ABPA) or allergic *Aspergillus sinusitis*, the recommended treatment is itraconazole, a prescription antifungal medication. Corticosteroids may also be helpful.

Invasive Aspergillosis

Invasive aspergillosis needs to be treated with prescription antifungal medication, usually voriconazole. Other antifungal medications used to treat aspergillosis include lipid amphotericin formulations, posaconazole, isavuconazole, itraconazole, caspofungin, and micafungin. Whenever possible, immunosuppressive medications should be discontinued or decreased. People who have severe cases of aspergillosis may need surgery. Other invasive forms of aspergillosis such as chronic pulmonary aspergillosis and cutaneous aspergillosis should be treated similarly to invasive aspergillosis. Aspergillomas ("fungus ball") might not need treatment.

Section 20.2

Blastomycosis

This section includes text excerpted from "About Blastomycosis,"
Centers for Disease Control and Prevention (CDC), August 13, 2018.

Blastomycosis is an infection caused by the fungus *Blastomyces*. The fungus lives in the environment, particularly in moist soil and in decomposing organic matter such as wood and leaves. In the United States, *Blastomyces* mainly lives in the midwestern, south-central, and southeastern states, particularly in areas surrounding the Ohio and Mississippi River valleys, the Great Lakes, and the Saint Lawrence River. The fungus also lives in Canada, and a few blastomycosis cases have been reported from Africa and India.

People can get blastomycosis after breathing in the microscopic fungal spores from the air, often after participating in activities that disturb the soil. Although most people who breathe in the spores do not get sick, some of those who do may have flu-like symptoms. In some people, such as those who have weakened immune systems, the infection can become severe, especially if it spreads from the lungs to other organs.

Symptoms of Blastomycosis

Approximately half of people who are infected with the fungus *Blastomyces* will show symptoms. The symptoms of blastomycosis are often similar to the symptoms of flu or other lung infections, and can include:

- Fever
- Cough
- Night sweats
- Muscle aches or joint pain
- Weight loss
- Chest pain
- Fatigue (extreme tiredness)

How Soon Do the Symptoms of Blastomycosis Appear?

Symptoms of blastomycosis usually appear between three weeks and three months after a person breathes in the fungal spores.

Severe Blastomycosis

In some people, particularly those who have weakened immune systems, blastomycosis can spread from the lungs to other parts of the body, such as the skin, bones and joints, and the central nervous system (CNS).

Risk and Prevention of Blastomycosis
Who Gets Blastomycosis

Anyone can get blastomycosis if they have been in an area where *Blastomyces* lives in the environment. People who participate in outdoor activities that expose them to wooded areas (such as forestry work, hunting, and camping) in these areas may be at higher risk for getting blastomycosis. People who have weakened immune systems may be more likely to develop severe blastomycosis than people who are otherwise healthy.

Is Blastomycosis Contagious?

No. Blastomycosis cannot spread between people or between people and animals.

How Can I Prevent Blastomycosis?

There is no vaccine to prevent blastomycosis, and it may not be possible to completely avoid being exposed to the fungus that causes blastomycosis in areas where it is common in the environment. People who have weakened immune systems may want to consider avoiding activities that involve disrupting soil in these areas.

Diagnosis and Testing of Blastomycosis
How Is Blastomycosis Diagnosed?

Healthcare providers use your medical and travel history, symptoms, physical examinations, and laboratory tests to diagnose blastomycosis. A doctor will likely test for blastomycosis by taking a blood sample or a urine sample and sending it to a laboratory.

Healthcare providers may do imaging tests such as chest x-rays or computed tomography (CT) scans of your lungs. They may also collect a sample of fluid from your respiratory tract or perform a tissue biopsy, in which a small sample of affected tissue is taken from the body and examined under a microscope. Laboratories may also see if *Blastomyces* will grow from body fluids or tissues (this is called a "culture").

Where Can I Get Tested for Blastomycosis?

Most healthcare providers can order a test for blastomycosis.

How Long Will It Take to Get My Test Results?

It depends on the type of test. Results from a blood test or a urine test are usually available in a few days. If your healthcare provider sends a sample to a laboratory to be cultured, the results could take a couple of weeks.

Treatment of Blastomycosis

Most people with blastomycosis will need treatment with prescription antifungal medication. Itraconazole is a type of antifungal medication that is typically used to treat mild to moderate blastomycosis. Amphotericin B is usually recommended for severe blastomycosis in the lungs or infections that have spread to other parts of the body. Depending on the severity of the infection and the person's immune status, the course of treatment can range from six months to one year.

Section 20.3

Coccidioidomycosis

This section includes text excerpted from "About Valley Fever (Coccidioidomycosis)," Centers for Disease Control and Prevention (CDC), January 2, 2019.

Valley fever is an infection caused by the fungus *Coccidioides*. The scientific name for valley fever is "coccidioidomycosis," and it is also sometimes called "San Joaquin Valley fever" or "desert rheumatism." The term "valley fever" usually refers to *Coccidioides* infection in the lungs, but the infection can spread to other parts of the body in severe cases (this is called "disseminated coccidioidomycosis").

The fungus is known to live in the soil in the southwestern United States and parts of Mexico and Central and South America. The fungus was also recently found in south-central Washington. People can get valley fever by breathing in the microscopic fungal spores from the air in these areas.

Most people who breathe in the spores do not get sick, but some people do. Usually, people who get sick with valley fever will get better on their own within weeks to months, but some people will need antifungal medication. Certain groups of people are at higher risk for developing the severe forms of the infection, and these people typically need antifungal treatment. It is difficult to prevent exposure to *Coccidioides* in areas where it is common in the environment, but people who are at higher risk for severe valley fever should try to avoid breathing in large amounts of dust if they are in these areas.

Symptoms of Valley Fever (Coccidioidomycosis)

Many people who are exposed to the fungus *Coccidioides* never have symptoms. Other people may have flu-like symptoms that go usually away on their own after weeks to months. If your symptoms last for more than a week, contact your healthcare provider.

Symptoms of valley fever include:

- Fatigue (tiredness)

- Cough

- Fever

- Shortness of breath

- Headache

- Night sweats

- Muscle aches or joint pain

- Rash on upper body or legs

In extremely rare cases, the fungal spores can enter the skin through a cut, wound, or splinter and cause a skin infection.

How Soon Do the Symptoms Appear?

Symptoms of valley fever may appear between one and three weeks after a person breathes in the fungal spores.

How Long Do the Symptoms Last?

The symptoms of valley fever usually last for a few weeks to a few months. However, some patients have symptoms that last longer than this, especially if the infection becomes severe.

Severe Valley Fever

Approximately 5 to 10 percent of people who get valley fever will develop serious or long-term problems in their lungs. In an even smaller percent of people (about 1%), the infection spreads from the lungs to other parts of the body, such as the central nervous system (CNS), skin, or bones and joints.

Risk and Prevention of Valley Fever (Coccidioidomycosis)
Who Gets Valley Fever

Anyone who lives in or travels to the southwestern United States (Arizona, California, Nevada, New Mexico, Texas, or Utah), or parts of Mexico or Central or South America can get valley fever. Valley fever can affect people of any age, but it is most common in adults aged 60 and older. Certain groups of people may be at higher risk for developing the severe forms of valley fever, such as:

- People who have weakened immune systems, for example, people who:
- Have human immunodeficiency virus (HIV)/acquired immunodeficiency syndrome (AIDS)
- Have had an organ transplant
- Are taking medications such as corticosteroids or Tumor Necrosis Factor (TNF)-inhibitors
- Pregnant women
- People who have diabetes
- People who are Black or Filipino

Is Valley Fever Contagious?

No. The fungus that causes valley fever, *Coccidioides*, cannot spread from the lungs between people or between people and animals. However, in extremely rare instances, a wound infection with *Coccidioides* can spread valley fever to someone else, or the infection can be spread through an organ transplant with an infected organ.

Traveling to an Endemic Area
Should I Worry about Valley Fever If I Am Traveling to an Area Where the Fungus Is Common?

The risk of getting valley fever is low when traveling to an area where *Coccidioides* lives in the environment, such as the southwestern United States, Mexico, or Central or South America. Your risk for infection could increase if you will be in a very dusty setting, but even then the risk is still low. If you have questions about your risk of getting valley fever while traveling, talk to your healthcare provider.

I Have Had It before Could I Get It Again?

Usually not. If you have already had valley fever, your immune system will most likely protect you from getting it again. Some people can have the infection come back again (a relapse) after getting better the first time, but this is very rare.

Coccidioides at My Workplace
What Should I Do If I Think I Have Been Exposed to **Coccidioides** *at My Workplace or in a Laboratory?*

If you think you have been exposed to *Coccidioides* at work or in a laboratory, you should contact your Occupational Health, Infection Control, Risk Management, or Safety/Security Department. If your workplace or laboratory does not have these services, you should contact your local city, county, or state health department. Recommendations about what to do in the event of a laboratory exposure have been published. There is no evidence showing that antifungal medication (i.e., prophylaxis) prevents people from getting sick with valley fever after a workplace exposure to *Coccidioides*. If you develop symptoms of valley fever, contact your healthcare provider.

How Can I Prevent Valley Fever?

It is very difficult to avoid breathing in the fungus *Coccidioides* in areas where it is common in the environment. People who live in these areas can try to avoid spending time in dusty places as much as possible. People who are at risk for severe valley fever (such as people who have weakened immune systems, pregnant women, people who have diabetes, or people who are Black or Filipino) may be able to lower their chances of developing the infection by trying to avoid breathing in the fungal spores.

The following are some common-sense methods that may be helpful to avoid getting valley fever. It is important to know that although these steps are recommended, they have not been proven to prevent valley fever.

- Try to avoid areas with a lot of dust like construction or excavation sites. If you cannot avoid these areas, wear an N95 respirator (a type of face mask) while you are there.

- Stay inside during dust storms and close your windows.

- Avoid activities that involve close contact to dirt or dust, including yard work, gardening, and digging.

- Use air filtration measures indoors.

- Clean skin injuries well with soap and water to reduce the chances of developing a skin infection, especially if the wound was exposed to dirt or dust.

- Take preventive antifungal medication if your healthcare provider says you need it.

Is There a Vaccine for Valley Fever?

No. Currently, there is no vaccine to prevent valley fever, but scientists have been trying to make one since the 1960s. Because people who have had valley fever are usually protected from getting it again, a vaccine could make the body's immune system think that it is already had valley fever, which would likely prevent a person from being able to get the infection.

Scientists have tried several different ways to make a valley fever vaccine. When one version of the vaccine was tested on humans in the 1980s, it did not provide good protection, and it also caused people to develop side effects such as swelling at the injection site. Since then, scientists have been looking at ways to make a vaccine with different ingredients that will provide better protection against valley fever and will not cause side effects. Studies of these new vaccines are ongoing, so it is possible that a vaccine to prevent valley fever could become available in the future.

How Is Valley Fever Diagnosed?

Healthcare providers rely on your medical and travel history, symptoms, physical examinations, and laboratory tests to diagnose valley fever. The most common way that healthcare providers test for valley fever is by taking a blood sample and sending it to a laboratory to look for *Coccidioides* antibodies or antigens.

Healthcare providers may do imaging tests such as chest x-rays or computed tomography (CT) scans of your lungs to look for valley fever pneumonia. They may also perform a tissue biopsy, in which a small sample of tissue is taken from the body and examined under a microscope. Laboratories may also see if *Coccidioides* will grow from body fluids or tissues (this is called a "culture").

Treatment of Valley Fever (Coccidioidomycosis)
How Is Valley Fever Treated?

For many people, the symptoms of valley fever will go away within a few months without any treatment. Healthcare providers choose to prescribe antifungal medication for some people to try to reduce the severity of symptoms or prevent the infection from getting worse. Antifungal medication is typically given to people who are at higher risk for developing severe valley fever. The treatment is usually three to six months of fluconazole or another type of antifungal medication. There are no over-the-counter (OTC) medications to treat valley fever. If you have valley fever, you should talk to your healthcare provider about whether you need treatment. The healthcare provider who diagnoses you with valley fever may suggest that you see other healthcare providers who specialize in treating valley fever.

People who have severe lung infections or infections that have spread to other parts of the body always need antifungal treatment and may need to stay in the hospital. For these types of infections, the course of treatment is usually longer than 6 months. Valley fever that develops into meningitis is fatal if it is not treated, so lifelong antifungal treatment is necessary for those cases.

If I Have Valley Fever, Should I Stay at Home?

Valley fever is not contagious, so you do not need to stay at home to avoid spreading the infection to other people. However, your healthcare provider may recommend that you rest at home to help your body fight off the infection.

Does Valley Fever Have Any Long-Term Effects?

Most people who have valley fever will make a full recovery. A small percent of people develop long-term lung infections that can take several years to get better. In very severe cases of valley fever, the nervous system can be affected and there may be long-term damage, but this is very rare.

Section 20.4

Cryptococcosis

This section includes text excerpted from "About
C. neoformans Infection," Centers for Disease Control
and Prevention (CDC), October 9, 2018.

Cryptococcus neoformans (*C. neoformans*) is a fungus that lives in the environment throughout the world. People can become infected with *C. neoformans* after breathing in the microscopic fungus, although most people who are exposed to the fungus never get sick from it.

Infection with the fungus *Cryptococcus* (either *C. neoformans* or *C. gattii*) is called "cryptococcosis." Cryptococcosis usually affects the lungs or the central nervous system (CNS), but it can also affect other parts of the body. Brain infections due to the fungus *Cryptococcus* are called "cryptococcal meningitis."

C. neoformans infections are rare in people who are otherwise healthy. Most cases of *C. neoformans* infection occur in people who have weakened immune systems, particularly those who have advanced human immunodeficiency virus (HIV)/acquired immunodeficiency syndrome (AIDS).

Symptoms of C. neoformans *Infection*

C. neoformans usually infects the lungs or the central nervous system (the brain and spinal cord), but it can also affect other parts of the body. The symptoms of the infection depend on the parts of the body that are affected.

In the Lungs

A *C. neoformans* infection in the lungs can cause a pneumonia-like illness. The symptoms are often similar to those of many other illnesses, and can include:

- Cough
- Shortness of breath
- Chest pain
- Fever

In the Brain (Cryptococcal Meningitis)

Cryptococcal meningitis is an infection caused by the fungus *Cryptococcus* after it spreads from the lungs to the brain. The symptoms of cryptococcal meningitis include:

- Headache
- Fever
- Neck pain
- Nausea and vomiting
- Sensitivity to light
- Confusion or changes in behavior

If you have symptoms that you think may be due to a *C. neoformans* infection, please contact your healthcare provider.

Infection Risk and Prevention of C. neoformans
Who Gets C. neoformans Infections

C. neoformans infections are rare among people who are otherwise healthy. Most cases of *C. neoformans* infection occur in people who have weakened immune systems, such as people who:

- Have advanced HIV/AIDS,
- Have had an organ transplant, or
- Are taking corticosteroids, medications to treat rheumatoid arthritis, or other medications that weaken the immune system

Is C. neoformans *Infection Contagious?*

No. The infection cannot spread between people or between people and animals.

How Can I Prevent a C. neoformans *Infection?*

It is difficult to avoid breathing in *C. neoformans* because it is thought to be common in the environment. Most people who breathe in *C. neoformans* never get sick from it. However, in people who have weakened immune systems, *C. neoformans* can stay hidden in the body and cause infection later when the immune system becomes too weak to fight it off. This leaves a window of time when the silent infection can be detected and treated early, before symptoms develop.

Detecting Silent Cryptococcal Infections in People Who Have Human Immunodeficiency Virus/Acquired Immunodeficiency Syndrome

One approach to prevent cryptococcal meningitis is called "targeted screening." Research suggests that *C. neoformans* is able to live in the body undetected, especially when a person's immune system is weaker than normal. In a targeted screening program, a simple blood test is used to detect cryptococcal antigen (an indicator of cryptococcal infection) in HIV-infected patients before they begin taking antiretroviral treatment (ART). A patient who tests positive for cryptococcal antigen can take fluconazole, an antifungal medication, to fight off the silent fungal infection and prevent it from developing into life-threatening meningitis.

How Is a C. neoformans *Infection Diagnosed?*

Healthcare providers rely on your medical history, symptoms, physical examinations, and laboratory tests to diagnose a *C. neoformans* infection.

Your healthcare provider will take a sample of tissue or body fluid (such as blood, cerebrospinal fluid (CBF), or sputum) and send the sample to a laboratory to be examined under a microscope, tested with an antigen test, or cultured. Your healthcare provider may also perform tests such as a chest x-ray or computed tomography (CT) scan of your lungs, brain, or other parts of the body.

How Are C. neoformans *Infections Treated?*

People who have *C. neoformans* infection need to take prescription antifungal medication for at least six months, often longer. The type of treatment usually depends on the severity of the infection and the parts of the body that are affected.

- For people who have asymptomatic infections (e.g., diagnosed via targeted screening) or mild-to-moderate pulmonary infections, the treatment is usually fluconazole.

- For people who have severe lung infections or infections in the central nervous system (brain and spinal cord), the recommended initial treatment is amphotericin B in combination with flucytosine. After that, patients usually need to take fluconazole for an extended time to clear the infection.

The type, dose, and duration of antifungal treatment may differ for certain groups of people, such as pregnant women, children, and people in resource-limited settings. Some people may also need surgery to remove fungal growths (cryptococcomas).

Section 20.5

Histoplasmosis

This section includes text excerpted from "Histoplasmosis," Centers for Disease Control and Prevention (CDC), August 13, 2018.

Histoplasmosis is an infection caused by a fungus called "*Histoplasma*." The fungus lives in the environment, particularly in soil that contains large amounts of bird or bat droppings. In the United States, *Histoplasma* mainly lives in the central and eastern states, especially areas around the Ohio and Mississippi River valleys. The fungus also lives in parts of Central and South America, Africa, Asia, and Australia.

People can get histoplasmosis after breathing in the microscopic fungal spores from the air. Although most people who breathe in the spores do not get sick, those who do may have a fever, cough, and fatigue. Many people who get histoplasmosis will get better on their own without medication, but in some people, such as those who have weakened immune systems, the infection can become severe.

Symptoms of Histoplasmosis

Most people who are exposed to the fungus *Histoplasma* never have symptoms. Other people may have flu-like symptoms that usually go away on their own.

Symptoms of histoplasmosis include:

- Fever

- Cough

- Fatigue (extreme tiredness)

- Chills

- Headache

- Chest pain

- Body aches

How Soon Do the Symptoms of Histoplasmosis Appear?

Symptoms of histoplasmosis may appear between 3 and 17 days after a person breathes in the fungal spores.

How Long Do the Symptoms of Histoplasmosis Last?

For most people, the symptoms of histoplasmosis will go away within a few weeks to a month. However, some people have symptoms that last longer than this, especially if the infection becomes severe.

Severe Histoplasmosis

In some people, usually those who have weakened immune systems, histoplasmosis can develop into a long-term lung infection, or it can spread from the lungs to other parts of the body, such as the central nervous system (the brain and spinal cord).

Risk and Prevention of Histoplasmosis
Who Gets Histoplasmosis

Anyone can get histoplasmosis if they have been in an area where *Histoplasma* lives in the environment. Histoplasmosis is often associated with activities that disturb soil, particularly soil that contains bird or bat droppings. Certain groups of people are at higher risk for developing the severe forms of histoplasmosis:

- People who have weakened immune systems, for example, people who:
  - Have human immunodeficiency virus (HIV)/acquired immunodeficiency syndrome (AIDS)
  - Have had an organ transplant
  - Are taking medications such as corticosteroids or Tumor Necrosis Factor (TNF)-inhibitors
- Infants
- Adults aged 55 and older

Is Histoplasmosis Contagious?

No. Histoplasmosis cannot spread from the lungs between people or between people and animals. However, in extremely rare cases, the infection can be passed through an organ transplant with an infected organ.

If I Have Already Had Histoplasmosis, Could I Get It Again?

It is possible for someone who is already had histoplasmosis to get it again, but the body's immune system usually provides some partial protection so that the infection is less severe the second time. In people who have weakened immune systems, histoplasmosis can remain hidden in the body for months or years and then cause symptoms later (also called a "relapse of infection").

How Can I Prevent Histoplasmosis?

It can be difficult to avoid breathing in *Histoplasma* in areas where it is common in the environment. In areas where *Histoplasma* is known to live, people who have weakened immune systems (for example, by

HIV/AIDS, an organ transplant, or medications such as corticosteroids or TNF-inhibitors) should avoid doing activities that are known to be associated with getting histoplasmosis, including:

- Disturbing material (for example, digging in soil or chopping wood) where there are bird or bat droppings

- Cleaning chicken coops

- Exploring caves

- Cleaning, remodeling, or tearing down old buildings

Large amounts of bird or bat droppings should be cleaned up by professional companies that specialize in the removal of hazardous waste.

What Are Public-Health Agencies Doing about Histoplasmosis?

- **Surveillance.** In some states, healthcare providers and laboratories are required to report histoplasmosis cases to public health authorities. Disease reporting helps government officials and healthcare providers understand how and why outbreaks occur and allows them to monitor trends in the number of histoplasmosis cases.

- **Developing better diagnostic tools.** The symptoms of histoplasmosis can be similar to those of other respiratory diseases. Faster, more reliable methods to diagnosis histoplasmosis are in development, which could help minimize delays in treatment, save money and resources looking for other diagnoses, and reduce unnecessary treatment for other suspected illnesses.

- **Building laboratory capacity.** Equipping laboratories in Latin America to be able to diagnose histoplasmosis and perform laboratory-based surveillance will help reduce the burden of HIV-associated histoplasmosis in these areas.

How Is Histoplasmosis Diagnosed?

Healthcare providers rely on your medical and travel history, symptoms, physical examinations, and laboratory tests to diagnose histoplasmosis. The most common way that healthcare providers test for histoplasmosis is by taking a blood sample or a urine sample and sending it to a laboratory.

Healthcare providers may do imaging tests such as chest x-rays or computed tomography (CT) scans of your lungs. They may also collect a sample of fluid from your respiratory tract or perform a tissue biopsy, in which a small sample of affected tissue is taken from the body and examined under a microscope. Laboratories may also see if *Histoplasma* will grow from body fluids or tissues (this is called a "culture").

How Is Histoplasmosis Treated?

For some people, the symptoms of histoplasmosis will go away without treatment. However, prescription antifungal medication is needed to treat severe histoplasmosis in the lungs, chronic histoplasmosis, and infections that have spread from the lungs to other parts of the body (disseminated histoplasmosis). Itraconazole is one type of antifungal medication that is commonly used to treat histoplasmosis. Depending on the severity of the infection and the person's immune status, the course of treatment can range from three months to one year.

Chapter 21

Inhalation Anthrax

When a person breathes in anthrax spores, they can develop inhalation anthrax. People who work in places, such as wool mills, slaughterhouses, and tanneries may breathe in the spores when working with infected animals or contaminated animal products from infected animals. Inhalation anthrax starts primarily in the lymph nodes in the chest before spreading throughout the rest of the body, ultimately causing severe breathing problems and shock.

Inhalation anthrax is considered to be the most deadly form of anthrax. Infection usually develops within a week after exposure, but it can take up to two months. Without treatment, only about 10 to 15 percent of patients with inhalation anthrax survive. However, with aggressive treatment, about 55 percent of patients survive.

How People Get Infected with Inhalation Anthrax

People get infected with anthrax when spores get into the body. When this happens, the spores can be activated and become anthrax bacteria. Then the bacteria can multiply, spread out in the body, produce toxins (poisons), and cause severe illness. This can happen when people breathe in spores, eat food or drink water that is contaminated with spores, or get spores in a cut or scrape in the skin.

This chapter includes text excerpted from "Inhalation Anthrax," Centers for Disease Control and Prevention (CDC), July 21, 2014. Reviewed August 2019.

Symptoms of Inhalation Anthrax

The symptoms of anthrax depend on the type of infection and can take anywhere from one day to more than two months to appear. All types of anthrax have the potential, if untreated, to spread throughout the body and cause severe illness and even death.

Inhalation anthrax symptoms can include:

- Fever and chills
- Chest discomfort
- Shortness of breath
- Confusion or dizziness
- Cough
- Nausea, vomiting, or stomach pains
- Headache
- Sweats (often drenching)
- Extreme tiredness
- Body aches

Diagnosis of Inhalation Anthrax

Doctors in the United States rarely see a patient with anthrax. The Centers for Disease Control and Prevention's (CDC) *Guidance and Case Definitions* are available to help doctors diagnose anthrax, take patient histories to determine how exposure may have occurred, and order necessary diagnostic tests.

If inhalation anthrax is suspected, chest x-rays or computed tomography (CT) scans can confirm if the patient has mediastinal widening or pleural effusion, which are x-ray findings typically seen in patients with inhalation anthrax.

The only ways to confirm an Anthrax diagnosis are:

- To measure antibodies or toxin in blood
- To test directly for *Bacillus anthracis* in a sample of:
  - Blood
  - Skin lesion swab
  - Spinal fluid

- Respiratory secretions

Samples must be taken before the patient begins taking antibiotics for treatment.

What to Do If You Think You Have Been Exposed to Inhalation Anthrax

If you think you may have been exposed to anthrax, you need to go to a doctor right away and explain why you think you may have been exposed. Doctors can prescribe antibiotics to prevent you from getting sick. If you already have symptoms of anthrax, it is important to get medical care as quickly as possible to have the best chances for a full recovery.

Anthrax is not contagious, which means you cannot catch it like the cold or flu.

Who Are at Risk of Getting Infected with Inhalation Anthrax?

Anyone who has come in contact with anthrax spores could be at risk of getting sick. Most people will never be exposed to anthrax. However, there are activities that can put some people at greater risk of exposure than others.

- People who handle animal products
- Veterinarians
- Livestock producers
- Travelers
- Laboratory professionals
- Mail handlers, military personnel, and response workers who may be exposed during a bioterror event involving anthrax spores

Recommendations for protecting workers are available from the CDC's National Institute for Occupational Safety and Health (NIOSH). This guidance covers the use of respirators, protective clothing, and the anthrax vaccine.

The anthrax vaccine is currently provided only to people who are at an increased risk of coming in contact with anthrax spores, such as members of the U.S. military, certain laboratory workers, and some people who handle animals or animal products (for example, farmers, veterinarians, and livestock handlers). The vaccine is not licensed for use in children under age 18, adults over age 65, or pregnant and nursing women.

Part Three

Inflammatory Respiratory Disorders

Chapter 22

Asthma

Chapter Contents

Section 22.1

Facts about Asthma

This section includes text excerpted from "Asthma,"
National Heart, Lung, and Blood Institute (NHLBI), May 19, 2019.

What Is Asthma?

Asthma is a chronic, or long-term, condition that intermittently inflames and narrows the airways in the lungs. The inflammation makes the airways swell. Asthma causes periods of wheezing, chest tightness, shortness of breath, and coughing. People who have asthma may experience symptoms that range from mild to severe and that may happen rarely or every day. When symptoms get worse, it is called an "asthma attack." Asthma affects people of all ages and often starts during childhood.

The goal of asthma management is to achieve control with an asthma action plan. An asthma action plan may include monitoring, avoiding triggers, and using medicines.

Causes of Asthma

The exact cause of asthma is unknown, and the causes may vary from person to person. However, asthma is often the result of a strong response of the immune system to an allergen in the environment. For example, exposure to an allergen, such as ragweed, may make your airways react strongly. Other people exposed to the same allergen may not react at all, or their response may be different. The reason one person reacts to an exposure while others do not is not completely understood, though it may be partially explained by genes.

Immune System

Asthma symptoms occur when the airways of the lungs narrow, which makes it more difficult to breathe. This narrowing is usually caused by inflammation, which makes the airways swell and may cause the cells of the airway to make excess mucus. Bronchospasm, or tightening of the muscles around the airways, also makes the airways narrow and results in trouble breathing.

Over time, if asthma remains active, the airway walls can become thicker.

Genes

Genes seem to play a role in making some people more susceptible to asthma. For example, some genes are involved in how your immune system responds to allergens. These genes can cause a stronger reaction in your airways when certain substances in the air end up there. The genes involved may be different in different people.

Environment

Environmental exposures that may lead to asthma include airborne allergens and virus infections in infancy or early childhood when the immune system is developing.

Risk Factors of Asthma

Asthma affects people of all ages, but it often starts during childhood. Sometimes asthma develops in adults, particularly women. This type of asthma is called "adult-onset" or "late-onset" asthma.

You may have an increased risk of asthma because of your environment or occupation, your family history or genes, other medical conditions, your race or ethnicity, or your sex.

Environment or Occupation

Environmental exposures, including those at work, may increase the risk of developing asthma or making asthma symptoms worse.

- Exposure to cigarette smoke during pregnancy or in a child's first few years increases the risk of the child developing asthma symptoms early in life. This exposure also may affect lung growth and development.

- Exposure to different microbes in the environment, especially early in life, can affect the development of the immune system. These effects on the immune system may either increase or protect against the risk of developing asthma.

- Exposures that occur in the workplace, such as chemical irritants or industrial dusts, may also be associated with an increased risk of developing asthma in susceptible people. This type of asthma is called "occupational asthma." It may develop over a period of years, and it often lasts even after you are no longer exposed.

- Poor air quality from pollution or allergens may worsen asthma. Pollutants include gases from heaters or vehicles. Allergens in the air include pollen, dust, or other air particles.

Family History and Genes

Genes and family history increase your risk of developing asthma.

- Having a parent who has asthma, especially if the mother has asthma, increases the risk that a child will develop asthma.
- The genes you inherit may play a role in the development of asthma because they affect how the immune system develops. More than one gene is likely involved.

Other Medical Conditions

Asthma is often linked to other medical conditions, such as:

- **Allergies.** Asthma is usually a type of allergic reaction. People who have asthma often have other types of allergies. They may have food allergies or get a runny or stuffy nose from pollen. You may be at higher risk for developing asthma if you had allergic reactions in early childhood to substances in the air, such as pollen, dander, mold, or dust. The more things you are allergic to, the higher your risk of asthma.
- **Obesity**
- **Respiratory infections and wheezing.** Young children who often have respiratory infections caused by viruses are at highest risk of developing asthma symptoms early in life.

Race or Ethnicity

African Americans and Puerto Ricans are at higher risk of asthma than people of other races or ethnicities. African American and Hispanic children are more likely to die from asthma-related causes than non-Hispanic White Americans.

Sex

Among children, more boys than girls have asthma. Among teens and adults, asthma is more common among women than men.

Screening and Prevention of Asthma

There is no routine screening for asthma, and there is no way to prevent asthma. Your doctor may recommend avoiding certain risk factors to help prevent asthma from getting worse or causing asthma attacks.

Signs, Symptoms, and Complications of Asthma

How often signs and symptoms of asthma occur may depend on how severe, or intense, the asthma is, and whether you are exposed to allergens. Some people have symptoms every day, while others have symptoms only a few days of the year. For some people, asthma may cause discomfort but does not interfere with daily activities. If you have more severe asthma, however, your asthma may limit what you are able to do.

When asthma is well controlled, it may not cause symptoms. When symptoms worsen, it is called an "asthma attack," "exacerbation," or "flare-up." Over time, uncontrolled asthma can damage the lungs.

Signs and Symptoms

Signs and symptoms of asthma may include:

- **Chest tightness**
- **Coughing**, especially at night or early morning
- **Shortness of breath**
- **Wheezing**, which causes a whistling sound when you exhale

Asthma attacks are episodes that occur when symptoms get much worse. Asthma attacks can happen suddenly and may be life-threatening. People who have severe asthma experience asthma attacks more often.

While other conditions can cause the same symptoms as asthma, the pattern of symptoms in people who have asthma usually has some of the following characteristics:

- They come and go over time, or within the same day.
- They start or get worse with viral infections, such as a cold.
- They are triggered by exercise, allergies, cold air, or hyperventilation from laughing or crying.
- They are worse at night or in the morning.

241

Diagnosis of Asthma

Your doctor may diagnose asthma based on your medical history, a physical exam, and results from diagnostic tests. Your history of asthma symptoms will help your doctor determine if you have mild, moderate, or severe asthma. The level of severity is used to determine the treatment you will receive.

Before diagnosing you with asthma, your doctor will rule out other medical reasons or conditions that could also cause similar signs and symptoms. You may need to see an asthma specialist, called a "pulmonologist," or an allergy specialist, called an "allergist."

Medical History

Your doctor may ask about any known allergies and the pattern of your symptoms. This includes how often symptoms occur, what seems to trigger your symptoms, when or where symptoms occur, and if your symptoms wake you up at night.

Physical Exam

During the physical exam, your doctor may:

- Listen to your breathing and look for signs of asthma, such as wheezing, a runny nose, or swollen nasal passages

- Look for allergic skin conditions, such as eczema

Diagnostic Tests

Several tests may be done to help determine if asthma is likely to be the cause of symptoms. These tests include:

- **Pulmonary function tests** such as spirometry, which involves breathing in and out through a tube connected to a computer. This measures how much and how fast the air moves when you breathe in and out with maximum effort.

- **Spirometry with bronchodilator (BD)** test to measure how much and how fast air moves in and out both before and after you take an inhaled medicine to relax the muscles in your airway.

- **Bronchoprovocation tests** to measure how your airways react to specific exposures. During this test, you inhale different concentrations of allergens or medicines that may tighten the muscles in your airways. Spirometry can also be done before and after the test.

- **Peak expiratory flow (PEF)** to measure how fast you can blow air out using maximum effort. This test can be done during spirometry or by breathing into a separate device, such as a tube.

Diagnosing Asthma in Children under Age Six

It can be hard to tell whether a child under 6 years old has asthma or another respiratory condition because they cannot perform a pulmonary function test such as spirometry. After checking a child's history and symptoms, the doctor may try asthma medicines for a few months to see how well a child responds. About 40 percent of children who wheeze when they get colds or respiratory infections are eventually diagnosed with asthma.

Allergy Tests

If you have a history of allergies, your doctor may test to find out which allergens in the environment, such as pet dander or pollen, affect you. This can be a skin test or a blood test.

Tests for Other Medical Conditions

Your doctor may want to test for other conditions if your symptoms include:

- A cough without other breathing issues

- Chest pain

- Coughing up mucus often

- Difficult and noisy breathing during exercise

- Shortness of breath with dizziness, light-headedness, or tingling in your hands or feet

Tests your doctor may use to rule out other medical conditions include:

- **Chest x-ray** to rule out lung infections, such as tuberculosis (TB), or a foreign substance, such as an object that was inhaled by accident

- **Electrocardiogram (EKG)** to rule out heart failure or arrhythmia while in emergency care

- **Laryngoscopy** to rule out vocal cord problems. The doctor can use this test to look at your upper airways and the vocal cords.

- **Sleep studies** to rule out sleep apnea

- **Tests that look at your esophagus and upper digestive system** to rule out gastroesophageal reflux disease (GERD). These tests may include endoscopy, in which a small camera is placed in the esophagus, or an x-ray of the digestive system. Tests may also measure the acid in your esophagus or measure how food or other substances move through the esophagus. Some people have both GERD and asthma.

Treatment of Asthma

If you are like most people who have asthma, treatment can manage your symptoms, allow you to resume normal activities, and prevent asthma attacks. Treatment usually depends on your age, asthma severity, and your response to a given treatment option. Your doctor may adjust your treatment until asthma symptoms are controlled.

Most people who have asthma are treated with daily medicine, called "long-term control medicines," along with inhalers containing medicine for short-term relief during an asthma attack or when symptoms worsen. An inhaler allows the medicine to go into the mouth and airways.

Control Medicines

Your doctor may prescribe control medicines to take daily to help prevent symptoms by reducing airway inflammation and preventing narrowing of the airways.

Control medicines include the following:

- **Corticosteroids** to reduce the body's inflammatory response. Your doctor may prescribe inhaled corticosteroids that you will need to take each day. If your symptoms get worse, your doctor may increase the dose of the inhaled corticosteroids to prevent severe asthma attacks or even give corticosteroids by mouth for short periods. Common side effects from inhaled corticosteroids include a hoarse voice or a mouth infection called "thrush."

A spacer or holding chamber on your inhaler can help avoid these side effects. Using high-dose inhaled corticosteroids more often or for longer periods may affect growth in young children. Oral corticosteroids also have more side effects than inhaled corticosteroids because more of the medicine goes outside the lungs.

- **Biologics**, such as omalizumab, mepolizumab, reslizumab, and benralizumab, to target specific parts of the body's response to allergens. Biologics are antibodies used in people who have severe asthma. These medicines are given by injection, either below the skin or in a vein, every few weeks.

- **Leukotriene modifiers** to reduce the effects of leukotrienes, which are released in the body as part of the response to allergens. Leukotrienes cause the airway muscles to tighten. These medicines block this response, allowing the airways to open, and reduce inflammation. You take these pills by mouth, alone or with corticosteroids, depending on what your doctor prescribes.

- **Mast cell stabilizers** such as cromolyn, to help prevent airway inflammation caused by exposure to allergens or other triggers. These medicines stop certain immune cells from releasing the signals that cause inflammation.

- **Inhaled long-acting beta2-agonists (LABAs)** keep the airways open by preventing narrowing of the airways. LABAs may be added to your inhaled corticosteroids to reduce narrowing and inflammation.

Short-Term Relief Medicines

Short-term relief medicines, also called "quick-relief medicines," help prevent symptoms or relieve symptoms during an asthma attack. They may be the only medicine needed for mild asthma or asthma that only happens with physical activity.

Your doctor will prescribe a quick-relief inhaler for you or your child to carry at all times.

Types of short-term relief medicines include:

- **Inhaled short-acting beta2-agonists (SABAs)** to quickly relax tight muscles around your airways. This allows the airways to open up so air can flow through them. Side effects can include tremors and rapid heartbeat. SABAs are usually the only medicine used to treat wheezing in children under five years old. If symptoms and medical history suggest asthma, doctors may treat it with inhaled corticosteroids for a trial period to see if they help. If symptoms do not improve, corticosteroids will be stopped to avoid side effects.

- **Oral and intravenous (IV) corticosteroids** to reduce inflammation caused by severe asthma symptoms

- **Short-acting anticholinergics** to help open the airways quickly. This medicine may be less effective than SABAs, but it is an option for people who may have side effects from SABAs.

Emergency Care

If you have a severe asthma attack and need emergency care, you may be treated with medicines, such as those listed above, given with a nebulizer or IV. You may also receive oxygen therapy or breathing assistance, either through a tube inserted in the airway or through noninvasive ventilation, which uses a mask with forced air that covers the face to support breathing.

Procedures

Your doctor may recommend a procedure called "bronchial thermoplasty" if you have severe asthma and other treatments are not working. In this procedure, your doctor will enter the airways through the mouth with a bronchoscope. This helps your doctor see inside the airways. Your doctor then will apply heat to the muscles along the airways to make them thinner and help prevent constriction.

Section 22.2

Allergic Asthma

This section includes text excerpted from "Allergic Asthma," Genetics Home Reference (GHR), National Institutes of Health (NIH), December 2018.

Asthma is a breathing disorder characterized by inflammation of the airways and recurrent episodes of breathing difficulty. These episodes, sometimes referred to as "asthma attacks," are triggered by irritation of the inflamed airways. In allergic asthma, the attacks occur when substances known as "allergens" are inhaled, causing an allergic reaction. Allergens are harmless substances that the body's immune system mistakenly reacts to as though they are harmful. Common allergens include pollen, dust, animal dander, and mold. The immune response leads to the symptoms of asthma. Allergic asthma is the most common form of the disorder.

A hallmark of asthma is bronchial hyperresponsiveness, which means the airways are especially sensitive to irritants and respond excessively. Because of this hyperresponsiveness, attacks can be triggered by irritants other than allergens, such as physical activity, respiratory infections, or exposure to tobacco smoke, in people with allergic asthma.

An asthma attack is characterized by tightening of the muscles around the airways (bronchoconstriction), which narrows the airway and makes breathing difficult. Additionally, the immune reaction can lead to swelling of the airways and overproduction of mucus. During an attack, an affected individual can experience chest tightness, wheezing, shortness of breath, and coughing. Over time, the muscles around the airways can become enlarged (hypertrophied), further narrowing the airways.

Some people with allergic asthma have another allergic disorder, such as hay fever (allergic rhinitis) or food allergies. Asthma is sometimes part of a series of allergic disorders, referred to as the atopic march. Development of these conditions typically follows a pattern, beginning with eczema (atopic dermatitis), followed by food allergies, then hay fever, and finally asthma. However, not all individuals with asthma have progressed through the atopic march, and not all individuals with one allergic disease will develop others.

Frequency of Allergic Asthma

Approximately 235 million people worldwide have asthma. In the United States, the condition affects an estimated 8 percent of the population. In nearly 90 percent of children and 50 percent of adults with asthma, the condition is classified as "allergic asthma."

Causes of Allergic Asthma

The cause of allergic asthma is complex. It is likely that a combination of multiple genetic and environmental factors contribute to development of the condition. Doctors believe genes are involved because having a family member with allergic asthma or another allergic disorder increases a person's risk of developing asthma.

Studies suggest that more than 100 genes may be associated with allergic asthma, but each seems to be a factor in only one or a few populations. Many of the associated genes are involved in the body's immune response. Others play a role in lung and airway function.

There is evidence that an unbalanced immune response underlies allergic asthma. While there is normally a balance between type 1 (or Th1) and type 2 (or Th2) immune reactions in the body, many individuals with allergic asthma predominantly have type 2 reactions. Type 2 reactions lead to the production of immune proteins called "IgE antibodies" and the generation of other factors that predispose to bronchial hyperresponsiveness. Normally, the body produces IgE antibodies in response to foreign invaders, particularly parasitic worms. For unknown reasons, in susceptible individuals, the body reacts to an allergen as if it is harmful, producing IgE antibodies specific to it. Upon later encounters with the allergen, IgE antibodies recognize it, which stimulates an immune response, causing bronchoconstriction, airway swelling, and mucus production.

Not everyone with a variation in one of the allergic asthma-associated genes develops the condition; exposure to certain environmental factors also contributes to its development. Studies suggest that these exposures trigger epigenetic changes to the DNA. Epigenetic changes modify DNA without changing the DNA sequence. They can affect gene activity and regulate the production of proteins, which may influence the development of allergies in susceptible individuals.

Inheritance Pattern of Allergic Asthma

Allergic asthma can be passed through generations in families, but the inheritance pattern is unknown. People with mutations in one or more of the associated genes inherit an increased risk of allergic asthma, not the condition itself. Because allergic asthma is a complex condition influenced by genetic and environmental factors, not all people with a mutation in an asthma-associated gene will develop the disorder.

Section 22.3

Exercise-Induced Bronchoconstriction and Asthma

This section includes text excerpted from "Exercise-Induced Bronchoconstriction and Asthma," Agency for Healthcare Research and Quality (AHRQ), U.S. Department of Health and Human Services (HHS), March 2010. Reviewed August 2019.

What Is Exercise-Induced Bronchoconstriction and Asthma?

Vigorous physical exercise can be followed by transient clinical signs and symptoms of asthma due to airway narrowing. The phenomenon was first recorded around 150 AD by Aretaeus of Cappadocia. Airway obstruction following exercise was first observed among individuals with underlying asthma from which the term "exercise-induced asthma" (EIA) was derived. Asthma is a chronic inflammatory disorder of the airways in which many cells and cellular elements play a role, and it is associated with bronchial (or airway) hyperresponsiveness. Similar post-exercise asthma-like symptoms have been observed in persons without the presence of co-existing asthma, particularly in athletes. In this population the phenomenon has been referred to as "exercise-induced bronchoconstriction" (EIB) and has been defined as "the airway obstruction that occurs in association with exercise without regard to the presence of chronic asthma." EIA is "the condition in which exercise induces symptoms of asthma in patients who have asthma."

The underlying mechanisms of EIB and EIA are multifactorial and complex. Whether the two phenomena have the same pathogenesis is still unknown and continues to be explored. In the early 1970s, it was recognized that the severity of the airway constriction was associated with the level of ventilation. In normal nasal breathing, inspired air is heated to body temperature and is completely saturated with water in the first few generations of the airways. There is a marked increase in minute ventilation during and following strenuous exercise and, as a result, the nose is unable to condition the increased volume of air. The added burden on the lower airways, down to the tenth generation and beyond, to warm and humidify the large volume of air triggers osmotic and thermal changes. Loss of water in the periciliary fluid layer of the airway produces a hyperosmotic environment that may stimulate degranulation of pulmonary mucosa mast cells with subsequent release of several inflammatory mediators, such as histamine, leukotrienes, prostaglandin, platelet-activating factors, and neuropeptides from sensory nerves. Theorists propose that the released mediators stimulate bronchial smooth muscle spasm and rapid rewarming leads to increased bronchial circulation and engorged capillary beds (or airway edema) that may intensify the obstruction.

The hallmark of EIB/EIA is that the acute airflow obstruction (measured by the forced expiratory volume in 1 second [FEV1]) peaks rapidly 3 to 15 minutes after exercise stops and then remits spontaneously within 20 to 60 minutes. It does not cause a prolonged deterioration in lung function. The nature and severity of episodes vary widely within and among individuals and can be influenced by multiple factors. Common clinical symptoms include coughing, wheezing, shortness of breath, excessive mucus production, chest tightness, chest pain, or an itching or scratching sensation in the chest. Less common symptoms include stomach pain, nausea; and near-death experiences. EIB/EIA has been shown to appear during prolonged exercise causing a lack of endurance despite conditioning. It may influence athletic performance and often results in a prolonged recovery time following exercise. A small subset of individuals experience a second, late-phase constriction 4 to 12 hours after the initial activity. This constriction is generally less severe than the first, but the magnitude of the two episodes are significantly correlated. No single factor predicts who will experience a late response, and these responses do not happen consistently in the same individuals.

Approximately 40 to 50 percent of individuals who have an initial episode of EIB/EIA experience a refractory period that is defined as "a period of diminished responsiveness when a second period of exercise follows in 1 to 4 hours." During this time the magnitude of the EIB/EIA response to an identical exercise task may be less than 50 percent of the initial response. This phenomenon is somewhat elusive as it can be present at some times but not at others. The cause is not fully understood but it has been suggested that depletion of catecholamines, increased circulation of prostaglandin, and degranulation of mast cell mediators play a role.

Table 22.1. Factors That May Influence the Severity of EIB/EIA

Factors	Decrease Exercise-Induced Bronchoconstriction (EIB)/Exercise-Induced Asthma (EIA)	Increase Exercise-Induced Bronchoconstriction (EIB)/Exercise-Induced Asthma (EIA)
Environmental conditions	• Warm temperatures (34 to 37°C) • High humidity (100%) • Absence of allergens • Low air pollution	• Cold temperatures, dry air • Airborne particles and pollutants, allergens, molds, dust • Irritants, such as automobile exhaust, sulfur dioxide, nitrogen dioxide, smoke, ozone, chlorine
Type, intensity, duration of exercise	• Short episodes of fast/slow running with brief rests • VO2 max <40% predicted <3 minutes continuous exercise	• Continuous activities that require near maximum aerobic capacity • VO2 max ≥60% predicted 6 to 8 minutes continuous exercise
Overall control of underlying asthma and BHR	• Good control: FEV1 >70 percent predicted fall in BHR	• Poor control: FEV1 <65 percent predicted increase in BHR
Physical conditioning	• Good physical conditioning • Warmup and cooldown sessions	• Poor physical conditioning • Sudden burst of activity • Fatigue • Emotional stress • Athletic overtraining
Respiratory tract infections, especially viral	• No respiratory tract infections	• Presence of respiratory tract infections • Sinusitis • Rhinitis

Table 22.1. Continued

Factors	Decrease Exercise-Induced Bronchoconstriction (EIB)/Exercise-Induced Asthma (EIA)	Increase Exercise-Induced Bronchoconstriction (EIB)/Exercise-Induced Asthma (EIA)
Time since last exercise	• If within 40 to 90 min may benefit from refractory period	• >2 to 3 hr
Concurrent medications	• Maintenance anti-inflammatory bronchodilator medication	• Salicylates • NSAIDs • β-blockers
Pre-exercise foods eaten	• None	• Peanuts, celery, shrimp, grain, carrots, bananas

Diagnosis of Exercise-Induced Bronchoconstriction and Asthma

Potential EIB/EIA can be detected by taking a thorough medical history. EIB/EIA is suspected when individuals, who otherwise have good lung function, complain of recurrent shortness of breath and symptoms of cough, wheeze, chest pain, or prolonged recovery time following exercise. These symptoms are independent of a person's conditioning level. If symptoms are relieved by inhaling a short-acting beta-agonist (SABA) or if symptoms are prevented by taking a SABA before exercise, a diagnosis of EIB/EIA is strongly supported. The degree of airway constriction can be measured objectively by a spectrum of pulmonary function tests; however, most clinicians and laboratories use the FEV1 or, very occasionally, the peak expiratory flow (PEF).

When a patient's history suggests EIB/EIA, measuring the change in FEV1 before and after a standardized exercise challenge test (ECT) on a treadmill or bicycle ergometer can assist in making the diagnosis. The American Thoracic Society (ATS) has published guidelines for conducting a standardized ECT, which include recommendations for environmental control, as well as the level and duration of intensity required to ensure a sufficiently vigorous challenge. Minute ventilation must reach the target level in the first four minutes of the challenge.

The standardized laboratory ECT has not always demonstrated sufficient sensitivity to identify EIB/EIA in elite athletes who perform in many venues and with widely varying intensity and duration, therefore, other surrogate tests have been recommended. Some of the current options include sport-specific challenges, the free running asthma screening test (FRAST), measures of direct bronchial responsiveness to methacholine (MCH) and indirect responsiveness to eucapnic voluntary hyperpnea (EVH) or mannitol.

In the general population, vigorous exercise should cause little to no prolonged decrease in airflow following exercise. A decrease of 10 percent from baseline has been shown to be a change greater than two standard deviations from the normal response. In 2001, prior to the Salt Lake City Olympics, the International Olympic Committee (IOC) Medical Commission met to determine the parameters for EIB/EIA. They accepted a cutpoint of a fall of 10 percent or more in FEV1, as suggested by the European Respiratory Society (ERS) and ATS guidelines. This decision was supported by a study indicating a coefficient of variation of six percent for repeated maneuvers of FEV1. However, the cutpoint value is a subject of ongoing debate. Two investigators have suggested that a fall in FEV1 of only 6.5 percent is appropriate. Some researchers claim that the 10 percent value is justified as this level of constriction could potentially limit exercise performance. A 10 percent fall is also supported by researchers who found this degree of constriction to have a specificity of 90 percent for identifying those with asthma.

Treatment of Exercise-Induced Bronchoconstriction and Asthma

The goal of treatment is to prevent or, at least, to reduce the severity of the bronchoconstriction and symptoms so that an individual can participate in any activity, regardless of its intensity and duration, without serious respiratory limitations. Through a combination of education, a commitment to fitness, pharmacologic intervention, and use of nonpharmacologic strategies, EIB/EIA can be successfully managed in the majority of cases. Different pharmaceutical agents that appear to operate on different phases of the response can provide at least partial relief from EIB/EIA. The most commonly used agents are inhaled SABA and long-acting beta-agonist (LABA) agents. Other agents include mast cell stabilizing agents (MCS), short-acting anticholinergics (SAAC), leukotriene receptor antagonists (LTRA), and inhaled corticosteroids (ICS). Theophyllines, antihistamines, calcium channel blockers, heparin, and furosemide have also been shown to have some degree of effectiveness. There are many unresolved issues with respect to the treatment of EIB/EIA with pharmaceutical agents. There is concern that the continuous use of the SABA and LABA agents to control asthma over the long term could lead to a decrease in efficacy when also used prophylactically to control EIA. A development of tolerance, or tachyphylaxis, to SABA or LABA agents may not only decrease their protective effect, but also shorten their duration of action. In the case of SABAs, a serious concern is that continuous use will decrease its impact as a rescue medication in the case of severe EIA.

Section 22.4

Other Types of Asthma

"Other Types of Asthma,"
© 2016 Omnigraphics. Reviewed August 2019.

There are many different types of asthma. Identifying a patient's specific type of asthma is a key to finding treatment methods that will control symptoms effectively. Cough-variant asthma is characterized by severe, unproductive coughing that lasts longer than six weeks. Because people with this type of asthma often do not experience wheezing or other classic asthma symptoms, cough-variant asthma is often misdiagnosed. Night-time or nocturnal asthma involves classic asthma symptoms that worsen at night and interfere with sleep. Nocturnal asthma is considered a serious condition because it is associated with higher mortality rates. Finally, a number of different health conditions can present symptoms that mimic asthma, so it is important for people experiencing such symptoms to undergo testing to obtain a definitive diagnosis.

Cough-Variant Asthma

A severe, persistent cough that does not produce any mucus can be a sign of cough-variant asthma. In fact, around 25 percent of people who seek medical attention for a chronic cough have cough-variant asthma. This type of asthma is often misdiagnosed because patients do not always have the classic symptoms of asthma, such as wheezing and shortness of breath. In children, however, cough-variant asthma often leads to the development of classic asthma symptoms.

Although the exact causes of cough-variant asthma are unknown, it often seems to develop following respiratory infections, vigorous exercise, or exposure to allergy triggers, such as strong fragrances or dust. Some people develop cough-variant asthma after they start taking beta-blockers, a class of drugs used to treat high blood pressure, heart disease, migraines, and eye problems such as glaucoma. Cough-variant asthma also tends to appear in people with aspirin sensitivity.

Cough-variant asthma is tricky to diagnose because there are many other possible causes of a cough, including bronchitis, sinusitis, post-nasal drip, chronic rhinitis, or acid reflux (heartburn). In addition, people with cough-variant asthma often have normal physical examinations and chest x-rays. To determine whether a persistent cough is related to asthma, doctors will likely perform a series of lung function tests.

One test that is typically used in the diagnosis of asthma is spirometry, which uses a device to measure the amount of air and the rate at which the patient can exhale. If this test does not indicate any impairment in lung function, the next option is a methacholine challenge. In this test, the patient inhales an aerosol mist containing methacholine, a drug that causes the airways to narrow and spasm. Although even healthy lungs will react to methacholine, a lower dosage is needed to trigger symptoms in people with asthma. A decline in lung function of 20 percent or more generally indicates that asthma is present.

Even without a conclusive diagnosis, patients with a persistent, dry cough may still be treated with asthma medications, such as inhalers containing albuterol or corticosteroids. If the symptoms improve with treatment, then the patient will be diagnosed with cough-variant asthma.

Night-Time (Nocturnal) Asthma

Night-time or nocturnal asthma is a common type of the disease characterized by symptoms that worsen at night. People with nocturnal asthma may be awakened from sleep by wheezing, shortness of breath, coughing, and a feeling of tightness in the chest. When experienced at night, these symptoms are potentially dangerous. In fact, studies have shown that a majority of asthma-related deaths occur at night. People with nocturnal asthma also tend to have more severe daytime asthma symptoms.

Night-time asthma sufferers may also experience health problems stemming from sleep disturbances. People who are unable to get adequate, quality sleep often feel tired and irritable during the day. They may also have trouble concentrating at work or at school. In fact, sleep disturbances due to asthma are one of the leading causes of children missing school. Studies have shown that children with nocturnal asthma may experience decreased mental function that affects their performance in school. When nocturnal asthma is treated effectively, however, sleep disturbance is reduced and mental function improves.

Causes of Nocturnal Asthma

Researchers have identified a number of factors that may contribute to the worsening of asthma symptoms at night.

- **Sleep-related airway changes.** Airways tend to narrow during sleep, which increases airflow resistance. As a result, airway function decreases gradually through the night. Although healthy people may not notice this effect, it can trigger symptoms in people with asthma. In fact, research has shown that people with asthma are more likely to experience breathing problems during sleep no matter when the sleep period occurs. Lung function test results tend to be worst around five hours after falling asleep, even for people who sleep during the daytime hours.

- **Sleep-related hormone changes.** The levels of certain hormones in the bloodstream tend to fluctuate according to a general pattern throughout the day and night. The changing hormone levels create the natural sleep-wake cycle, or circadian rhythms, and can also exert a powerful effect on asthma symptoms. The hormone epinephrine, for instance, reaches its lowest level in most people around 4:00 a.m. This hormone helps keep airways open by relaxing muscles surrounding the bronchial tubes. In addition, epinephrine suppresses histamines and other substances that cause the body to produce mucus.

- **Mucus drainage or sinusitis.** The increased production of mucus in the sinuses at night, combined with the narrowing of airways during sleep, can cause coughing and breathing problems in people with asthma. Sinusitis due to a viral or bacterial infection can also irritate sensitive airways and increase nocturnal asthma symptoms.

- **Reclining position.** Lying down may also contribute to night-time asthma symptoms. Reclining allows mucus secretions to drain from the sinuses and accumulate in the airways. In addition, it increases the volume of blood and decreases the volume of air in the lungs, which contributes to airway resistance.

- **Exposure to allergens.** About half of people who have an asthma attack immediately following exposure to an allergen will experience a second airway obstruction three to eight hours later. Known as a "late phase response," this second episode can be more severe and prolonged than the initial one. Research indicates that exposure to allergens in the evening increases a patient's susceptibility to a late phase response at night.

- **Cooling of the airways.** Whether from sleeping in an air-conditioned bedroom in summer or turning the thermostat down in winter, breathing cold, dry air can result in the loss of heat from the airways. The cooling of the airways at night is considered a contributing factor to nocturnal asthma.

- **Heartburn.** Gastroesophageal reflux disease (GERD), commonly known as "acid reflux" or "heartburn," occurs when stomach acid flows back into the esophagus and larynx. In people with frequent heartburn, stomach acid can irritate the lower esophagus and lead to bronchial spasm and airway constriction. Stomach acid that reaches the throat can also drip down into the lungs, causing airway irritation and increased mucus production. Since lying down often makes heartburn worse, it can be related to nocturnal asthma.

Treatment of Nocturnal Asthma

Night-time asthma can interfere with sleep and create serious health risks. The keys to managing asthma symptoms that worsen at night include finding the right asthma medications and determining when to use them to ensure quality sleep. Daily medications, such as inhaled corticosteroids, can help reduce inflammation of the airways and thus prevent night-time symptoms. But some short-term medications cannot cover a long enough time period to allow patients to sleep through the night. In such cases, a long-acting inhaled corticosteroid or bronchodilator may help alleviate symptoms.

For people whose nocturnal asthma may be triggered by allergens, it is important to avoid exposure to common allergens, such as dust mites or animal dander, especially in the evening hours. Regulating the temperature and humidity of the bedroom and elevating the head of the bed may also be helpful. Finally, people with GERD can often get relief from nocturnal asthma symptoms by taking medication that reduces acid production in the stomach.

Health Conditions That May Mimic Asthma

The most common symptoms of asthma—such as wheezing, coughing, and shortness of breath—can also be caused by other health conditions. Some of the illnesses with symptoms that may mimic asthma include:

- **Respiratory illnesses.** Many common respiratory illnesses can cause coughing, wheezing, and difficulty breathing, from the common cold to influenza. Sinusitis, or inflammation of the sinuses related to a viral or bacterial infection, often coexists with asthma. Other possible culprits include respiratory syncytial virus (RSV), which can cause pneumonia in children, and pulmonary aspergillosis, a fungal infection of the lungs.

- **Lung diseases.** A variety of lung conditions may present symptoms similar to asthma, including accidental aspiration of food, water, or other matter into the lungs; obstruction of the airway by an esophageal tumor or enlarged thyroid gland; injury to the lungs or airways; or lung cancer (bronchogenic carcinoma). Chronic obstructive pulmonary disease (COPD) refers to several lung diseases that are often related to cigarette smoking, such as emphysema and chronic bronchitis. COPD is characterized by wheezing and difficulty breathing.

- **Heart conditions.** Shortness of breath can also be an indication of heart disease. Congestive heart failure occurs when the heart does not circulate blood properly, leading to a buildup of fluid in the lungs. Myocardial ischemia occurs when the heart muscle does not receive adequate oxygen, usually because of a blockage in a coronary artery. Chest pain is the most common symptom, but shortness of breath with exercise may also occur.

- **Vocal cord dysfunction.** Vocal cord dysfunction is a condition in which the muscles of the larynx tighten and close, which can cause wheezing and difficulty breathing. This condition is most common among young women. The most extreme case is vocal cord paralysis, which involves a total loss of function in those muscles.

- **GERD.** The heartburn associated with gastroesophageal reflux disease can irritate the airways and cause symptoms that mimic asthma.

Diagnosing Asthma

Since so many other health conditions present similar symptoms, diagnosing asthma can be difficult. Doctors will typically begin by reviewing the patient's medical history and family history, including any history of breathing problems, allergies, or lung conditions. They will also inquire whether the patient has ever smoked, as smoking is a significant risk factor in many of the heart and lung diseases that can mimic asthma. Doctors will also ask for a detailed description of the patient's symptoms, including when and how often they usually occur. In addition to conducting a physical examination, doctors will likely perform a number of different tests to confirm or rule out various conditions, such as allergy tests, blood tests, chest and sinus x-rays, and lung function tests. If the diagnosis is asthma, determining the specific type is necessary in order to treat it effectively.

References

1. "Cough-Variant Asthma," WebMD Asthma Health Center, 2015.

2. "Nocturnal (Night-Time) Asthma," WebMD Asthma Health Center, 2015.

3. "Health Conditions That Mimic Asthma," WebMD Asthma Health Center, 2015.

Section 22.5

Acetaminophen Use and the Risk of Developing Asthma

This section includes text excerpted from "Acetaminophen May Increase the Risk of Developing Asthma," National Institute of Environmental Health Sciences (NIEHS), November 25, 2008. Reviewed August 2019.

There is a growing body of scientific literature suggesting a causal link between the use of the nonsteroidal anti-inflammatory drug (NSAID) acetaminophen and the rise in the incidence of asthma in children. A new epidemiologic study, supported by the National Institute of Environmental Health Sciences (NIEHS), conducted with 345 pregnant women adds to the growing evidence.

There are plausible biological and associative links between acetaminophen and asthma. Acetaminophen became the drug of choice for pain and fever relief in the 1980s after several studies reported a link between Reyes syndrome and aspirin use. In 1986, the U.S. Food and Drug Agency (FDA) placed warning labels regarding the Reyes Syndrome link on acetaminophen bottles. Shortly afterward, pediatricians nationwide started noticing a rise in asthma incidence. Acetaminophen, unlike aspirin and ibuprofen, decreases the level of the antioxidant glutathione in the lungs and other tissues.

In the NIEHS-funded work, women were recruited during their first trimester of pregnancy. Use of acetaminophen during pregnancy was determined by a questionnaire and related to respiratory outcomes in their newborns during their first year of life. Use of acetaminophen in the second and third trimesters was significantly related to wheezing in the first year. While wheezing is a known symptom of asthma in young children, it alone does not constitute a diagnosis of asthma.

The findings in this report are consistent with previous literature showing increases in asthma symptoms after exposure to acetaminophen. The researchers will continue to follow these children until they reach 5 years of age enabling them to provide more precise estimates of asthma incidence. The researchers point out that this is only the second study suggesting that exposure to acetaminophen late in pregnancy may affect the subsequent development of allergic symptoms in the child. Confirmation of these finding in larger cohorts could have substantial public health implications in defining factors attributable to the development of asthma.

Chapter 23

Bronchiectasis

What Is Bronchiectasis?

Bronchiectasis is a condition in which damage to the airways causes them to widen and become flabby and scarred. The airways are tubes that carry air in and out of your lungs.

Bronchiectasis usually is the result of an infection or other condition that injures the walls of your airways or prevents the airways from clearing mucus. Mucus is a slimy substance that the airways produce to help remove inhaled dust, bacteria, and other small particles.

In bronchiectasis, your airways slowly lose their ability to clear out mucus. When mucus cannot be cleared, it builds up and creates an environment in which bacteria can grow. This leads to repeated, serious lung infections. Each infection causes more damage to your airways. Over time, the airways lose their ability to move air in and out. This can prevent enough oxygen from reaching your vital organs.

Bronchiectasis can lead to serious health problems, such as respiratory failure, atelectasis, and heart failure.

This chapter includes text excerpted from "Bronchiectasis," National Heart, Lung, and Blood Institute (NHLBI), November 3, 2011. Reviewed August 2019.

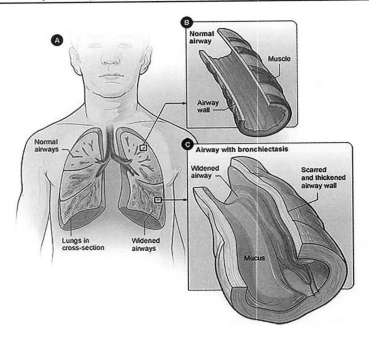

Figure 23.1. *Lungs with Normal Airways and Airway with Bronchiectasis*

Figure A shows a cross-section of the lungs with normal airways and with widened airways. Figure B shows a cross-section of a normal airway. Figure C shows a cross-section of an airway with bronchiectasis.

Other Names

- Acquired bronchiectasis
- Congenital bronchiectasis

Causes of Bronchiectasis

Damage to the walls of the airways usually is the cause of bronchiectasis. A lung infection may cause this damage. Examples of lung infections that can lead to bronchiectasis include:

- Severe pneumonia
- Whooping cough or measles (uncommon in the United States due to vaccination)
- Tuberculosis
- Fungal infections

Conditions that damage the airways and raise the risk of lung infections also can lead to bronchiectasis. Examples of such conditions include:

- **Cystic fibrosis.** This disease leads to almost half of the cases of bronchiectasis in the United States.

- **Immunodeficiency disorders**, such as common variable immunodeficiency and, less often, human immunodeficiency virus (HIV) and acquired immunodeficiency syndrome (AIDS)

- **Allergic bronchopulmonary aspergillosis.** This is an allergic reaction to a fungus called *"Aspergillus."* The reaction causes swelling in the airways.

- **Disorders that affect cilia function**, such as primary ciliary dyskinesia (PCD). Cilia are small, hair-like structures that line your airways. They help clear mucus (a slimy substance) out of your airways.

- **Chronic (ongoing) pulmonary aspiration.** This is a condition in which you inhale food, liquids, saliva, or vomited stomach contents into your lungs. Aspiration can inflame the airways, which can lead to bronchiectasis.

- **Connective tissue diseases**, such as rheumatoid arthritis (RA), Sjögren syndrome, and Crohn disease

Other conditions, such as an airway blockage, also can lead to bronchiectasis. Many things can cause a blockage, such as a growth or a noncancerous tumor. An inhaled object, such as a piece of a toy or a peanut, also can cause an airway blockage.

A problem with how the lungs form in a fetus may cause congenital bronchiectasis. This condition affects infants and children.

Risk Factors of Bronchiectasis

People who have conditions that damage the lungs or increase the risk of lung infections are at risk for bronchiectasis. Such conditions include:

- **Cystic fibrosis.** This disease leads to almost half of the cases of bronchiectasis in the United States.

- **Immunodeficiency disorders**, such as common variable immunodeficiency and, less often, human immunodeficiency virus (HIV) and acquired immunodeficiency syndrome (AIDS)

- **Allergic bronchopulmonary aspergillosis.** This is an allergic reaction to a fungus called "aspergillus." The reaction causes swelling in the airways.

- **Disorders that affect cilia function,** such as PCD. Cilia are small, hair-like structures that line your airways. They help clear mucus (a slimy substance) out of your airways.

Bronchiectasis can develop at any age. Overall, two-thirds of people who have the condition are women. However, in children, the condition is more common in boys than in girls.

Screening and Prevention of Bronchiectasis

To prevent bronchiectasis, it is important to prevent lung infections and lung damage that can cause it. Avoiding toxic fumes, gases, smoke, and other harmful substances also can help protect your lungs.

Childhood vaccines for measles and whooping cough prevent infections related to these illnesses. These vaccines also reduce complications from these infections, such as bronchiectasis. Proper treatment of lung infections in children also may help preserve lung function and prevent lung damage that can lead to bronchiectasis.

Stay alert to keep children (and adults) from inhaling small objects (such as pieces of toys and food that might stick in a small airway). If you think you, your child, or someone else has inhaled a small object, seek prompt medical care.

In some cases, treating the underlying cause of bronchiectasis can slow or prevent its progression.

Signs, Symptoms, and Complications of Bronchiectasis

The initial airway damage that leads to bronchiectasis often begins in childhood. However, signs and symptoms may not appear until months or even years after you start having repeated lung infections.

The most common signs and symptoms of bronchiectasis are:

- A daily cough that occurs over months or years

- Daily production of large amounts of sputum (spit). Sputum, which you cough up and spit out, may contain mucus (a slimy substance), trapped particles, and pus.

- Shortness of breath and wheezing (a whistling sound when you breathe)

- Chest pain

- Clubbing (the flesh under your fingernails and toenails gets thicker)

If your doctor listens to your lungs with a stethoscope, he or she may hear abnormal lung sounds.

Over time, you may have more serious symptoms. You may cough up blood or bloody mucus and feel very tired. Children may lose weight or not grow at a normal rate.

Complications of Bronchiectasis

Severe bronchiectasis can lead to other serious health conditions, such as respiratory failure and atelectasis.

Respiratory failure is a condition in which not enough oxygen passes from your lungs into your blood. The condition also can occur if your lungs cannot properly remove carbon dioxide (a waste gas) from your blood.

Respiratory failure can cause shortness of breath, rapid breathing, and air hunger (feeling like you cannot breathe in enough air). In severe cases, signs and symptoms may include a bluish color on your skin, lips, and fingernails; confusion; and sleepiness.

Atelectasis is a condition in which one or more areas of your lungs collapse or do not inflate properly. As a result, you may feel short of breath. Your heart rate and breathing rate may increase, and your skin and lips may turn blue.

If bronchiectasis is so advanced that it affects all parts of your airways, it may cause heart failure. Heart failure is a condition in which the heart cannot pump enough blood to meet the body's needs.

The most common signs and symptoms of heart failure are shortness of breath or trouble breathing, tiredness, and swelling in the ankles, feet, legs, abdomen, and veins in the neck.

Diagnosis of Bronchiectasis

Your doctor may suspect bronchiectasis if you have a daily cough that produces large amounts of sputum (spit).

To find out whether you have bronchiectasis, your doctor may recommend tests to:

- Identify any underlying causes that require treatment

- Rule out other causes of your symptoms

- Find out how much your airways are damaged

Diagnostic Tests and Procedures
Chest Computed Tomography Scan

A chest computed tomography scan, or chest CT scan, is the most common test for diagnosing bronchiectasis.

This painless test creates precise pictures of your airways and other structures in your chest. A chest CT scan can show the extent and location of lung damage. This test gives more detailed pictures than a standard chest x-ray.

Chest X-Ray

This painless test creates pictures of the structures in your chest, such as your heart and lungs. A chest x-ray can show areas of abnormal lung and thickened, irregular airway walls.

Other Tests

Your doctor may recommend other tests, such as:

- **Blood tests.** These tests can show whether you have an underlying condition that can lead to bronchiectasis. Blood tests also can show whether you have an infection or low levels of certain infection-fighting blood cells.

- **A sputum culture.** Lab tests can show whether a sample of your sputum contains bacteria (such as the bacteria that cause tuberculosis) or fungi.

- **Lung function tests.** These tests measure how much air you can breathe in and out, how fast you can breathe air out, and how well your lungs deliver oxygen to your blood. Lung function tests help show how much lung damage you have.

- A sweat test or other tests for cystic fibrosis.

Bronchoscopy

If your bronchiectasis does not respond to treatment, your doctor may recommend bronchoscopy. Doctors use this procedure to look inside the airways.

During bronchoscopy, a flexible tube with a light on the end is inserted through your nose or mouth into your airways. The tube is called a "bronchoscope." It provides a video image of your airways. You will be given medicine to numb your upper airway and help you relax during the procedure.

Bronchoscopy can show whether you have a blockage in your airways. The procedure also can show the source of any bleeding in your airways.

Treatment of Bronchiectasis

Bronchiectasis often is treated with medicines, hydration, and chest physical therapy (CPT). Your doctor may recommend surgery if the bronchiectasis is isolated to a section of lung or you have a lot of bleeding.

If the bronchiectasis is widespread and causing respiratory failure, your doctor may recommend oxygen therapy.

The goals of treatment are to:

- Treat any underlying conditions and lung infections.

- Remove mucus (a slimy substance) from your lungs. Maintaining good hydration helps with mucus removal.

- Prevent complications.

Early diagnosis and treatment of the underlying cause of bronchiectasis may help prevent further lung damage.

In addition, any disease associated with the bronchiectasis, such as cystic fibrosis or immunodeficiency, also should be treated.

Medicines

Your doctor may prescribe antibiotics, bronchodilators, expectorants, or mucus-thinning medicines to treat bronchiectasis.

Antibiotics

Antibiotics are the main treatment for the repeated lung infections that bronchiectasis causes. Oral antibiotics often are used to treat these infections.

For hard-to-treat infections, your doctor may prescribe intravenous (IV) antibiotics. These medicines are given through an IV line inserted into your arm. Your doctor may help you arrange for a home care provider to give you IV antibiotics at home.

Expectorants and Mucus-Thinning Medicines

Your doctor may prescribe expectorants and mucus thinners to help you cough up mucus.

Expectorants help loosen the mucus in your lungs. They often are combined with decongestants, which may provide extra relief. Mucus thinners, such as acetylcysteine, loosen the mucus to make it easier to cough up.

For some of these treatments, little information is available to show how well they work.

Hydration

Drinking plenty of fluids, especially water, helps prevent airway mucus from becoming thick and sticky. Good hydration helps keep airway mucus moist and slippery, which makes it easier to cough up.

Chest Physical Therapy

Chest physical therapy (CPT) also is called "physiotherapy" or "chest clapping" or "percussion." This technique is generally performed by a respiratory therapist but can be done by a trained member of the family. It involves the therapist pounding your chest and back over and over with his or her hands or a device. Doing this helps loosen mucus from your lungs so you can cough it up.

You can sit with your head tilted down or lie on your stomach with your head down while you do CPT. Gravity and force help drain the mucus from your lungs.

Some people find CPT hard or uncomfortable to do. Several devices can help with CPT, such as:

- An electric chest clapper, known as a "mechanical percussor."

- An inflatable therapy vest that uses high-frequency airwaves to force mucus toward your upper airways so you can cough it up.

- A small handheld device that you breathe out through. It causes vibrations that dislodge the mucus.

- A mask that creates vibrations to help break loose mucus from your airway walls.

Some of these methods and devices are popular with patients and doctors, but little information is available on how well they actually work. Choice is usually based on convenience and cost.

Several breathing techniques also are used to help move mucus to the upper airway so it can be coughed up. These techniques include forced expiration technique (FET) and active cycle breathing (ACB).

Forced expiration technique involves forcing out a couple of breaths and then doing relaxed breathing. ACB is FET that involves deep breathing exercises.

Other Treatments

Depending on your condition, your doctor may recommend bronchodilators, inhaled corticosteroids, oxygen therapy, or surgery.

Bronchodilators

Bronchodilators relax the muscles around your airways. This helps open your airways and makes breathing easier. Most bronchodilators are inhaled medicines. You will use an inhaler or a nebulizer to breathe in a fine mist of medicine.

Inhaled bronchodilators work quickly because the medicine goes straight to your lungs. Your doctor may recommend that you use a bronchodilator right before you do CPT.

Inhaled Corticosteroids

If you also have wheezing or asthma with your bronchiectasis, your doctor may prescribe inhaled corticosteroids (used to treat inflammation in the airways).

Oxygen Therapy

Oxygen therapy can help raise low blood oxygen levels. For this treatment, you will receive oxygen through nasal prongs or a mask. Oxygen therapy can be done at home, in a hospital, or in another health facility.

Surgery

Your doctor may recommend surgery if no other treatments have helped and only one part of your airway is affected. If you have major bleeding in your airway, your doctor may recommend surgery to remove part of your airway or a procedure to control the bleeding.

In very rare instances of severe bronchiectasis, your doctor may recommend that you receive a lung transplant replacing your diseased lungs with a healthy set of lungs.

Living with Bronchiectasis

Early diagnosis and treatment of bronchiectasis can prevent further damage to your lungs. People who have bronchiectasis should have ongoing care and try to follow a healthy lifestyle.

Ongoing Care

If you have bronchiectasis, work closely with your doctor to learn how to improve your quality of life. This involves learning as much as you can about bronchiectasis and any underlying conditions that you have.

Take steps to avoid lung infections. Ask your doctor about getting flu and pneumonia vaccines. Wash your hands often to lower your risk of getting viruses and bacterial infections.

Healthy Lifestyle

Following a healthy lifestyle is important for overall health and well-being. For example, if you smoke, try to quit. Smoking harms nearly every organ in your body, including your lungs.

Talk with your doctor about programs and products that can help you quit smoking. Also, try to avoid secondhand smoke.

If you have trouble quitting smoking on your own, consider joining a support group. Many hospitals, workplaces, and community groups offer classes to help people quit smoking.

You also can protect your airways by avoiding toxic fumes, gases, and other harmful substances.

A healthy lifestyle also involves following a healthy diet. A healthy diet includes a variety of vegetables and fruits. It also includes whole grains, fat-free or low-fat dairy products, and protein foods, such as lean meats, poultry without skin, seafood, processed soy products, nuts, seeds, beans, and peas.

A healthy diet is low in sodium (salt), added sugars, solid fats, and refined grains. Solid fats are saturated fat and trans-fatty acids. Refined grains come from processing whole grains, which results in a loss of nutrients (such as dietary fiber).

Staying hydrated is also important. Drinking plenty of fluids, especially water, helps prevent airway mucus from becoming thick and sticky.

Try to be as physically active as you can. Physical activity, such as walking and swimming, can help loosen mucus. Ask your doctor what types and amounts of activity are safe for you.

Emotional Support

People who have chronic lung diseases are more prone to depression, anxiety, and other emotional problems. Talk about how you feel with your healthcare team. Talking to a professional counselor also can help. If you are very depressed, your doctor may recommend medicines or other treatments that can improve your quality of life.

Joining a patient support group may help you adjust to living with bronchiectasis. You can see how other people who have the same symptoms have coped with them. Talk with your doctor about local support groups or check with an area medical center.

Support from family and friends also can help relieve stress and anxiety. Let your loved ones know how you feel and what they can do to help you.

Chapter 24

Chronic Obstructive Pulmonary Disease

Chapter Contents

Section 24.1

What Is Chronic Obstructive Pulmonary Disease?

This section includes text excerpted from "COPD," National Heart, Lung, and Blood Institute (NHLBI), June 25, 2019.

Chronic obstructive pulmonary disease (COPD); chronic bronchitis; or emphysema is a progressive disease that makes it hard to breathe. Progressive means the disease gets worse over time.

Chronic obstructive pulmonary disease can cause coughing that produces large amounts of a slimy substance called "mucus," wheezing, shortness of breath, chest tightness, and other symptoms.

Cigarette smoking is the leading cause of COPD. Most people who have COPD smoke or used to smoke. However, up to 25 percent of people with COPD never smoked. Long-term exposure to other lung irritants—such as air pollution, chemical fumes, or dusts—also may contribute to COPD. A rare genetic condition called "alpha-1 antitrypsin" (AAT) deficiency can also cause the disease

To understand COPD, it helps to understand how the lungs work. The air that you breathe goes down your windpipe into tubes in your lungs called "bronchial tubes" or "airways." Within the lungs, your bronchial tubes branch many times into thousands of smaller, thinner

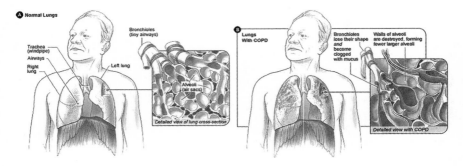

Figure 24.1. *Normal Lungs and Lungs with Chronic Obstructive Pulmonary Syndrome*

Figure A shows the location of the lungs and airways in the body. The inset image shows a detailed cross-section of the bronchioles and alveoli. Figure B shows lungs damaged by COPD. The inset image shows a detailed cross-section of the damaged bronchioles and alveolar walls.

tubes called "bronchioles." These tubes end in bunches of tiny round air sacs called "alveoli."

Small blood vessels called "capillaries" run along the walls of the air sacs. When air reaches the air sacs, oxygen passes through the air sac walls into the blood in the capillaries. At the same time, a waste product called "carbon dioxide" (CO_2) gas moves from the capillaries into the air sacs. This process, called "gas exchange," brings in oxygen for the body to use for vital functions and removes the CO_2.

The airways and air sacs are elastic or stretchy. When you breathe in, each air sac fills up with air, like a small balloon. When you breathe out, the air sacs deflate and the air goes out.

In COPD, less air flows in and out of the airways because of one or more of the following:

- The airways and air sacs lose their elastic quality.

- The walls between many of the air sacs are destroyed.

- The walls of the airways become thick and inflamed.

- The airways make more mucus than usual and can become clogged.

Most people who have COPD have both emphysema and chronic bronchitis, but the severity of each condition varies from person to person. Thus, the general term COPD is more accurate. Some well-known facts about COPD are:

- Chronic obstructive pulmonary disease is a major cause of disability, and it is the fourth leading cause of death in the United States. Over 16 million people are diagnosed with COPD. Many more people may have the disease and not even know it.

- Chronic obstructive pulmonary disease develops slowly. Symptoms often worsen over time and can limit your ability to do routine activities. Severe COPD may prevent you from doing even basic activities, such as walking, cooking, or taking care of yourself.

- Chronic obstructive pulmonary disease is diagnosed in middle-aged or older adults, most of the time. The disease is not contagious, meaning it cannot be passed from person to person.

- Chronic obstructive pulmonary disease has no cure yet, and doctors do not know how to reverse the damage to the lungs. However, treatments and lifestyle changes can help you feel better, stay more active, and slow the progress of the disease.

Causes of Chronic Obstructive Pulmonary Disease

Long-term exposure to lung irritants that damage the lungs and the airways usually is the cause of COPD. In the United States, the most common irritant that causes COPD is cigarette smoke. Pipe, cigar, and other types of tobacco smoke also can cause COPD, especially if the smoke is inhaled. Breathing in secondhand smoke, which is in the air from other people smoking; air pollution; or chemical fumes or dust from the environment or workplace also can contribute to COPD.

Rarely, a genetic condition called "alpha-1 antitrypsin" (AAT) deficiency may play a role in causing COPD. People who have this condition have low blood levels of AAT—a protein made in the liver. Having a low level of the AAT protein can lead to lung damage and COPD if you are exposed to smoke or other lung irritants. If you have AAT deficiency and also smoke, COPD can worsen very quickly.

Some people who have asthma can develop COPD. Asthma is a chronic lung disease that inflames and narrows the airways. Treatment usually can reverse the inflammation and narrowing that occurs in asthma.

Risk Factors of Chronic Obstructive Pulmonary Disease

The main risk factor for COPD is smoking. Up to 75 percent of people who have COPD smoke or used to smoke. People who have a family history of COPD are more likely to develop the disease if they smoke.

Long-term exposure to other lung irritants also is a risk factor for COPD. Examples of other lung irritants include air pollution, chemical fumes, and dust from the environment or workplace, and secondhand smoke, which is smoke in the air from other people smoking.

Most people who have COPD are at least 40 years old when symptoms begin. Although uncommon, people younger than 40 can have COPD. This may occur, for example, if a person has a predisposing health issue, such as the genetic condition known as "alpha-1 antitrypsin" (AAT) deficiency.

Screening and Prevention of Chronic Obstructive Pulmonary Disease

You can take steps to prevent COPD before it starts. If you already have COPD, you can take steps to prevent complications and slow the progression of the disease.

Prevent Chronic Obstructive Pulmonary Disease

Smoking is the leading cause of COPD. If you smoke, talk with your doctor about programs and products that can help you quit. If you have trouble quitting smoking on your own, consider joining a support group. Many hospitals, workplaces, and community groups offer classes to help people quit smoking. Ask your family members and friends to support you in your efforts to quit. Also, try to avoid lung irritants that can contribute to COPD, such as air pollution, chemical fumes, dust, and secondhand smoke, which is smoke in the air from other people smoking. For free help and support to quit smoking, you may call the National Cancer Institute's (NCI) Smoking Quitline at 877-448-7848.

Prevent Complications and Slow the Progression of Chronic Obstructive Pulmonary Disease

If you have COPD, the most important step you can take is to quit smoking. Quitting can help prevent complications and slow the progression of the disease. You also should avoid exposure to lung irritants such as air pollution, chemical fumes, dust, and secondhand smoke, which is smoke in the air from other people smoking.

Follow your treatments for COPD exactly as your doctor prescribes. They can help you breathe easier, stay more active, and avoid or manage severe symptoms. Talk with your doctor about whether and when you should get the flu, or influenza, and pneumonia vaccines. These vaccines can lower your chances of getting these illnesses, which are major health risks for people who have COPD.

Signs, Symptoms, and Complications of Chronic Obstructive Pulmonary Disease

At first, COPD may cause no symptoms or only mild symptoms. As the disease gets worse, symptoms usually become more severe. Common signs and symptoms of COPD include:

- An ongoing cough or a cough that produces a lot of mucus; this is often called "smoker's cough"

- Shortness of breath, especially with physical activity

- Wheezing or a whistling or squeaky sound when you breathe

- Chest tightness

If you have COPD, you may often have colds or other respiratory infections such as the flu, or influenza. Not everyone who has the symptoms described above has COPD. Likewise, not everyone who has COPD has these symptoms. Some of the symptoms of COPD are similar to the symptoms of other diseases and conditions. Your doctor can determine if you have COPD.

If your symptoms are mild, you may not notice them, or you may adjust your lifestyle to make breathing easier. For example, you may take the elevator instead of the stairs.

Over time, symptoms may become severe enough to cause you to see a doctor. For example, you may become short of breath during physical exertion. The severity of your symptoms will depend on how much lung damage you have. If you keep smoking, the damage will occur faster than if you stop smoking. Severe COPD can cause other symptoms, such as swelling in your ankles, feet, or legs; weight loss; and lower muscle endurance.

Some severe symptoms may require treatment in a hospital. You—or, if you are unable, family members or friends—should seek emergency care if you are experiencing the following:

- You are having a hard time catching your breath or talking.

- Your lips or fingernails turn blue or gray, a sign of a low oxygen level in your blood.

- People around you notice that you are not mentally alert.

- Your heartbeat is very fast.

- The recommended treatment for symptoms that are getting worse is not working.

Diagnosis of Chronic Obstructive Pulmonary Disease

Your doctor will diagnose COPD based on your signs and symptoms, your medical and family histories, and test results. Your doctor may ask whether you smoke or have had contact with lung irritants, such as secondhand smoke, air pollution, chemical fumes, or dust. If you have an ongoing cough, let your doctor know how long you have had it, how much you cough, and how much mucus comes up when you cough. Also, let your doctor know whether you have a family history of COPD. Your doctor will examine you and use a stethoscope to listen for wheezing or other abnormal chest sounds. He or she also may recommend one or more tests to diagnose COPD.

Pulmonary Function Tests

Pulmonary function tests measure how much air you can breathe in and out, how fast you can breathe air out, and how well your lungs deliver oxygen to your blood. The main test for COPD is spirometry. Other lung function tests, such as a lung diffusion capacity test, also might be used.

Spirometry

During this painless test, the technician will ask you to take a deep breath in. Then, you will blow as hard as you can into a tube connected to a small machine. The machine is called a "spirometer." The machine measures how much air you breathe out. It also measures how fast you can blow air out. The patient takes a deep breath and blows as hard as possible into a tube connected to a spirometer. The spirometer measures the amount of air breathed out. It also measures how fast the air was blown out. Your doctor may have you inhale, or breathe in, medicine that helps open your airways and then blow into the tube again. He or she can then compare your test results before and after taking the medicine. Spirometry can detect COPD before symptoms develop. Your doctor also might use the test results to find out how severe your COPD is and to help set your treatment goals. The test results also may help find out whether another condition, such as asthma or heart failure, is causing your symptoms.

Other Tests

Your doctor may recommend other tests, such as:

- **A chest x-ray or chest CT scan.** These tests create pictures of the structures inside your chest, such as your heart, lungs, and blood vessels. The pictures can show signs of COPD. They also may show whether another condition, such as heart failure, is causing your symptoms.

- **An arterial blood gas test.** This blood test measures the oxygen level in your blood using a sample of blood taken from an artery. The results from this test can show how severe your COPD is and whether you need oxygen therapy.

Treatment of Chronic Obstructive Pulmonary Disease

Chronic obstructive pulmonary disease has no cure yet. However, lifestyle changes and treatments can help you feel better, stay more active, and slow the progress of the disease.

The goals of COPD treatment include:

- Relieving your symptoms

- Slowing the progress of the disease

- Improving your exercise tolerance or your ability to stay active

- Preventing and treating complications

- Improving your overall health

To assist with your treatment, your family doctor may advise you to see a pulmonologist. This is a doctor who specializes in treating lung disorders.

Lifestyle Changes
Quit Smoking and Avoid Lung Irritants

Quitting smoking is the most important step you can take to treat COPD. Talk with your doctor about programs and products that can help you quit. If you have trouble quitting smoking on your own, consider joining a support group. Many hospitals, workplaces, and community groups offer classes to help people quit smoking. Ask your family members and friends to support you in your efforts to quit. Also, try to avoid secondhand smoke and places with dust, fumes, or other toxic substances that you may inhale.

Other Lifestyle Changes

If you have COPD, especially more severe forms, you may have trouble eating enough because of symptoms such as shortness of breath and fatigue. As a result, you may not get all of the calories and nutrients you need, which can worsen your symptoms and raise your risk for infections. Talk with your doctor about following an eating plan that will meet your nutritional needs. Your doctor may suggest eating smaller, more frequent meals; resting before eating; and taking vitamins or nutritional supplements. Also, talk with your doctor about what types of activity are safe for you. You may find it hard to remain active with your symptoms. However, physical activity can strengthen the muscles that help you breathe and improve your overall wellness.

Medicines
Bronchodilators

Bronchodilators relax the muscles around your airways. This helps open your airways and makes breathing easier. Depending on the severity of your COPD, your doctor may prescribe short-acting or long-acting bronchodilators. Short-acting bronchodilators last about 4 to 6 hours and should be used only when needed. Long-acting bronchodilators last about 12 hours or more and are used every day. Most bronchodilators are taken using a device called an "inhaler." This device allows the medicine to go straight to your lungs. Not all inhalers are used the same way. Ask your healthcare providers to show you the correct way to use your inhaler.

If your COPD is mild, your doctor may only prescribe a short-acting inhaled bronchodilator. In this case, you may use the medicine only when symptoms occur. If your COPD is moderate or severe, your doctor may prescribe regular treatment with short- and long-acting bronchodilators.

Combination Bronchodilators Plus Inhaled Glucocorticosteroids (Steroids)

In general, using inhaled steroids alone is not a preferred treatment. If your COPD is more severe, or if your symptoms flare up often, your doctor may prescribe a combination of medicines that includes a bronchodilator and an inhaled steroid. Steroids help reduce airway inflammation. Your doctor may ask you to try inhaled steroids with the bronchodilator for a trial period of six weeks to three months to see whether the addition of the steroid helps relieve your breathing problems.

Vaccines
Flu Shots

The flu, or influenza, can cause serious problems for people who have COPD. Flu shots can reduce your risk of getting the flu. Talk with your doctor about getting a yearly flu shot.

Pneumococcal Vaccine

This vaccine lowers your risk for pneumococcal pneumonia and its complications. People who have COPD are at higher risk for pneumonia than people who do not have COPD. Talk with your doctor about whether you should get this vaccine.

Pulmonary Rehabilitation

Pulmonary rehabilitation or rehab is a broad program that helps improve the well-being of people who have chronic breathing problems. Rehab may include an exercise program, disease management training, and nutritional and psychological counseling. The program's goal is to help you stay active and carry out your daily activities. Your rehab team may include doctors, nurses, physical therapists, respiratory therapists, exercise specialists, and dietitians. These health professionals will create a program that meets your needs.

Oxygen Therapy

If you have severe COPD and low levels of oxygen in your blood, oxygen therapy can help you breathe better. For this treatment, oxygen is delivered through nasal prongs or a mask.

You may need extra oxygen all the time or only at certain times. For some people who have severe COPD, using extra oxygen for most of the day can help them:

- Do tasks or activities while experiencing fewer symptoms

- Protect their hearts and other organs from damage

- Sleep more during the night and improve alertness during the day

- Live longer

Surgery

Surgery may benefit some people who have COPD. Surgery usually is a last resort for people who have severe symptoms that have not improved from taking medicines. Surgeries for people who have COPD that is mainly related to emphysema include bullectomy and lung volume reduction surgery (LVRS). A lung transplant might be an option for people who have very severe COPD.

Bullectomy

When the walls of the air sacs are destroyed, larger air spaces called "bullae" form. These air spaces can become so large that they interfere with breathing. In a bullectomy, doctors remove one or more very large bullae from the lungs.

Lung Volume Reduction Surgery

In LVRS, surgeons remove damaged tissue from the lungs. This helps the lungs work better. In carefully selected patients, LVRS can improve breathing and quality of life.

Lung Transplant

During a lung transplant, doctors remove your damaged lung and replace it with a healthy lung from a donor. A lung transplant can improve your lung function and quality of life. However, lung transplants have many risks, such as infections and rejection of the transplanted lung.

If you have very severe COPD, talk with your doctor about whether a lung transplant is an option. Ask your doctor about the benefits and risks of this type of surgery.

Managing Complications

Chronic obstructive pulmonary disease symptoms usually worsen slowly over time. However, they can worsen suddenly. For instance, a cold, flu, or lung infection may cause your symptoms to quickly worsen. You may have a much harder time catching your breath. You also may have chest tightness, coughing, changes in the color or amount of your sputum or spit, and a fever. Call your doctor right away if your symptoms worsen suddenly. He or she may prescribe antibiotics to treat the infection, along with other medicines, such as bronchodilators and inhaled steroids, to help you breathe. Some severe symptoms may require treatment in a hospital.

Section 24.2

What Is Alpha-1 Antitrypsin Deficiency?

This section includes text excerpted from
"Alpha-1 Antitrypsin Deficiency," National Heart, Lung,
and Blood Institute (NHLBI), November 15, 2013.
Reviewed August 2019.

Alpha-1 antitrypsin (AAT) deficiency, is a condition that raises your risk for lung disease (especially if you smoke) and other diseases. Some people who have severe AAT deficiency develop emphysema—often when they are only in their forties or fifties. Emphysema is a serious lung disease in which damage to the airways makes it hard to breathe. A small number of people who have AAT deficiency develop cirrhosis and other serious liver diseases. Cirrhosis is a disease in which the liver becomes scarred. The scarring prevents the organ from working well. In people who have AAT deficiency, cirrhosis and other liver diseases usually occur in infancy and early childhood. A very small number of people who have AAT deficiency have a rare skin disease called "necrotizing panniculitis." This disease can cause painful lumps under or on the surface of the skin. This section focuses on AAT deficiency as it relates to lung disease. Some well-known facts about alpha-1 antitrypsin deficiency are:

- People who have AAT deficiency may not have serious complications, and they may live close to a normal lifespan.

- Among people with AAT deficiency who have a related lung or liver disease, about 3 percent die each year.

- Smoking is the leading risk factor for life-threatening lung disease if you have AAT deficiency. Smoking or exposure to tobacco smoke increases the risk of earlier lung-related symptoms and lung damage. If you have severe AAT deficiency, smoking can shorten your life by as much as 20 years.

- AAT deficiency has no cure, but treatments are available. Treatments often are based on the type of disease you develop.

Causes of Alpha-1 Antitrypsin Deficiency

Alpha-1 antitrypsin deficiency is an inherited disease. "Inherited" means it is passed from parents to children through genes. Children who have AAT deficiency inherit two faulty *AAT* genes, one from each parent. These genes tell cells in the body how to make AAT proteins.

In AAT deficiency, the AAT proteins made in the liver are not the right shape. Thus, they get stuck in the liver cells. The proteins cannot get to the organs in the body that they protect, such as the lungs. Without the AAT proteins protecting the organs, diseases can develop. The most common faulty gene that can cause AAT deficiency is called *"PiZ."* If you inherit two *PiZ* genes (one from each parent), you will have AAT deficiency. If you inherit a *PiZ* gene from one parent and a normal *AAT* gene from the other parent, you will not have AAT deficiency. However, you might pass the *PiZ* gene to your children. Even if you inherit two faulty *AAT* genes, you may not have any related complications. You may never even realize that you have AAT deficiency.

Risk Factors of Alpha-1 Antitrypsin Deficiency

Alpha-1 antitrypsin deficiency occurs in all ethnic groups. However, the condition occurs most often in White people of European descent. AAT deficiency is an inherited condition. "Inherited" means the condition is passed from parents to children through genes. If you have bloodline relatives with known AAT deficiency, you are at increased risk for the condition. Even so, it does not mean that you will develop one of the diseases related to the condition. Some risk factors make it more likely that you will develop lung disease if you have AAT deficiency. Smoking is the leading risk factor for serious lung disease if you have AAT deficiency. Your risk for lung disease also may go up if you are exposed to dust, fumes, or other toxic substances.

Screening and Prevention of Alpha-1 Antitrypsin Deficiency

You cannot prevent AAT deficiency because the condition is inherited (passed from parents to children through genes). If you inherit two faulty *AAT* genes, you will have AAT deficiency. Even so, you may never develop one of the diseases related to the condition. You can take steps to prevent or delay lung diseases related to AAT deficiency. One important step is to quit smoking. If you do not smoke, do not start. Talk with your doctor about programs and products that can help you quit smoking. If you have trouble quitting smoking on your own, consider joining a support group. Many hospitals, workplaces, and community groups offer classes to help people quit smoking. Also, try to avoid secondhand smoke and places with dust, fumes, or other toxic substances that you may inhale. Check your living and working spaces for things that may irritate your lungs. Examples include flower and tree pollen, ash, allergens, air pollution, wood-burning stoves, paint fumes, and fumes from cleaning products and other household items.

If you have a lung disease related to AAT deficiency, ask your doctor whether you might benefit from augmentation therapy. This is a treatment in which you receive infusions of AAT protein. Augmentation therapy raises the level of AAT protein in your blood and lungs.

Signs, Symptoms, and Complications of Alpha-1 Antitrypsin Deficiency

The first lung-related symptoms of AAT deficiency may include shortness of breath, less ability to be physically active, and wheezing. These signs and symptoms most often begin between the ages of 20 and 40. Other signs and symptoms may include repeated lung infections, tiredness, a rapid heartbeat upon standing, vision problems, and weight loss. Some people who have severe AAT deficiency develop emphysema—often when they are only in their forties or fifties. Signs and symptoms of emphysema include problems breathing, wheezing, and a chronic (ongoing) cough. At first, many people who have AAT deficiency are diagnosed with asthma. This is because wheezing also is a symptom of asthma. Also, people who have AAT deficiency respond well to asthma medicines.

Diagnosis of Alpha-1 Antitrypsin Deficiency

Alpha-1 antitrypsin deficiency usually is diagnosed after you develop a lung or liver disease that is related to the condition. Your doctor may suspect AAT deficiency if you have signs or symptoms of a serious lung condition, especially emphysema, without any obvious cause. He or she also may suspect AAT deficiency if you develop emphysema when you are 45 years old or younger.

Specialists Involved

Many doctors may be involved in the diagnosis of AAT deficiency. These include primary care doctors, pulmonologists (lung specialists), and hepatologists (liver specialists). To diagnose AAT deficiency, your doctor will:

- Ask about possible risk factors. Risk factors include smoking and exposure to dust, fumes, and other toxic substances.

- Ask about your medical history. A common sign of AAT deficiency is if you have a lung or liver disease without any obvious causes or risk factors. Another sign is if you have emphysema at an unusually early age (45 years or younger).

- Ask about your family's medical history. If you have bloodline relatives who have AAT deficiency, you are more likely to have the condition.

Diagnostic Tests

Your doctor may recommend tests to confirm a diagnosis of AAT deficiency. He or she also may recommend tests to check for lung- or liver-related conditions. A genetic test is the most certain way to check for AAT deficiency. This test will show whether you have faulty AAT genes. A blood test also may be used. This test checks the level of AAT protein in your blood. If the level is a lot lower than normal, it is likely that you have AAT deficiency.

Lung-Related Tests

If you have a lung disease related to AAT deficiency, your doctor may recommend lung function tests and high-resolution computed tomography scanning, also called "CT scanning." Lung function tests measure how much air you can breathe in and out, how fast you can breathe air out, and how well your lungs deliver oxygen to your blood. These tests may show how severe your lung disease is and how well treatment is working. High-resolution CT scanning uses x-rays to create detailed pictures of parts of the body. A CT scan can show whether you have emphysema or any other lung disease and how severe it is.

Treatment of Alpha-1 Antitrypsin Deficiency

Alpha-1 antitrypsin deficiency has no cure, but its related lung diseases have many treatments. Most of these treatments are the same as the ones used for a lung disease called "chronic obstructive pulmonary disease" (COPD). If you have symptoms related to AAT deficiency, your doctor may recommend:

- **Inhaled bronchodilators and inhaled steroids.** These medicines help open your airways and make breathing easier. They also are used to treat asthma and COPD.

- **Flu and pneumococcal vaccines** to protect you from illnesses that could make your condition worse. Prompt treatment of lung infections also can help protect your lungs.

- **Pulmonary rehabilitation (rehab).** Rehab involves treatment by a team of experts at a special clinic. In rehab, you will learn how to manage your condition and function at your best.

- **Extra oxygen**, if needed

- **A lung transplant.** A lung transplant may be an option if you have severe breathing problems. If you have a good chance of surviving the transplant surgery, you may be a candidate for it.

- **Augmentation therapy** is a treatment used only for people who have AAT-related lung diseases. This therapy involves getting infusions of the AAT protein. The infusions raise the level of the protein in your blood and lungs. Not enough research has been done to show how well this therapy works. However, some research suggests that this therapy may slow the development of AAT deficiency in people who do not have severe disease. People who have AAT deficiency and develop related liver or skin diseases will be referred to doctors who treat those diseases.

Future Treatments

Researchers are working on possible treatments that will target the faulty *AAT* genes and replace them with healthy genes. These treatments are in the early stages of development. Researchers also are studying therapies that will help misshapen AAT proteins move from the liver into the bloodstream. They are also studying a type of augmentation therapy in which the AAT protein is inhaled instead of injected into a vein.

Living with Alpha-1 Antitrypsin Deficiency

People who have AAT deficiency do not always develop serious lung or liver diseases. This means that you can have AAT deficiency and not even know it. If you already know you have AAT deficiency, you probably also have a related lung or liver disease. Ongoing medical care and lifestyle changes can help you manage your health.

Ongoing Medical Care

If you have AAT deficiency, you will need ongoing medical care. Talk with your doctor about how often you should schedule medical visits. Take all of your medicines as prescribed, and follow your treatment plan. Get flu and pneumococcal vaccines to protect you from illnesses that may worsen your condition. If you have a lung infection, get treatment right away. You also should get treatment right away for any breathing problems. If treatment includes pulmonary rehabilitation, work with your healthcare team to learn how to manage your condition and function at your best.

Lifestyle Changes
Quit Smoking and Avoid Lung Irritants

If you smoke, quit. If you do not smoke, do not start. Smoking is the leading risk factor for life-threatening lung disease if you have AAT deficiency.

Talk with your doctor about programs and products that can help you quit smoking. If you have trouble quitting smoking on your own, consider joining a support group. Many hospitals, workplaces, and community groups offer classes to help people quit smoking.

Also, try to avoid secondhand smoke and other lung irritants, such as dust, fumes, or toxins. Check your living and working spaces for things that may irritate your lungs. Examples include flower and tree pollen, ash, allergens, air pollution, wood-burning stoves, paint fumes, and fumes from cleaning products and other household items. Because AAT deficiency is inherited, your children may have the condition or carry the gene for it. Advise them to avoid smoking and to stay away from places where they might inhale irritants or toxins.

Follow a Healthy Diet

A healthy diet is an important part of a healthy lifestyle. A healthy diet includes a variety of vegetables and fruits. It also includes whole grains, fat-free or low-fat dairy products, and protein foods, such as lean meats, poultry without skin, seafood, processed soy products, nuts, seeds, beans, and peas.

A healthy diet is low in sodium (salt), added sugars, solid fats, and refined grains. Solid fats are saturated fat and trans fatty acids. Refined grains come from processing whole grains, which results in a loss of nutrients (such as dietary fiber). Also, talk with your doctor about whether it is safe for you to drink alcohol.

291

Be Physically Active

Try to do physical activity regularly. Talk with your doctor about how much and what types of activity are safe for you.

Reduce Stress

Learning how to manage stress, relax, and cope with problems can improve your emotional and physical health. Relaxation techniques—such as meditation, yoga, breathing exercises, and muscle relaxation—can help you cope with stress.

Emotional Issues and Support

Living with AAT deficiency may cause fear, anxiety, depression, and stress. Talk about how you feel with your healthcare team. Talking to a professional counselor also can help. If you are very depressed, your doctor may recommend medicines or other treatments that can improve your quality of life.

Joining a patient support group may help you adjust to living with AAT deficiency. You can see how other people who have the same symptoms have coped with them. Talk with your doctor about local support groups or check with an area medical center.

Support from family and friends also can help relieve stress and anxiety. Let your loved ones know how you feel and what they can do to help you.

Chapter 25

Idiopathic Pulmonary Fibrosis

What Is Idiopathic Pulmonary Fibrosis?

Idiopathic pulmonary fibrosis (IPF) is a serious chronic disease that affects the tissue surrounding the air sacs, or alveoli, in your lungs. This condition occurs when that lung tissue becomes thick and stiff for unknown reasons. Over time, these changes can cause permanent scarring in the lungs, called "fibrosis," that make it progressively more difficult to breathe.

Your risk for IPF is higher if you smoke or have a family history of IPF, and the risk increases with age. The most common symptoms of IPF are shortness of breath and cough. Some people may not have symptoms at first, but signs and symptoms can develop and get worse as the disease progresses.

The way IPF advances varies from person to person, and scarring may happen slowly or quickly. In some people, the disease stays the same for years. In other people, the condition rapidly declines. Many people with IPF also experience what are known as "acute exacerbations," where symptoms suddenly become much more severe. Other complications of IPF include pulmonary hypertension (PH) and respiratory failure, which happens when the lungs cannot deliver enough

This chapter includes text excerpted from "Idiopathic Pulmonary Fibrosis," National Heart, Lung, and Blood Institute (NHLBI), May 13, 2015. Reviewed August 2019.

oxygen into the bloodstream without support. This prevents the brain and other organs from getting the oxygen they need.

There is currently no cure for IPF. However, certain medicines may slow the progression of IPF, which may extend the lifespan and improve the quality of life (QOL) for people who have the disease.

Causes of Idiopathic Pulmonary Fibrosis

Idiopathic pulmonary fibrosis is a type of interstitial lung disease. It is caused by lung tissue becoming thick and stiff and eventually forming scar tissue within the lungs. The scarring, or fibrosis, seems to result from a cycle of damage and healing that occurs in the lungs. Over time, the healing process stops working correctly and scar tissue forms. What causes these changes in the first place is unknown.

To understand IPF it helps to understand how the lungs work. In IPF, the scarring makes it difficult to breathe and deliver oxygen from

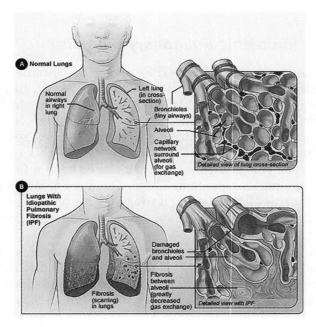

Figure 25.1. *Normal Lungs and Lungs with Idiopathic Pulmonary Fibrosis*

Figure A shows the location of the lungs and airways in the body. The inset image shows a detailed view of the lung's airways and air sacs in cross-section. Figure B shows fibrosis (scarring) in the lungs. The inset image shows a detailed view of the fibrosis and how it damages the airways and air sacs.

the lungs to the rest of the body. In healthy lungs, oxygen passes easily through the walls of the air sacs, called "alveoli," into your capillaries and bloodstream. However, in IPF, the scarring makes the walls of the alveoli thicker. The thickened walls of the alveoli make it harder for oxygen to pass into the blood.

Risk Factors of Idiopathic Pulmonary Fibrosis

You may have an increased risk for IPF because of your age, family history, and genetics, lifestyle habits, or your sex.

Age

The risk of developing IPF increases as you age and usually occurs in people older than 50. IPF is diagnosed most often in people who are in their 60s or 70s.

Family History and Genetics

Your risk for IPF is higher if a first-degree relative, such as a parent or sibling, has IPF. The specific genes you inherit may make you more likely to develop IPF, especially if those genes contain certain changes or mutations. To date, mutations in more than 10 different genes have been linked to an increased risk for IPF.

Your genes can put you at risk for IPF in a few ways.

Lifestyle Habits

Smoking is a common risk factor among people who have Idiopathic pulmonary fibrosis.

Sex

Idiopathic pulmonary fibrosis is more common among men than women.

Screening and Prevention of Idiopathic Pulmonary Fibrosis

There are no screening methods to determine who may develop IPF. If you have certain risk factors, especially a family history of IPF, your doctor may recommend you have a pulmonary function test or an imaging test, such as a high-resolution chest computed tomography (CT) scan, to look for scarring in the lungs.

Signs, Symptoms, and Complications of Idiopathic Pulmonary Fibrosis

The signs and symptoms of IPF develop over time. Symptoms may be different between people and may develop slowly or quickly.

Signs and Symptoms

The most common signs and symptoms are:

- **Shortness of breath** that gets worse over time. At first, you may be short of breath only during exercise. Over time, you may feel breathless even at rest.
- **A dry cough that gets worse.** You may have repeated bouts of coughing that you cannot control.

Other signs and symptoms may include:

- **Aching muscles and joints**
- **Clubbing,** which is a widening and rounding of the tips of the fingers or toes
- **Fatigue**
- **Gradual, unintended weight loss**
- **Generally feeling unwell**
- **Rapid, shallow breathing**

Complications

Complications of IPF may include the following:

- Depression and anxiety
- Lung cancer
- Pulmonary hypertension
- Respiratory failure
- Sleep problems or disorders

Diagnosis for Idiopathic Pulmonary Fibrosis

Your doctor will diagnose IPF based on your symptoms, your medical and family history, your risk factors, and the results from tests and procedures. Idiopathic means that your doctors cannot determine a cause of your disease at the time of diagnosis. They will rule out other medical reasons or conditions that may be causing your symptoms before diagnosing you with IPF. This may be done by doing other tests and talking to specialists.

Medical History and Physical Exam

To help determine whether you have IPF and rule out other possible causes of lung problems, your doctor may ask about your medical history and possible risk factors.

Your doctor may look for signs of IPF during a physical exam, such as:

- Blue hands and feet from not enough oxygen in the blood

- Clubbing of the fingers or toes

- High-pitched crackles when listening to your lungs

Diagnostic Tests and Procedures

To diagnose IPF, your doctor may have you undergo some of the following tests and procedures.

- **High-resolution chest CT scan,** or HRCT, to take pictures of the inside of your lungs and look for scarring or inflammation. CT scans can also help distinguish between types of lung diseases. For IPF, doctors look for a pattern where the lungs look similar to a honeycomb.

- **Lung biopsy** to see if your lung tissue shows signs of inflammation, scarring, or other changes. This procedure is sometimes used to verify the diagnosis of IPF. It usually is done by thoracoscopic surgery, in which small incisions are made and a small camera is used to direct surgical instruments.

- **Chest x-ray** to take pictures of the lungs and look for evidence of inflammation or damage, such as scarring. An x-ray does not provide as much detail as a high-resolution CT scan.

Tests for Other Medical Conditions

Your doctor may perform some tests and procedures to help rule out other conditions that may cause lung disorders, including the following:

- **Blood tests,** such as an antibody test to look for signs of an autoimmune disease that can cause lung scarring.

- **Bronchoalveolar lavage (BAL)** to look at the types of cells in your lung fluid. Sometimes it may be used when the types of cells can help distinguish between IPF and other lung diseases.

- **Pulmonary function tests** to see if you show signs of reduced breathing capacity or abnormal blood oxygen levels. These tests help assess the severity of your lung disease, and they can help monitor whether your condition is stable or worsening over time.

- **Genetic testing,** if you have a family history of interstitial lung disease or signs of early aging.

Treatment of Idiopathic Pulmonary Fibrosis

There is currently no cure for IPF. Your doctor may recommend medicines, pulmonary rehabilitation, procedures, or other treatments to slow the progression of IPF and help improve your QOL.

Medicines

Your doctor may recommend the following medicines:

- **Kinase inhibitors,** such as Nintedanib or Pirfenidone, to help slow the decline in lung function from IPF. They may also help to prevent an acute exacerbation, which is an unexpected and sudden worsening of symptoms over a period of days or weeks and may prolong survival.

- **Antacids** to help treat gastroesophageal reflux disease (GERD). Treating GERD may help prevent acid from getting into the lungs from reflux, making IPF worse.

Other Treatments

Your doctor may recommend other treatments to treat IPF, including:

- **Oxygen therapy** to decrease shortness of breath and improve the ability to exercise.

- **Ventilator** support to help with breathing.

Surgery

A lung transplant may be an option for some people who have advanced IPF. The major complications of a lung transplant are infection and rejection of the new organ by the body. You will have to take medicines for the rest of your life to reduce the risk of rejection following a lung transplant.

Chapter 26

Interstitial Lung Disease

Interstitial lung disease (ILD) describes a large group of disorders associated with progressive scarring of the lung tissue. The tissue between the air sacs in the lung is called the "interstitium." This is the area most affected by the scarring. Since the scarring is also caused by fibrosis, interstitial lung disease may also be called "pulmonary fibrosis."*

Pulmonary fibrosis is a condition in which the tissue deep in your lungs becomes scarred over time. This tissue gets thick and stiff. That makes it hard for you to catch your breath, and your blood may not get enough oxygen. Causes of pulmonary fibrosis include environmental pollutants, some medicines, some connective tissue diseases, and interstitial lung disease.

The scarring associated with interstitial lung disease may progress to where it affects the ability to breathe and get enough oxygen into the bloodstream.

What Causes Interstitial Lung Disease

Interstitial lung disease can be caused by many things. Long-term exposure to hazardous materials, such as asbestos can cause interstitial lung disease. Some types of autoimmune diseases, such as

---

This chapter includes text excerpted from "Interstitial Lung Disease," U.S. Department of Veterans Affairs (VA), September 16, 2015. Reviewed August 2019.

rheumatoid arthritis can be associated with interstitial lung disease. In most cases, the causes remain unknown.

In ILD, the lung becomes damaged and the walls between the air sacs become inflamed and scarring results. Once lung scarring occurs, it is generally irreversible.

What Are the Symptoms of Interstitial Lung Disease?

Individual symptoms may vary, but the most common symptoms include:

- Shortness of breath—especially with exercise

- Fatigue

- Dry cough

- Weight loss

What Can a Patient Do to Help with Interstitial Lung Disease?

Identifying and determining the cause of interstitial lung disease can be very challenging. Specific treatments by your doctor will be based on the suspected etiology of the ILD, your age, the extent of disease and your personal preferences.

Being actively involved in the treatment discussions with the doctor is very important. Also staying as healthy as possible is important, including:

- Do not smoke. And avoid having people smoke around you.

- Eat well.

- Make sure you get your annual flu vaccination and discuss with your doctor if you should receive the pneumonia vaccine.

- Stay active.

Chapter 27

Occupational Lung Disorders

Chapter Contents

Section 27.1

Asbestos-Related Disease

This section includes text excerpted from "Asbestos Toxicity," Agency for Toxic Substances and Disease Registry (ATSDR), Centers for Disease Control and Prevention (CDC), August 9, 2016.

According to the American Thoracic Society, "asbestos has been the largest cause of occupational cancer in the United States and a significant cause of disease and disability from nonmalignant disease." It has been estimated that the cumulative total number of asbestos-associated deaths in the United States may exceed 200,000 by the year 2030.

Depending on the level and duration of exposure, inhalation of asbestos fibers can cause different diseases, such as:

* Asbestosis

* Asbestos-related pleural abnormalities

* Lung and laryngeal carcinoma

* Malignant mesothelioma of the pleura or peritoneum

Any combination of these diseases can be present in a single patient. Clinically, it is important to distinguish nonmalignant conditions from malignant diseases; differential diagnosis will be discussed further in later sections of this document.

Asbestosis

Asbestosis is a diffuse interstitial fibrosis of lung tissue resulting from inhalation of asbestos fibers. Asbestos fibers inhaled deep into the lung become lodged in the tissue, eventually resulting in diffuse alveolar and interstitial fibrosis. The fibrosis usually first occurs in the respiratory bronchioles, particularly in the subpleural portions of the lower lobes. The fibrosis can progress to include the alveolar walls. Fibrosis tends to progress even after exposure ceases. This fibrosis can lead to:

* Reduced lung volumes

* Decreased lung compliance

* Impaired gas exchange

- Restrictive pattern of impairment
- Obstructive features due to small airways disease
- Progressive exertional dyspnea with an insidious onset

Asbestosis is characterized by the following radiographic changes: fine, irregular opacities in both lung fields (especially in the bases) and septal lines that progress to honeycombing and sometimes, in more severe disease, obscuration of the heart border and hemidiaphragm—the so-called shaggy heart sign. Radiographic changes depend on the:

- Duration
- Frequency
- Intensity of exposure

Patients with asbestosis may have elevated levels of antinuclear antibody and rheumatoid factors and a progressive decrease in total lymphocyte count with advancing fibrosis.

Asbestosis has no unique pathognomonic signs or symptoms, but the diagnosis is made by the constellation of clinical, functional, and radiographic findings as outlined by the American Thoracic Society. These criteria include:

- Sufficient history of exposure to asbestos
- The appearance of disease with a consistent time interval from first exposure
- Clinical picture, such as the insidious onset of dyspnea on exertion, bibasilar end-inspiratory crackles not cleared by coughing
- Functional tests showing restrictive (occasionally obstructive) pattern with reduced diffusing capacity (DLco)
- Characteristic radiographic appearance
- Exclusion of other causes of interstitial fibrosis or obstructive disease, such as usual interstitial pneumonia, connective tissue disease, drug-related fibrosis

The table below describes the natural history associated with asbestosis.

Table 27.1. Natural History of Asbestosis

Parameter	Typical Findings
Sufficient exposures	Usually associated with high-level occupational exposures
Latency periods	Radiographic changes: commonly less than 20 years Clinical manifestations: commonly 20 to 40 years Asbestosis appears earliest in those with the highest exposure levels.
Risk of asbestosis	Asbestosis develops in around 50% of adults with occupational asbestos exposure.
Co-morbid conditions	Increased risk for asbestos-related lung cancer and mesothelioma, though both can occur without asbestos
Mortality and morbidity	Severe asbestosis may lead to respiratory failure over 1 to 2 decades. Many patients with asbestosis die of other causes such as asbestos-associated lung cancer (38%), mesothelioma (9%), and other causes (32%)

Asbestos-Related Pleural Abnormalities

Asbestos-related pleural abnormalities encompass four types of pleural changes.

- Pleural plaques

- Nonmalignant asbestos pleural effusions

- Diffuse pleural thickening

- Rounded atelectasis (folded lung)

The pleura are more sensitive to asbestos than the lung parenchyma, so the effects of asbestos exposure show here first and occur at much lower doses than the fibrotic changes in the lung.

Pleural plaques are well-circumscribed areas of thickening, usually located bilaterally on the parietal pleura. They are usually asymptomatic, though they can cause small reductions in lung function. On rare occasions (less than 1%), pleural plaques can cause pleuritic pain requiring medical pain management. Pleural plaques are the most common manifestations of asbestos exposure; by occupation, the highest rate (58%) has been reported in insulation workers. The presence of pleural plaques in the general environmentally exposed population in developed societies is in the range of 0.5 percent to 8 percent. Indeed, they are considered a biomarker of asbestos exposure, depending more on length from first exposure, than on cumulative exposure. Pleural plaques can also form following exposure to:

- Ceramic fibers
- Talc
- Silicates
- Erionite, a rare zeolite

Nonmalignant asbestos pleural effusions are small and often bloody unilateral effusions. These effusions are among the earliest manifestations of asbestos exposure; they can occur within 10 years of exposure. They are usually asymptomatic. Rarely, they can cause pain, fever, and dyspnea. These effusions typically last for months, and may occasionally recur. Their presence can precede the occurrence of diffuse pleural thickening.

Diffuse pleural thickening is a noncircumscribed fibrous thickening of the visceral pleura with areas of adherence to the parietal pleura and obliteration of the pleural space. It can be associated with more extensive asbestos exposure than pleural plaque. In fact, diffuse pleural thickening has been reported in 10% of patients with asbestosis. Diffuse pleural thickening can occur after nonmalignant pleural effusions. The fibrotic areas are ill-defined, involving costophrenic angles, apices, lung bases, and interlobar fissures. Diffuse pleural thickening can be associated with mild (or, rarely, moderate to severe) restrictive pulmonary function deficits, such as decreased ventilatory capacity. When this occurs, the patient may experience progressive dyspnea and chest pain.

Rounded atelectasis (or folded lung) occurs when portions of lung tissue are caught in bands of fibrous pleural tissue with in-drawing of the bronchi and vessels. This produces a distinctive radiographic appearance: a rounded pleural mass with bands of lung tissue radiating outwards. This condition is usually asymptomatic, though some patients develop dyspnea or dry cough. The course is usually stable or slowly progressive. Folded lung is the least common asbestos-related nonmalignant pleural disease; it is not only associated with asbestosis exposure but can occur following other exposures and medical conditions. However, asbestos exposure is the leading cause of rounded atelectasis, accounting for 29 percent to 86 percent of cases. It can rarely also co-occur with lung cancer.

The differential causes of rounded atelectasis includes:

- Exposure to mineral dusts, such as asbestos, and occupational exposures to silica and mixed mineral dusts

307

- Exudative pleural effusions, such as:
  - Empyema
  - Tuberculous effusions
  - Hemothorax
  - Postcardiac surgery
  - Chronic hemodialysis
- Other medical conditions, such as:
  - Legionella pneumonia
  - Histoplasmosis
  - End-stage renal disease
  - Pneumothorax
  - Childhood cancer

Table 27.2 shows typical findings and natural history associated with asbestos-related nonmalignant pleural abnormalities.

Lung Carcinoma

Most lung cancers are associated with exposure to tobacco smoke. According to the 2004 Surgeon General Report on smoking, men with a lifetime of smoking have a 16 percent higher risk of dying from lung cancer than those who do not smoke. Lung cancer currently accounts for 28 percent of all cancer deaths in the United States.

Exposure to asbestos is associated with all major histological types of lung carcinoma (adenocarcinoma, squamous cell carcinoma, and small-cell carcinoma). It is estimated that 4 percent to 12 percent of lung cancers are related to occupational levels of exposure to asbestos. It is estimated that 20 percent to 25 percent of heavily exposed asbestos workers will develop bronchogenic carcinomas. Whether asbestos exposure will lead to lung cancer depends on several factors:

- Level, duration, and frequency of asbestos exposure (cumulative exposure)
- Time elapsed since exposure occurred
- Age when exposure occurred
- History of tobacco use
- Individual susceptibility factors not yet determined

Table 27.2. Natural History and Findings of Asbestos-Related Pleural Abnormalities

Parameter	Pleural Plaques	Pleural Effusions	Diffuse Pleural Thickening	Rounded Atelectasis
Typical Exposures	Can occur with short low-level exposures or high-level occupational exposures		Usually associated with moderate to high level exposures. Less specific for asbestos exposure than pleural plaques	May occur with occupational and environmental exposures. Has other causes besides asbestos exposure.
Average Latency Periods	20 to 30 years	10 years	15 years	N/A
Co-morbid Conditions	Since the presence of these plaques is an indicator of asbestos exposure, there is an increased incidence of asbestos-related diseases associated with them.	Other asbestos-related diseases.	Other asbestos-related diseases. Can follow nonmalignant pleural effusions.	Follows nonmalignant pleural effusions; can co-exist with other asbestos-related diseases or its other causes
Mortality and Morbidity	Not fatal/usually asymptomatic; incidental finding	Not fatal. Clinical presentation ranges from asymptomatic to pleuritic chest pain and fever.	Not fatal. If severe, can cause dyspnea. Usually no significant functional impairment unless very extensive.	Not fatal. Usually asymptomatic; if severe, chest pain, dyspnea, and cough. Usually no functional impairment unless accompanied by other asbestos-related disease.

Most asbestos-related lung cancers reflect the dual influence of asbestos exposure and smoking. It has been known for over 25 years, that smoking and asbestos exposure have a multiplicative effect on the risk of lung cancer. The presence of asbestosis is an indicator of high-level asbestos exposure, but lung cancer can occur without asbestosis.

One of the best known sets of criteria to guide the clinician regarding whether asbestos contributed to lung cancer in an asbestos-exposed individual is the Helsinki criteria. For these criteria, some of the markers for attributing asbestos exposure as a contributing factor to lung cancer are

- The presence of asbestosis—serves as marker for significant exposures to asbestos

- Estimated cumulative exposure to asbestos of at least 25 fiber-years (if known)

- By history, at least 1 year of heavy occupational exposure or 5 to 10 years of moderate exposure

- Lag time of at least 10 years since first exposure

Table 27.3 shows typical findings associated with lung carcinoma.

Table 27.3. Findings Associated with Lung Carcinoma

Parameter	Typical Findings
Typical exposures	Large cumulative exposure (short-term, high-level exposures or long-term, moderate-level exposures)
Latency periods	20 to 30 years
Clinical presentation	Only 5 percent to 15 percent of patients are asymptomatic when diagnosed. Most present with cough, hemoptysis, wheeze, dyspnea.
Co-morbid conditions	Asbestosis, other asbestos-related diseases. Paraneoplastic syndromes associated with lung cancer.
Mortality	Same as lung carcinoma with other causes – 14% five-year survival rate

Pleural Mesothelioma

Diffuse malignant mesothelioma is a tumor arising from the thin serosal membrane of the body cavities:

- Pleura

- Peritoneum

- Pericardium

- Tunica vaginalis testis

- Outer surface of ovaries

It is a rare neoplasm, accounting for less than 5 percent of pleural malignancies. There are three histological types of malignant mesothelioma:

- Epithelial

- Mixed

- Sarcomatous

Of malignant mesotheliomas, 80 percent affect the pleura, and 20 percent affect the peritoneum. A 2003 report of mesothelioma incidence in Australia reported pleural mesotheliomas at 93.2 percent, peritoneal mesotheliomas at 6.5 percent and mesotheliomas of other rare sites at 0.3 percent. Peritoneal mesothelioma is discussed in the next section.

In most cases of pleural mesothelioma, the tumor is rapidly invasive locally. Patients with malignant pleural mesothelioma can have a sudden onset of pleural effusion and/or pleural thickening, dyspnea, and chest pain. By the time symptoms appear, the disease is most often rapidly fatal.

Pleural mesothelioma is a signal tumor for asbestos exposure; other causes are uncommon. The risk of mesothelioma depends on the amount of asbestos exposure. All types of asbestos can cause mesothelioma, but some researchers believe that the amphibole form is more likely to induce mesothelioma than the serpentine form.

In 2007, about 2,700 people in the United States died of mesothelioma. According to the National Cancer Institute's (NCI) Surveillance Epidemiology and End Results (SEER) data, there was an increase in the incidence of mesothelioma in the United States from the early 1970s to the mid-1990s, as the disease developed in people exposed during peak asbestos exposure years (1940 to 1970). Mesothelioma incidence has probably started to decline in the United States, although it may still be increasing in Europe and Australia because of more abundant and prolonged use of asbestos in these countries than in the United States.

Table 27.4 shows few typical findings associated with pleural mesothelioma.

Table 27.4. Findings Associated with Pleural Mesothelioma

Parameter	Typical Findings
Typical exposures	Short-term, high-level exposures or chronic low-level exposures, especially to amphibole asbestos; incidence increases in dose-related manner
Latency periods	10 to 57 years (30 to 40 years typical)
Clinical presentation	Frequently presents with chest pain accompanied by pleural mass or pleural effusion on chest radiograph
Mortality	High. The typical 1-year survival rate is less than 30%. Median survival time is 8 to 14 months after diagnosis.

Section 27.2

Silica-Related Disease

This section includes text excerpted from "Protect Yourself Silicosis," Occupational Safety and Health Administration (OSHA), September 22, 2005. Reviewed August 2019.

Silicosis is caused by exposure to respirable crystalline silica dust. Crystalline silica is a basic component of soil, sand, granite, and most other types of rock, and it is used as an abrasive blasting agent. Silicosis is a progressive, disabling, and often fatal lung disease. Cigarette smoking adds to the lung damage caused by silica.

Effects of Silicosis

- **Lung cancer.** Silica has been classified as a human lung carcinogen.

- **Bronchitis/chronic obstructive pulmonary disorder (COPD)**

- **Tuberculosis (TB).** Silicosis makes an individual more susceptible to TB.

- **Scleroderma,** a disease affecting skin, blood vessels, joints, and skeletal muscles

- **Possible renal disease**

Symptoms of Silicosis

- Shortness of breath; possible fever
- Fatigue; loss of appetite
- Chest pain; dry, nonproductive cough
- Respiratory failure, which may eventually lead to death

Sources of Exposure

- Sandblasting for surface preparation
- Crushing and drilling rock and concrete
- Masonry and concrete work (e.g., building and road construction and repair)
- Mining/tunneling; demolition work
- Cement and asphalt pavement manufacturing

Preventing Silicosis

- Use all available engineering controls, such as blasting cabinets and local exhaust ventilation. Avoid using compressed air for cleaning surfaces
- Use water sprays, wet methods for cutting, chipping, drilling, sawing, grinding, etc.
- Substitute noncrystalline silica blasting material
- Use respirators approved for protection against silica; if sandblasting, use abrasive blasting respirators
- Do not eat, drink, or smoke near crystalline silica dust
- Wash hands and face before eating, drinking, or smoking away from exposure area

Section 27.3

Work-Related Asthma

This section includes text excerpted from "Work-Related Asthma," Centers for Disease Control and Prevention (CDC), May 11, 2017.

Work-related asthma is asthma triggered by an exposure at work. Many asthma triggers can be found in the workplace. Over 300 known or suspected substances in the workplace can cause or worsen asthma. Avoiding triggers can prevent asthma from getting worse.

Worsening asthma or new onset asthma in a worker should raise questions about workplace causes. Asthma symptoms can develop shortly after exposure, or they can develop months or years after repeated exposures to harmful substances.

What Causes Work-Related Asthma

Work-related asthma is associated with exposure to worksite irritants, allergens, and physical conditions called "triggers." Some examples of asthma triggers are:

- Animal dander and insects

- Chlorine-based cleaning products

- Cigarette smoke

- Cockroach droppings

- Cold air

- Dust from wood, grain, flour, or green coffee beans

- Dust mites

- Gases such as ozone

- Indoor dampness and mold

- Irritant chemicals

- Metal dust

- Physical exertion

- Pollen and plants

- Strong fumes

- Vapors from chemicals (e.g., ammonia, isocyanates, and solvents)

- Wood smoke

What Are the Symptoms of Work-Related Asthma?
How Do I Know If I Have Work-Related Asthma?

Symptoms for work-related asthma tend to get better on weekends, vacations, or other times when away from work. However, in some cases, symptoms do not improve until an extended time away from the exposure or trigger.

Work-related asthma can be diagnosed by your doctor. Tell your doctor about work exposures and possible asthma triggers, including your job, tasks, and the materials you use. Also consider logging when and where your symptoms occur to help determine any patterns. Your doctor will ask you questions about your symptoms and will conduct a physical examination. The doctor might also order one or more of the following tests:

- Breathing tests (e.g., peak flow readings and spirometry)

- Allergy tests, such as skin or blood tests

If your doctor is concerned about something other than asthma, she or he might order other tests, such as x-rays or imaging tests.

Symptoms

The symptoms of work-related asthma are the same as symptoms for nonwork-related asthma. They include:

- Wheezing

- Coughing

- Chest tightness

- Shortness of breath

Asthma symptoms can come and go, and some workers might not have all symptoms. Workers can get work-related asthma even when using personal protective equipment such as respirators or face masks. Sometimes, these breathing problems start at work and continue even after the worker leaves work and exposure has stopped.

How Is Work-Related Asthma Treated?

The most important step of treating asthma is stopping or reducing exposure to asthma triggers causing symptoms. You should work with your doctor to develop a personal asthma control plan. Asthma is often treated with two general types of medicine:

- **Quick-relief rescue inhalers** (e.g., albuterol, levalbuterol) to open the airways. People use these medicines to treat asthma attacks or flare-ups.

- **Long-term control medicines** to reduce inflammation in the airways. People use these medicines to help keep asthma symptoms from occurring. When these medicines are working well, quick relief medicine is not used as much.

How Are Work-Related Asthma Exposures Identified and Prevented?

The following guidelines can help employers and employees develop and maintain a worksite safe from asthma triggers. Minimizing exposure to work-related asthma triggers can help employees to be healthier.

Employers

The hierarchy of controls is an approach that groups actions by their likely effectiveness in removing or reducing hazards. The preferred approach includes the following:

- Eliminate or substitute hazardous processes or materials. When developing a project, take necessary precautions to prevent potentially harmful exposures and reduce the need for additional controls in the future.

- Install engineering controls to reduce exposure or shield employees. For example, isolate or enclose processes, and install local exhaust ventilation to capture exposures at the source.

- Implement administrative controls, such as work practices or policies that reduce or prevent hazardous exposures.

- Train workers on potential workplace hazards, what precautions they should take to protect themselves, and workplace policies for reporting their concerns.

- Establish a no-smoking policy in the workplace. Tobacco smoke is a trigger for some people with asthma.

Some employers might want to consider establishing a medical surveillance plan to monitor for asthma through questionnaires and routine lung function testing (spirometry). A surveillance plan might identify workers with asthma at earlier stages of disease, when workers are more responsive to treatment.

Personal protective equipment (PPE) might also be needed. PPE is the least effective means of controlling hazardous exposures and should not be the sole method for controlling hazardous exposures. Rather, PPE should be used until effective engineering and administrative controls are in place. Proper use of PPE requires a comprehensive program and a high level of employee involvement and commitment. Additionally, the right personal protective equipment must be chosen for each hazard.

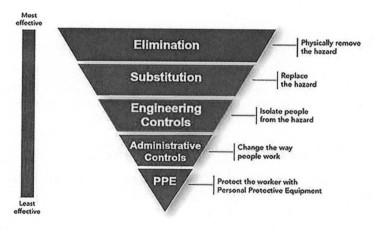

Figure 27.1. *Hierarchy of Controls*

Employees

Employees should be attentive to their work environment, especially those with breathing problems. Follow the steps below if you feel you have work-related asthma symptoms:

- Identify and avoid exposure to asthma triggers.

- Participate in your employer's asthma surveillance plan, if available.

- Report new or worsening breathing problems to your doctor and the designated person at your workplace.

- Immediately report if personal protective equipment or engineering controls malfunction to your supervisor.

- If you have asthma, take your medications as prescribed and regularly see your doctor.

- Get a flu shot every year.

- If you smoke, talk to your doctor or employer about resources to help you quit smoking.

Section 27.4

Chronic Beryllium Disease

This section includes text excerpted from "Beryllium Disease," Genetic and Rare Diseases Information Center (GARD), National Center for Advancing Translational Sciences (NCATS), October 20, 2014. Reviewed August 2019.

What Is Chronic Beryllium Disease?

Chronic beryllium disease (CBD) is a granulomatous, interstitial lung disease that occurs in individuals who develop beryllium sensitization (BeS), a cell-mediated immune response to environmental and occupational beryllium exposure. BeS precedes the lung disease that may present with chronic dry cough, fatigue, weight loss, chest pain, and increasing dyspnea.

Epidemiology

The number of workers exposed to beryllium has been estimated at 1 million in the United States, although no accurate figure exists for the United States or globally. The prevalence of sensitization in those exposed ranges from 1 to 20 percent. CBD among those with BeS ranges from 15 to 100 percent.

Clinical Description

Patients with CBD can range from those who are asymptomatic to those with severe lung dysfunction. Manifestations occur a few months to a many years after exposure to beryllium and include chronic dry cough, dyspnea on exertion, chest pain, fatigue, fever, night sweats, and weight loss. Additional extrapulmonary manifestations of dermatitis and skin granulomas have been reported. Progressive pulmonary fibrosis can eventually lead to cor pulmonale and respiratory failure. An increased risk of lung cancer among workers exposed to high levels of beryllium has also been observed.

Etiology

Chronic beryllium disease is caused by occupational exposure to beryllium and beryllium-containing alloys (usually by inhalation of dust or fumes but also via contact with skin). Over time, in a subset of individuals, a cell-mediated immune response to beryllium may occur, causing the development of sensitized T cells that accumulate within the lungs and eventually form granulomas which can lead to fibrosis. A genetic variant in the HLA-DPB1 gene (6p21.3) with the presence of a glutamic acid at amino acid position 69 has been associated with the development of BeS and CBD.

Diagnostic Methods

Diagnosis is based on a history of exposure to beryllium, characteristic clinical findings and laboratory testing. BeS can be detected with the beryllium lymphocyte proliferation test (BeLPT) where mononuclear cells from peripheral blood or bronchoalveolar lavage are exposed to beryllium in vitro. Increased proliferation of lymphocytes compared to control cells indicates BeS. Granulomatous and/or mononuclear cell infiltrates in lung tissue, are indicative of CBD. Chest x-ray, CT scan of the lungs, exercise tolerance testing and pulmonary function tests can also aid in the diagnosis.

Differential Diagnosis

The main differential diagnoses are sarcoidosis (most common) and tuberculosis as well as other occupational lung diseases (i.e., silicosis).

Management and Treatment of Chronic Beryllium Disease

There is no cure for CBD. Treatment involves cessation of beryllium exposure and use of corticosteroids (prednisone). The early symptomatic disease may be treated with inhaled corticosteroids along with a short-acting bronchodilator. Methotrexate and other immunosuppressive therapies can reduce steroid side effects. The efficacy of corticosteroids may be limited and relapses can occur after cessation of therapy or when dose is lowered. Those with advanced disease and major breathing difficulties may require oxygen supplementation. In severe cases, a lung transplant may be suggested. Patients should refrain from smoking. CBD may be prevented by providing exposed workers with respiratory protective devices and protective clothing and by minimizing exposure through use of workplace administration and engineering controls. The BeLPT is used to identify patients early on and to define workplace areas for modification in order to ultimately reduce additional BeS and CBD cases.

Prognosis of Chronic Beryllium Disease

Prognosis varies, with some patients remaining clinically stable for many years and some experiencing a gradual worsening of symptoms over time. A debilitating course resulting in respiratory failure is also possible but regular monitoring and treatment can slow down the disease process.

Section 27.5

Byssinosis

"Byssinosis," © 2019 Omnigraphics.
Reviewed August 2019.

Byssinosis is caused by occupational exposure to dust that affects the lungs. The condition is said to occur when dust particles from cotton and hemp obstruct the small air tubes in the lungs and cause the disorder. Other names for byssinosis are "Monday fever," "brown lung disease," "mill fever," or "cotton workers' lung."

Symptoms of Byssinosis

Symptoms of byssinosis generally begin at the start of the work week and grow worse by the end of the week as exposure to the dust particles increases. As exposure to the dust particles increases, one might experience symptoms during the entire week. Symptoms include asthma, chronic obstructive lung disease, tightness in the chest, wheezing, and coughing. Severe cases include flu-like symptoms, such as:

- Fever
- Muscle and joint pain
- Shivering
- Tiredness
- Dry cough

Causes and Risk Factors of Byssinosis

Industry workers are the most affected by byssinosis. Inhalation of raw flax, hemp, and cotton dust causes this disease. Smoking, a history of asthma, and allergies increase the risk of developing byssinosis.

Diagnosing Byssinosis

Your doctor might inquire about your recent activities and work environment to determine if you have been exposed to textile dust. The doctor will perform a physical examination followed by a chest x-ray and a computed tomography (CT) scan to check the lungs. Lung health is often checked using pulmonary function tests.

A peak flow meter is given to the patient to test the lungs throughout the workweek. This meter detects how quick air is expelled from the lungs. If there is a change in breathing during a week or a day, it will help the doctor determine where and when one is getting exposed to cotton dust.

Treating Byssinosis

Bronchodilators are prescribed to relieve mild-to-moderate symptoms and help to open constricted airways.

Inhaled corticosteroids may be prescribed for severe cases. These drugs help in reducing lung inflammation. However, they also cause fungal infections in the mouth and throat that can be reduced by rinsing the mouth after inhalation. Supplemental oxygen therapy might be needed for patients with low blood oxygen levels. A nebulizer or any other respiratory treatment might be recommended for chronic byssinosis. Certain physical activities and breathing exercises help to improve lung health. As hemp, cotton, and flax dust can cause irreversible damage to your lungs over a period of years, you might require a change of occupation.

Recovering from Byssinosis

The foremost treatment for byssinosis is avoiding inhalation of and exposure to textile particle dust. A treatment plan can be created with the help of a primary doctor, a lung specialist, and an occupational medical expert.

Finding Support

Managing byssinosis can be easy with the assistance of pulmonologists. The correct use of inhaled medicines can be learned from a respiratory therapist or nurse. Some patients may require oxygen for serious and permanent lung damage.

Preventing Byssinosis

Byssinosis is not a chronic or life-threatening disease, and can be prevented by wearing a mask while you work near dust. According to the guidelines created by the Occupational Safety and Health Administration (OSHA), U.S. industries have a legal obligation to protect their employees from dangerous products at work. The employer should provide protective gear to every employee.

Prognosis of Byssinosis

As far as byssinosis is considered, it is not a terminal or chronic disease, because the person who is affected gets better when exposure to the dust decreases. However, it is important to know the cause of the disease in order to prevent it from recurring after treatment.

Questions for Your Doctor about Byssinosis

Ask your doctor to answer the following questions so that you can better manage byssinosis.

- Is the diagnosis confirmed?

- Are there symptoms of any other disease such as asthma or chronic obstructive pulmonary disease?

- Should the occupational exposure be completely avoided?

- How should one monitor her or his lung function?

- How frequently should the prescribed medicines be used?

When to Contact a Medical Professional

The following list provides a list of times when you should call a medical professional:

- You have the symptoms of byssinosis.

- You suspect that you have breathing problems because of dust particles of cotton, hemp, or fiber.

- You have symptoms of pneumonia.

- You develop a cough, shortness of breath, fever, or other signs of a lung infection or think you have the flu.

References

1. Wint, Carmella, and Boskey, Elizabeth. "Byssinosis: Brown Lungs and What You Need to Know about Them," Healthline, February 23, 2016.

2. "Byssinosis," MedlinePlus, A.D.A.M. Encylopedia, July 17, 2019.

3. "Byssinosis," American Lung Association, December 11, 2015.

4. "Byssinosis," Chest Foundation, January 2018.

Section 27.6

Hypersensitivity Pneumonitis (Hot Tub Lung)

This section includes text excerpted from "Hypersensitivity Pneumonitis," National Heart, Lung, and Blood Institute (NHLBI), June 12, 2017.

Also known as "extrinsic allergic alveolitis," "bird fancier's lung," "farmer's lung," "hot tub lung," "humidifier lung."

Hypersensitivity pneumonitis is a rare immune system disorder that affects the lungs. It occurs in some people after they breathe in certain substances they encounter in the environment. These substances trigger their immune systems, causing short- or long-term inflammation, especially in a part of the lungs called the "interstitium." This inflammation makes it harder for the lungs to function properly and may even permanently damage the lungs. If diagnosed, some types of hypersensitivity pneumonitis are treatable by avoiding exposure to the environmental substances or with medicines such as cortico-steroids that reduce inflammation. If the condition goes untreated or is not well controlled over time, the chronic inflammation can cause irreversible scarring of the lungs that may severely impair their ability to function.

Causes of Hypersensitivity Pneumonitis

Hypersensitivity pneumonitis is caused by repeated exposure to environmental substances that cause inflammation in the lungs when inhaled. These substances include certain:

- Bacteria and mycobacteria

- Fungi or molds

- Proteins

- Chemicals

Where Can These Substances Be Found in the Environment?

Common environmental sources of substances that can cause hyper-sensitivity pneumonitis are:

- Animal furs
- Air conditioner, humidifier, and ventilation systems
- Bird droppings and feathers
- Contaminated foods such as cheese, grapes, barley, sugarcane
- Contaminated industry products or materials such as sausage casings and corks
- Contaminated metalworking fluid
- Hardwood dusts
- Hay or grain animal feed
- Hot tubs

Because this condition is caused by different substances found in many environmental sources, doctors once thought they were treating different lung diseases. Research has helped understand hypersensitivity pneumonitis is triggered by different causative substances.

Why Does Hypersensitivity Pneumonitis Only Occur in Some People?

If you have hypersensitivity pneumonitis, your body's immune system reacts strongly to certain substances. Differences in our immune systems may explain why some people have strong reactions after breathing in certain substances, while others who breathe those same substances do not.

Risk Factors of Hypersensitivity Pneumonitis

Certain factors affect your risk of developing hypersensitivity pneumonitis. These factors include age, environment or occupation, family history and genetics, lifestyle habits, other medical conditions, and sex or gender.

Age

Although hypersensitivity pneumonitis can occur at any age, people tend to be diagnosed with this condition between 50 and 55 years of age. Hypersensitivity pneumonitis is a common type of chronic interstitial lung disease in children.

Environment or Occupation

Repeated exposure to certain substances that cause the condition, possibly while working in occupations where environmental sources are common, can increase your risk of developing hypersensitivity pneumonitis. Certain occupations—such as farmers or people who breed animals or birds, cheese washers, woodworkers, and wine makers—have a greater chance of exposure to causative substances. However, you may be exposed to environmental sources in your home or elsewhere. Even having pets such as birds in the home can increase your risk of hypersensitivity pneumonitis.

Alone, environmental exposure to causative substances is not enough to cause hypersensitivity pneumonitis. An estimated 85 to 95 percent of people exposed to causative substances either never develop hypersensitivity pneumonitis or they experience a mild immune reaction with no obvious signs or symptoms or disease.

Family History and Genetics

Genetics is thought to predispose some people to have strong immune responses and develop hypersensitivity pneumonitis after repeat exposures to a causative substance. In some populations, family history of pulmonary fibrosis or hypersensitivity pneumonitis may increase the risk of developing hypersensitivity pneumonitis. When hypersensitivity pneumonitis occurs in relatives it is called "familial hypersensitivity pneumonitis."

Researchers are beginning to map genetic variations in immune system proteins that may increase the risk for developing hypersensitivity pneumonitis. These differences may explain why immune cells respond differently between people who do or do not develop hypersensitivity pneumonitis after the same exposure to a causative substance.

Lifestyle Habits

Smoking is not thought to increase the risk of developing hypersensitivity pneumonitis. However, smoking can worsen chronic hypersensitivity pneumonitis and cause complications. If you have hypersensitivity pneumonitis, learn why doctors recommend quitting smoking.

Other Medical Conditions

Some viral infections later in life may increase the risk of developing hypersensitivity pneumonitis.

Sex or Gender

Men and women can have hypersensitivity pneumonitis. Some small studies found this condition to be slightly more common in women.

Screening and Prevention of Hypersensitivity Pneumonitis

As of now there are no screening methods to determine who will or will not develop hypersensitivity pneumonitis. you avoid common environmental sources of substances known to cause this condition. If you are at risk for hypersensitivity pneumonitis, your doctor may recommend you avoid common environmental sources of substances known to cause this condition.

Signs and symptoms vary between acute, subacute, and chronic types of hypersensitivity pneumonitis. If your condition is not diagnosed or well controlled by treatment, it can lead to irreversible lung damage and other potentially fatal complications.

Signs and Symptoms

Figure 27.2 shows the common signs and symptoms of acute, subacute, and chronic hypersensitivity pneumonitis.

Type of Hypersensitivity Pneumonitis	Signs and Symptoms								
	Flu-like Illness (fever, chills, muscle or joint pain, headache)	Rales	Cough	Chronic Bronchitis	Shortness of Breath	Anorexia or Weight Loss	Fatigue	Lung Fibrosis	Clubbing of Fingers or Toes
Acute	✓	✓	✓						
Subacute		✓	✓	✓	✓	✓			
Chronic			✓	✓	✓	✓	✓	✓	✓

Figure 27.2. *Common Signs and Symptoms of Acute, Subacute, and Chronic Hypersensitivity Pneumonitis*

Signs and symptoms of acute, subacute, and chronic hypersensitivity pneumonitis may include flu-like illness including fever, chills, muscle or joint pain, or headaches; rales; cough; chronic bronchitis; shortness of breath; anorexia or weight loss; fatigue; fibrosis of the lungs; and clubbing of fingers or toes.

While some signs and symptoms occur in several types of hypersensitivity pneumonitis, they may vary in severity. The exact signs and symptoms you experience also may vary.

Complications

Hypersensitivity pneumonitis may cause the following potentially fatal complications if the condition is not diagnosed or well controlled by treatment. Irreversible lung damage and permanently reduced lung function because of severe fibrosis and impaired ability to oxygenate the blood during normal breathing. Pulmonary hypertension due to damage of blood vessels in the lungs.

Heart failure because inflammation makes it harder for the heart to pump blood to and through the lungs.

Diagnosis of Hypersensitivity Pneumonitis

To diagnose hypersensitivity pneumonitis, your doctor will collect your medical history to understand your symptoms and see if you have an exposure history to possible causative substances. Your doctor will perform a physical exam and may order diagnostic tests and procedures. Based on this information, your doctor may able to determine whether you have acute, subacute, or chronic hypersensitivity pneumonitis.

Diagnostic Tests and Procedures

To diagnose hypersensitivity pneumonitis, your doctor may order:

- **Blood tests** to detect high levels of white blood cells and other immune cells and factors in your blood that indicate your immune system is activated and causing inflammation somewhere in your body.

- **Bronchoalveolar lavage (BAL)** to collect fluid from your lungs that can be tested for high levels of white blood cells and other immune cells. High levels of these cells mean your body is making an immune response in your lungs, but low levels do not rule out hypersensitivity pneumonitis.

- **Computed tomography (CT)** to image the lungs and look for inflammation or damage such as fibrosis. CT scans, particularly high-resolution ones, can help distinguish between types of hypersensitivity pneumonitis.

- **Inhalation challenge tests** to see if a controlled exposure to a suspected causative substance triggers your immune system and the onset of common signs and symptoms such as an increase in temperature, increase in white blood cell levels, rales that are heard during a physical exam, or reduced lung function. A positive test can confirm an inhaled substance triggers your immune system. A negative test does not rule out that you have hypersensitivity pneumonitis, because it may mean a different untested environmental substance is causing your condition. Before having this test, talk to your doctor about the benefits and possible risks of this procedure.

- **Lung biopsies** to see if your lung tissue shows signs of inflammation, fibrosis, or other changes known to occur in hypersensitivity pneumonitis.

- **Lung function tests** to see if you show signs of restriction such as reduced breathing capacity or abnormal blood oxygen levels and check if you have obstructed airways. These tests help assess the severity of your lung disease and when repeated they can help monitor whether your condition is stable or worsening over time. Lung function tests may be normal between acute flares.

- **Precipitin tests** to see if you have antibodies in your blood that recognize and bind to a causative substance. While a positive test means that you have been exposed to a substance, it cannot confirm you have hypersensitivity pneumonitis. This is because some people without this condition also have antibodies in their blood to these substances. If you have antibodies to a substance, your doctor may have you perform an inhalation challenge test to see if a new exposure to the same substance can activate your immune system and cause a new acute flare.

- **Chest x-rays** to image the lungs and look for inflammation or damage such as fibrosis in your lungs.

Treatment of Hypersensitivity Pneumonitis

Treatments for hypersensitivity pneumonitis usually include avoidance strategies and medicines. Occasionally, lung transplants are used to treat severe chronic disease in some patients.

Avoidance Strategies

If your doctor is able to identify the environmental substance that causes your hypersensitivity pneumonitis, he or she will recommend that you adopt the following avoidance strategies.

- Remove the causative substance if possible

- Replace workplace or other products with available alternatives that do not contain the substance responsible for your condition

- Alter work processes so you do not continue to breathe in the causative substance

- Stay away from known sources of your causative substance

Medicines

If avoidance strategies do not work for your condition, your doctor may prescribe corticosteroids or other immunosuppressive medicines to treat your condition. The choice, dose, and duration of these medicines will depend on your condition and medical history. Acute and subacute types of hypersensitivity pneumonitis usually respond well to these treatments.

Depending on your condition, your doctor also may prescribe some of the following supportive therapies.

- Oxygen therapy as needed for low levels of oxygen in the blood.

- Bronchodilators to relax the muscles in the airways and open your airways to make breathing easier.

- Opioids to control shortness of breath or chronic cough that is resistant to other treatments. Regular (e.g. several times a day, for several weeks or more) or longer use of opioids can lead to physical dependence and possibly addiction.

Lung Transplants

If your condition is not adequately controlled by avoidance strategies or medicines and you develop serious complications, you may be a candidate for a lung transplant. During this procedure, healthy donor lung will be transplanted into you to replace the damaged lung. Two important things to know:

- This procedure is not a cure. This is because your immune system will be the same after the procedure. This means that if you are exposed again to the substances that triggers your immune system, new inflammation may damage the transplanted donor lung tissue.

- This procedure is not for everyone. Even if you are a candidate for this procedure, it may be difficult to find a matching organ donor. Lung transplants are serious medical procedures with their own risks. Talk to your doctor about what procedures are right for you.

Living with Hypersensitivity Pneumonitis

If you have hypersensitivity pneumonitis, you can take steps to control the condition and prevent complications by receiving routine follow-up care, monitoring your condition, preventing new acute flares and complications, and learning about and preparing for serious complications.

Receive Routine Follow-Up Care

In addition to treatments you are using to control your condition, your doctor may recommend other medical care to improve your quality of life, vaccines to prevent lung infections, and lifestyle changes such as physical activity and quitting smoking to improve overall health and avoid some complications.

- **Other medical care.** Your doctor may evaluate how your condition is affecting your activity level and mental health. To improve your quality of life, your doctor may recommend other treatments to address pain, fatigue, or mental-health concerns that you may have.

- **Vaccines.** Remember that your condition causes you to have reduced lung function, particularly if you have subacute or chronic hypersensitivity pneumonitis. Your doctor may recommend that you receive routine pneumococcal and flu (influenza) vaccines to avoid lung infections that can further impair your reduced lung function.

- **Physical activity.** Patients with hypersensitivity pneumonitis benefit from regular exercise. Before starting any exercise program, ask your doctor about what level of physical activity is right for you.

- **Quit smoking.** If you smoke, quit. Although smoking does not increase the risk of developing hypersensitivity pneumonitis, some studies suggest smoking can worsen disease and shorten survival for people with chronic hypersensitivity pneumonitis compared to nonsmokers with chronic hypersensitivity pneumonitis. Another study reported lung cancer in patients who smoked and had chronic hypersensitivity pneumonitis.

Monitor Your Condition

If you have been diagnosed with subacute or chronic hypersensitivity pneumonitis, your doctor may recommend follow-up testing to see how well your treatment is working and if your disease is improving, stable, or worse. To monitor your condition, your doctor may recommend repeating tests used earlier to diagnose hypersensitivity pneumonitis such as chest x-rays, computed tomography (CT) scans, or lung function tests.

Your doctor may determine your disease is worse if you have new or more severe fibrosis or lung function problems. High-resolution CT scans may be more informative than lung function tests at assessing disease progression.

There is a growing recognition that disease tends to be worse, such as greater lung fibrosis, if it starts in childhood or early adult life. Therefore, more careful monitoring may be required for younger patients with hypersensitivity pneumonitis.

Prevent New Acute Flares and Serious Complications Over Your Lifetime

To help prevent new acute flares and complications, your doctor may recommend tests to identify the substances causing your condition, as well as additional screening tests to prevent potentially fatal complications.

- **Identification of substances causing your condition.** If you do not know the environmental substances causing your condition, your doctor may recommend diagnostic precipitin and inhalation challenge tests. Identification can help avoid the environmental sources of the substances causing your condition. Successful avoidance strategies can help you live a longer, prevent new acute flares, and slow or stop progression to chronic disease with serious complications.

- **Screening for serious complications.** If you have been diagnosed with chronic hypersensitivity pneumonitis, your doctor may recommend echocardiography and right-heart catheterization to evaluate pulmonary artery pressure and screen for pulmonary hypertension. Pulmonary hypertension can occur in people who have chronic hypersensitivity pneumonitis, particularly in patients with more severe disease who have poorer lung function and reduced exercise capacity.

Learn the Warning Signs of Serious Complications and Have a Plan

Always notify your doctor if your symptoms suddenly worsen. Your doctor will need to rule out other causes including infection and order repeat chest imaging tests. If these chest imaging tests show new findings without evidence of another cause, your doctor may modify your hypersensitivity pneumonitis treatment plan to better control your condition. Talk to your doctor and agree on a clinical decision plan to help you know when to seek urgent medical care.

Chapter 28

Pleurisy and Other Pleural Disorders

What Is Pleurisy and Other Pleural Disorders?

Pleurisy is a condition in which the pleura is inflamed. The pleura is a membrane that consists of two large, thin layers of tissue. One layer wraps around the outside of your lungs. The other layer lines the inside of your chest cavity.

Between the layers of tissue is a very thin space called the "pleural space." Normally this space is filled with a small amount of fluid— about four teaspoons full. The fluid helps the two layers of the pleura glide smoothly past each other as you breathe in and out.

Pleurisy occurs if the two layers of the pleura become irritated and inflamed. Instead of gliding smoothly past each other, they rub together every time you breathe in. The rubbing can cause sharp pain.

Many conditions can cause pleurisy, including viral infections.

Pleurisy is a condition in which the pleura is inflamed. The pleura is a membrane that consists of two large, thin layers of tissue. One layer wraps around the outside of your lungs. The other layer lines the inside of your chest cavity.

Between the layers of tissue is a very thin space called the "pleural space." Normally this space is filled with a small amount of fluid—about

This chapter includes text excerpted from "Pleurisy and Other Pleural Disorders," National Heart, Lung, and Blood Institute (NHLBI), October 10, 2011. Reviewed August 2019.

four teaspoons full. The fluid helps the two layers of the pleura glide smoothly past each other as you breathe in and out.

Pleurisy occurs if the two layers of the pleura become irritated and inflamed. Instead of gliding smoothly past each other, they rub together every time you breathe in. The rubbing can cause sharp pain.

Many conditions can cause pleurisy, including viral infections.

Other Pleural Disorders

Pneumothorax

Air or gas can build up in the pleural space. When this happens, it is called a "pneumothorax." Lung disease or acute lung injury can cause a pneumothorax.

Some lung procedures also can cause a pneumothorax. Examples include lung surgery, drainage of fluid with a needle, bronchoscopy and mechanical ventilation.

Sometimes the cause of a pneumothorax is not known.

The most common symptoms of a pneumothorax are a sudden pain in one side of the lung and shortness of breath. The air or gas in the pleural space also can put pressure on the lung and cause it to collapse.

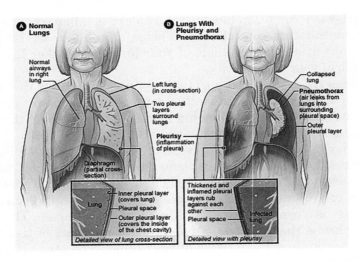

Figure 28.1. *Normal Lungs and Lungs with Pleurisy and Pneumothorax*

Figure A shows the location of the lungs, airways, pleura, and diaphragm (a muscle that helps you breathe). The inset image shows a detailed view of the two pleural layers and pleural space. Figure B shows lungs with pleurisy and a pneumothorax. The inset image shows a detailed view of an infected lung with thickened and inflamed pleural layers.

A small pneumothorax may go away without treatment. A large pneumothorax may require a procedure to remove air or gas from the pleural space. A very large pneumothorax can interfere with blood flow through your chest and cause your blood pressure to drop. This is called a "tension pneumothorax."

Pleural Effusion

In some cases of pleurisy, excess fluid builds up in the pleural space. This is called a "pleural effusion." A lot of extra fluid can push the pleura against your lung until the lung, or part of it collapses. This can make it hard for you to breathe. Sometimes the extra fluid gets infected and turns into an abscess. When this happens, it is called an "empyema."

You can develop a pleural effusion even if you do not have pleurisy. For example, pneumonia, heart failure, cancer, or pulmonary embolism can lead to a pleural effusion.

Hemothorax

Blood also can build up in the pleural space. This condition is called "hemothorax." An injury to your chest, chest or heart surgery, or lung or pleural cancer can cause a hemothorax. A hemothorax can put pressure on the lung and cause it to collapse. A hemothorax also can cause shock. In shock, not enough blood and oxygen reach your body's vital organs.

Causes of Pleurisy and Other Pleural Disorders
Pleurisy

Many conditions can cause pleurisy. Viral infections are likely the most common cause. Other causes of pleurisy include:

- Bacterial infections, such as pneumonia and tuberculosis, and infections from fungi or parasites

- Pulmonary embolism, a blood clot that travels through the blood vessels to the lungs

- Autoimmune disorders, such as lupus and rheumatoid arthritis

- Cancer, such as lung cancer, lymphoma, and mesothelioma

- Chest and heart surgery, especially coronary artery bypass grafting

- Lung diseases, such as lymphangioleiomyomatosis (LAM) or asbestosis

- Inflammatory bowel disease

- Familial Mediterranean fever, an inherited condition that often causes fever and swelling in the abdomen or lungs

Other causes of pleurisy include chest injuries, pancreatitis (an inflamed pancreas), and reactions to certain medicines. Reactions to certain medicines can cause a condition similar to lupus. These medicines include procainamide, hydralazine, and isoniazid.

Sometimes doctors cannot find the cause of pleurisy.

Pneumothorax

Lung diseases or acute lung injury can make it more likely that you will develop a pneumothorax (a buildup of air or gas in the pleural space). Such lung diseases may include chronic obstructive pulmonary disease (COPD), tuberculosis, and LAM.

Surgery or a chest injury also may cause a pneumothorax.

You can develop a pneumothorax without having recognized lung disease or chest injury. This is called a "spontaneous pneumothorax." Smoking increases your risk of spontaneous pneumothorax. Having a family history of the condition also increases your risk.

Pleural Effusion

The most common cause of a pleural effusion (a buildup of fluid in the pleural space) is heart failure. Lung cancer, LAM, pneumonia, tuberculosis, and other lung infections also can lead to a pleural effusion.

Sometimes kidney or liver disease can cause fluid to build up in the pleural space. Asbestosis, sarcoidosis and reactions to some medicines also can lead to a pleural effusion.

Hemothorax

An injury to the chest, chest or heart surgery, or lung or pleural cancer can cause a hemothorax (buildup of blood in the pleural space). A hemothorax also can be a complication of an infection (for example, pneumonia), tuberculosis, or spontaneous pneumothorax.

Signs, Symptoms, and Complications of Pleurisy and Other Pleural Disorders

Pleurisy

The main symptom of pleurisy is a sharp or stabbing pain in your chest that gets worse when you breathe in deeply or cough or sneeze. The pain may stay in one place or it may spread to your shoulders or back. Sometimes the pain becomes a fairly constant dull ache.

Depending on what is causing pleurisy, you may have other symptoms, such as:

- Shortness of breath or rapid, shallow breathing
- Coughing
- Fever and chills
- Unexplained weight loss

Pneumothorax

The symptoms of pneumothorax include:

- Sudden, sharp chest pain that gets worse when you breathe in deeply or cough
- Shortness of breath
- Chest tightness
- Easy fatigue (tiredness)
- A rapid heart rate
- A bluish tint to the skin caused by lack of oxygen

Other symptoms of pneumothorax include flaring of the nostrils; anxiety, stress, and tension; and hypotension (low blood pressure).

Pleural Effusion

Pleural effusion often has no symptoms.

Hemothorax

The symptoms of hemothorax often are similar to those of pneumothorax. They include:

- Chest pain

- Shortness of breath

- Respiratory failure

- A rapid heart rate

- Anxiety

- Restlessness

Diagnosis of Pleurisy and Other Pleural Disorders

Your doctor will diagnose pleurisy or another pleural disorder based on your medical history, a physical exam, and test results.

Your doctor will want to rule out other causes of your symptoms. She or he also will want to find the underlying cause of pleurisy or other pleural disorder so it can be treated.

Medical History

Your doctor may ask detailed questions about your medical history. She or he likely will ask you to describe any pain, especially:

- What it feels like

- Where it is located and whether you can feel it in your arms, jaw, or shoulders

- When it started and whether it goes away and then comes back

- What makes it better or worse

Your doctor also may ask whether you have other symptoms, such as shortness of breath, coughing, or palpitations. Palpitations are feelings that your heart is skipping a beat, fluttering, or beating too hard or fast.

Your doctor also may ask whether you have ever:

- Had heart disease

- Smoked

- Traveled to places where you may have been exposed to tuberculosis (TB)

- Had a job that exposed you to asbestos. Asbestos is a mineral that, at one time, was widely used in many industries

Your doctor also may ask about medicines you take or have taken. Reactions to some medicines can cause pleurisy or other pleural disorders.

Physical Exam

Your doctor will listen to your breathing with a stethoscope to find out whether your lungs are making any abnormal sounds.

If you have pleurisy, the inflamed layers of the pleura make a rough, scratchy sound as they rub against each other when you breathe. Doctors call this a pleural friction rub. If your doctor hears the friction rub, she or he will know that you have pleurisy.

If you have a pleural effusion, fluid buildup in the pleural space will prevent a friction rub. But if you have a lot of fluid, your doctor may hear a dull sound when she or he taps on your chest. Or, she or he may have trouble hearing any breathing sounds.

Muffled or dull breathing sounds also can be a sign of a pneumothorax (a buildup of air or gas in the pleural space).

Diagnostic Tests

Depending on the results of your physical exam, your doctor may recommend tests.

Chest X-Ray

A chest x-ray is a painless test that creates a picture of the structures in your chest, such as your heart, lungs, and blood vessels. This test may show air or fluid in the pleural space.

A chest x-ray also may show what is causing a pleural disorder—for example, pneumonia, a fractured rib, or a lung tumor. Sometimes a chest x-ray is taken while you lie on your side. This position can show fluid that did not appear on an x-ray taken while you were standing.

Chest Computerized Tomography Scan

A chest computed tomography scan, or chest CT scan (chest computerized tomography scan) is a painless test that creates precise pictures of the structures in your chest. This test provides a computer-generated picture of your lungs that can show pockets of fluid. A chest CT scan also may show signs of pneumonia, a lung abscess, a tumor, or other possible causes of pleural disorders.

341

Ultrasound

This test uses sound waves to create pictures of your lungs. An ultrasound may show where fluid is located in your chest. The test also can show some tumors.

Chest Magnetic Resonance Imaging

A chest magnetic resonance imaging scan, or chest magnetic resonance imaging (MRI), uses radio waves, magnets, and a computer to create detailed pictures of the structures in your chest. This test can show pleural effusions and tumors. This test is also called a "magnetic resonance" (MR) scan or a "nuclear magnetic resonance" (NMR) scan.

Blood Tests

Blood tests can show whether you have an illness that increases your risk of pleurisy or another pleural disorder. Such illnesses include bacterial or viral infections, pneumonia, pancreatitis (an inflamed pancreas), kidney disease, or lupus.

Arterial Blood Gas Test

For this test, a blood sample is taken from an artery, usually in your wrist. The blood's oxygen and carbon dioxide levels are checked. This test shows how well your lungs are taking in oxygen.

Thoracentesis

Once your doctor knows whether fluid has built up in the pleural space and where it is, she or he can remove a sample for testing. This is done using a procedure called "thoracentesis." During the procedure, your doctor inserts a thin needle or plastic tube into the pleural space and draws out the excess fluid. After the fluid is removed from your chest, it is sent for testing.

The risks of thoracentesis—such as pain, bleeding, and infection—usually are minor. They get better on their own, or they are easily treated. Your doctor may do a chest x-ray after the procedure to check for complications.

Fluid Analysis

The fluid removed during thoracentesis is examined under a microscope. It is checked for signs of infection, cancer, or other conditions that can cause fluid or blood to build up in the pleural space.

Biopsy

Your doctor may suspect that tuberculosis or cancer has caused fluid to build up in your pleural space. If so, she or he may want to look at a small piece of the pleura under a microscope.

To take a tissue sample, your doctor may do one of the following procedures:

- Insert a needle into your chest to remove a small sample of the pleura's outer layer

- Insert a tube with a light on the end (endoscope) into tiny cuts in your chest wall so that she or he can see the pleura. Your doctor can then snip out small pieces of tissue. This procedure must be done in a hospital. You will be given medicine to make you sleep during the procedure.

- Snip out a sample of the pleura through a small cut in your chest wall. This is called an "open pleural biopsy." It is usually done if the sample from the needle biopsy is too small for an accurate diagnosis. This procedure must be done in a hospital. You will be given medicine to make you sleep during the procedure.

Treatment of Pleurisy and Other Pleural Disorders

Pleurisy and other pleural disorders are treated with procedures, medicines, and other methods. The goals of treatment include:

- Relieving symptoms

- Removing the fluid, air, or blood from the pleural space (if a large amount is present)

- Treating the underlying condition

Relieving Symptoms

To relieve pleurisy symptoms, your doctor may recommend:

- Acetaminophen or anti-inflammatory medicines (such as ibuprofen) to control pain

- Codeine-based cough syrups to control coughing

- Lying on your painful side. This might make you more comfortable.

343

- Breathing deeply and coughing to clear mucus as the pain eases. Otherwise, you may develop pneumonia.

- Getting plenty of rest

Removing Fluid, Air, or Blood from the Pleural Space

Your doctor may recommend removing fluid, air, or blood from your pleural space to prevent lung collapse.

The procedures used to drain fluid, air, or blood from the pleural space are similar.

- During a thoracentesis, your doctor will insert a thin needle or plastic tube into the pleural space. An attached syringe will draw fluid out of your chest. This procedure can remove more than 6 cups of fluid at a time.

- If your doctor needs to remove a lot of fluid, she or he may use a chest tube. Your doctor will inject a painkiller into the area of your chest wall where the fluid is. She or he will then insert a plastic tube into your chest between two ribs. The tube will be connected to a box that suctions out the fluid. Your doctor will use a chest x-ray to check the tube's position.

- Your doctor also can use a chest tube to drain blood and air from the pleural space. This process can take several days. The tube will be left in place, and you will likely stay in the hospital during this time.

Sometimes the fluid in the pleural space contains thick pus or blood clots. It may form a hard skin or peel, which makes the fluid harder to drain. To help break up the pus or blood clots, your doctor may use a chest tube to deliver medicines called "fibrinolytics" to the pleural space. If the fluid still would not drain, you may need surgery.

If you have a small, persistent air leak into the pleural space, your doctor may attach a one-way valve to the chest tube. The valve allows air to exit the pleural space, but not reenter. Using this type of valve may allow you to continue your treatment from home.

Treat the Underlying Condition

The fluid sample that was removed during thoracentesis will be checked under a microscope. This can tell your doctor what is causing the fluid buildup, and she or he can decide the best way to treat it.

If the fluid is infected, treatment will involve antibiotics and drainage. If you have tuberculosis or a fungal infection, treatment will involve long-term use of antibiotics or antifungal medicines.

If tumors in the pleura are causing fluid buildup, the fluid may quickly build up again after it is drained. Sometimes antitumor medicines will prevent further fluid buildup. If they do not, your doctor may seal the pleural space. Sealing the pleural space is called "pleurodesis." For this procedure, your doctor will drain all of the fluid out of your chest through a chest tube. Then she or he will push a substance through the chest tube into the pleural space. The substance will irritate the surface of the pleura. This will cause the two layers of the pleura to stick together, preventing more fluid from building up.

Chemotherapy or radiation treatment also may be used to reduce the size of the tumors.

If heart failure is causing fluid buildup, treatment usually includes diuretics (medicines that help reduce fluid buildup) and other medicines.

Chapter 29

Sarcoidosis

Sarcoidosis is a rare condition in which groups of immune cells form lumps, called "granulomas," in various organs in the body. Inflammation, which may be triggered by infection or exposure to certain substances, is thought to play a role in the formation of granulomas.

Sarcoidosis can affect any organ. Most often it affects the lungs and lymph nodes in the chest. You may experience fatigue, which is extreme tiredness, or fever, but you may also experience other signs and symptoms depending on the organ that is affected. Your doctor will diagnose sarcoidosis in part by ruling out other diseases that have similar symptoms.

Determining whether treatment is needed and what type depends on your signs and symptoms, which organs are affected, and how well those organs are working. Medicines used to treat sarcoidosis help reduce inflammation or suppress the immune system. Many people recover with few or no long-term problems. Sometimes the disease causes permanent scarring in the affected organs. When scarring happens in the lungs, this is called "pulmonary fibrosis."

Causes of Sarcoidosis

Sarcoidosis is a condition in which immune cells form lumps, called "granulomas," in your organs. Inflammation is thought to cause

---

This chapter includes text excerpted from "Sarcoidosis," National Heart, Lung, and Blood Institute (NHLBI), March 29, 2018.

granulomas to form and may lead to temporary or permanent scarring at the site of the granulomas. Your inherited genes or certain environmental factors may trigger the inflammation that leads to granulomas.

Genetics

Studies suggest that people get sarcoidosis because of genes that make you susceptible to the disease. Some of the genes that are related to sarcoidosis are associated with the immune system.

Environmental Factors

Environmental factors, such as infection or exposure to certain substances, can trigger changes in the immune system and lead to sarcoidosis. Studies suggest that these triggers may cause sarcoidosis only in people with genes that make them susceptible to the disease.

Risk Factors for Sarcoidosis

You may have an increased risk for sarcoidosis because of your age, your family history and genetics, or your race. Some risk factors, such as occupation, can be changed. Most risk factors, such as age, family history and genetics, race and ethnicity, and sex, cannot be changed.

Age

You can be diagnosed with sarcoidosis at any age, but sarcoidosis is most commonly diagnosed in people age 55 and older.

Environment or Occupation

Your risk for sarcoidosis may be higher if you have repeated exposure to environmental substances that cause inflammation, such as insecticides or mold, or if you work in healthcare or as a firefighter. Working in these occupations may expose you to substances that trigger the formation of granulomas.

Family History and Genetics

You have a higher risk of sarcoidosis if you have a close relative with sarcoidosis.

Other Medical Conditions

Sarcoidosis sometimes occurs after lymphoma, a type of blood cancer.

Race or Ethnicity

People of any race can get sarcoidosis, but it is more common in people of African or Scandinavian descent.

Sex

Both men and women can develop sarcoidosis, but it is more common in women. You may have an increased risk for sarcoidosis because of your age, your family history and genetics, or your race. Some risk factors, such as occupation, can be changed. Most risk factors, such as age, family history and genetics, race and ethnicity, and sex, cannot be changed.

Age

You can be diagnosed with sarcoidosis at any age, but sarcoidosis is most commonly diagnosed in people age 55 and older.

Environment or Occupation

Your risk for sarcoidosis may be higher if you have repeated exposure to environmental substances that cause inflammation, such as insecticides or mold, or if you work in healthcare or as a firefighter. Working in these occupations may expose you to substances that trigger the formation of granulomas.

Family History and Genetics

You have a higher risk of sarcoidosis if you have a close relative with sarcoidosis.

Other Medical Conditions

Sarcoidosis sometimes occurs after lymphoma, a type of blood cancer.

Race or Ethnicity

People of any race can get sarcoidosis, but it is more common in people of African or Scandinavian descent.

Sex

Both men and women can develop sarcoidosis, but it is more common in women.

Screening and Prevention of Sarcoidosis

Currently, there are no screening methods to determine who will develop sarcoidosis. If you are at risk for sarcoidosis, your doctor may recommend you try to avoid insecticides, mold, or other environmental sources of substances known to trigger the formation of granulomas.

Signs, Symptoms, and Complications of Sarcoidosis

Many people who have sarcoidosis have no signs or symptoms. Some people experience general signs and symptoms of sarcoidosis, such as fever and weight loss. Others will experience signs and symptoms that will depend on which organs are affected. If inflammation continues, some people may develop permanent scarring, which can lead to life-threatening serious heart or lung complications.

Signs and Symptoms

Many people have general signs and symptoms, such as:

- Depression
- Fatigue
- Fever
- Malaise, or a feeling of discomfort or illness
- Pain and swelling in the joints
- Weight loss

Sarcoidosis most often affects the lungs and the lymph nodes in the chest. Some people with sarcoidosis in the lungs may wheeze, cough, feel short of breath, or have chest pain. However, people with sarcoidosis in the lungs do not always have lung-related symptoms.

If sarcoidosis affects other organs or parts of your body, you may have other symptoms related to those organs:

- Abdominal pain
- A larger-than-normal spleen

- Anemia

- Burning, itchy, or dry eyes

- Fainting

- Heart palpitations

- Joint pain

- Muscle weakness

- Problems with a liver that is larger than normal, including itching, vomiting, nausea, jaundice, or abdominal pain

- Problems with the nervous system, including headaches, dizziness, vision problems, seizures, mood swings, disturbed behavior, hallucinations, delusions, back pain, or pain associated with particular nerves

- Skin changes, including erythema nodosum or lupus pernio, a condition that causes skin sores that usually affect the face, especially the nose, cheeks, lips, and ears. The sores associated with lupus pernio tend to last a long time. Lupus pernio occurs mostly in African Americans and can return after sarcoidosis treatment is over.

- Swelling of the salivary glands

- Swollen or tender lymph nodes in other areas of the body besides the chest, such as in your neck, chin, armpits, or groin

Lofgren syndrome occurs in some people when they first have sarcoidosis, especially women between ages 30 and 40. Lofgren syndrome usually goes away completely within two years. It may include:

- Erythema nodosum

- Fever

- Joint pain

- Swollen lymph nodes

Complications

If sarcoidosis is untreated or if the treatment does not work, inflammation can continue and scarring may develop. Sarcoidosis can cause serious and life-threatening damage to the organs it affects, including:

351

- **Blindness**
- **Blood and bone marrow problems,** including lower-than-usual numbers of red or white blood cells
- **Endocrine conditions,** including hypercalcemia, diabetes insipidus, and amenorrhea
- **Heart complications,** including arrhythmia, heart failure, sudden cardiac arrest, cardiomyopathy
- **Kidney conditions,** such as kidney stones or kidney failure
- **Cirrhosis**
- **Lung diseases,** such as pulmonary hypertension and pulmonary fibrosis
- **Problems with the nervous system,** including brain tumors, meningitis, hydrocephalus, psychiatric problems, and nerve pain

Diagnosis of Sarcoidosis

Your doctor will diagnose sarcoidosis based on your symptoms, a physical exam, imaging tests, or a biopsy of an affected organ. The doctor will also perform tests to rule out other diseases that have similar signs and symptoms.

Diagnostic Tests and Procedures

To diagnose sarcoidosis and determine which organs are affected, your doctor may have you undergo some of the following tests and procedures:

- Biopsy of the lungs, liver, skin, or other affected organs to check for granulomas
- Blood tests, including complete blood counts, to check hormone levels and to test for other conditions that may cause sarcoidosis
- Bronchoscopy, which may include rinsing an area of the lung to get cells or using a needle to take cells from the lymph nodes in the chest
- Chest x-ray to look for granulomas in the lungs and heart and determine the stage of the disease. Often, sarcoidosis is found because a chest x-ray is performed for another reason.
- Neurological tests, such as electromyography, evoked potentials, spinal taps, or nerve conduction tests, to detect problems with the nervous system caused by sarcoidosis

- Eye exam to look for eye damage, which can occur without symptoms in a person with sarcoidosis

- Gallium scan, which uses a radioactive material called "gallium" to look for inflammation, usually in the eyes or lymph nodes.

- High-resolution computed tomography (CT) scan to look for granulomas

- Magnetic resonance imaging (MRI) to help find granulomas.

- Positron emission tomography (PET) scan, a type of imaging that can help find granulomas

- Pulmonary function tests to check whether you have breathing problems

- Ultrasound to look for granulomas

Tests for Other Medical Conditions

To help diagnose sarcoidosis, your doctor may need to perform tests or ask questions to rule out other medical conditions that have similar signs and symptoms as sarcoidosis.

- Blood tests to help the doctor distinguish between sarcoidosis and cancer or infections

- A bronchoscopy to find signs that may suggest an infection or cancer

- Questions about environmental exposure to help determine whether the granulomas are related to sarcoidosis or another condition. Exposure to beryllium, for example, can cause granulomas similar to sarcoidosis even though they are actually associated with chronic beryllium disease

- A urinalysis to help the doctor rule out other conditions that resemble sarcoidosis

Stages of Sarcoidosis

Doctors use stages to describe the various imaging findings of sarcoidosis of the lung or lymph nodes of the chest. There are four stages of sarcoidosis, and they indicate where the granulomas are located. In each of the first three stages, sarcoidosis can range from mild to severe. Stage IV is the most severe and indicates permanent scarring in the lungs.

- **Stage I:** Granulomas are located only in the lymph nodes.
- **Stage II:** Granulomas are located in the lungs and lymph nodes.
- **Stage III:** Granulomas are located in the lungs only.
- **Stage IV:** Pulmonary fibrosis.

Treatment of Sarcoidosis

The goal of treatment is remission, a state in which the condition is not causing problems. Not everyone who is diagnosed with sarcoidosis needs treatment. Sometimes the condition goes away on its own. Whether you need treatment—and what type you need—will depend on your signs and symptoms, which organs are affected, and whether those organs are working well. Some people do not respond to treatment.

Medicines

Because inflammation is thought to be involved in sarcoidosis, your doctor may prescribe medicines to reduce inflammation or treat an overactive immune system that may be causing too much inflammation in the body. Some of the medicines include:

- **Corticosteroids to reduce inflammation.** The corticosteroid prednisone is the most commonly used treatment for sarcoidosis. Corticosteroids can be taken as pills or be injected, inhaled, or taken as eye drops or other topical medicines. Corticosteroids can have serious side effects with long-term use.

- **Disease-modifying antirheumatic drugs (DMARDs)** to treat an overactive immune system. Examples of DMARDs include methotrexate, azathioprine, and leflunomide. Potential side effects include liver damage.

- **Monoclonal antibodies** to treat an overactive immune system. Examples include infliximab, adalimumab, rituximab, and golimumab.

- **Antibiotics** to treat sarcoidosis of the skin. Side effects of common antibiotics, such as minocycline, tetracycline, and doxycycline, include dizziness and gastrointestinal problems.

- **Antimalarials** to treat sarcoidosis of the skin, lungs, or nervous system. These medicines are typically used to fight malaria. Side effects include eye damage.

- **Colchicine** to treat joint pain from sarcoidosis. This medicine is usually prescribed for gout. Side effects include nausea, vomiting, diarrhea, and stomach cramps or pain.

- **Corticotropin** to treat an overactive immune system. This is a type of hormone therapy. Side effects include changes to appetite or mood.

- **Pentoxifylline** to block the release of TNF-a, a substance in white blood cells that can cause granulomas. This medicine is normally prescribed to improve blood flow. Side effects include nausea.

Part Four

Other Conditions
That Affect Respiration

Chapter 30

Pulmonary Edema

What Is Pulmonary Edema?

Pulmonary edema, also known as "lung congestion," is a medical condition in which excess fluid accumulates in the lungs. The lungs are made up of alveoli, small sacs that expand and contract with each breath. The function of alveoli is to take in oxygen and release carbon dioxide during breathing. In healthy people, this exchange of oxygen and carbon dioxide occurs naturally and without problems. For people with pulmonary edema, the alveoli accumulate fluid that prevents the exchange of oxygen and carbon dioxide. This fluid prevents oxygen from being released into the bloodstream, causing a feeling of shortness of breath.

Pulmonary edema is usually classified as cardiogenic (related to a heart problem, also known as "congestive heart failure") or noncardiogenic (caused by a health problem not related to the heart). Cardiogenic pulmonary edema (CPE) is the more common form of pulmonary edema and affects an estimated two percent of Americans.

What Causes Pulmonary Edema

Cardiogenic pulmonary edema develops when the heart is unable to move enough blood from the lungs into the bloodstream. This causes uneven pressure inside the chambers of the heart, which in turn causes

"Pulmonary Edema," © 2017 Omnigraphics. Reviewed August 2019.

fluid to be pushed back into the lungs. This fluid fills the alveoli and prevents the lungs from functioning properly.

Cardiogenic pulmonary edema can be caused by:

- Heart attack

- Heart disease

- Abnormal heart valve function

- Abnormal arterial function

- Uncontrolled hypertension (high blood pressure)

Noncardiogenic pulmonary edema develops when the blood vessels in the lungs become damaged, causing fluid to leak from the blood vessels into the alveoli. This fluid leakage can be caused by a variety of factors, including:

- Abnormal thyroid function

- Kidney failure

- Lung damage or pulmonary embolism

- Adult respiratory distress syndrome (ARDS)

- Bacterial or viral infection (pneumonia, hantavirus, and dengue virus)

- Major bodily injury or trauma (head injury, seizure, and brain hemorrhage)

- Use/abuse of certain drugs (aspirin, chemotherapy, cocaine, and heroin)

- Inhaled toxins (ammonia, chlorine gas, and smoke inhalation)

- Inhaled water (when swimming or nearly drowning)

- Exposure to an altitude above 8,000 feet without proper acclimation

What Are the Symptoms of Pulmonary Edema?

Pulmonary edema symptoms may begin suddenly or develop gradually over time. Symptoms include:

- Shortness of breath (the most common symptom)

- Difficulty breathing when lying flat that improves upon sitting up or standing

- Gasping for breath, wheezing, gurgling, and feeling of drowning
- Inability to speak due to shortness of breath
- Difficulty breathing with exertion or exercise
- Coughing up blood, and bloody froth
- Chest pain, irregular or rapid heartbeat
- Fatigue
- Swelling of abdomen or legs
- Unnatural skin tone, grey or blue appearance
- Excessive sweating
- Anxiety, restlessness
- Decreased alertness, impaired thought, and poor decision-making
- Headache
- Vomiting

What Are the Complications Associated with Pulmonary Edema?

If left untreated, pulmonary edema can result in severe complications. Hypertension due to pulmonary edema can increase pressure on the pulmonary artery, causing the heart to weaken and fail. This, in turn, can lead to swelling of the legs and abdomen, liver congestion and swelling, and accumulation of fluid in the membranes surrounding the lungs. These complications can be fatal if uncontrolled.

What Is the Diagnosis of Pulmonary Edema?

A doctor or other healthcare provider can diagnose pulmonary edema using a variety of assessments and tests. A physical exam is performed to check for abnormal heart sounds, rapid or irregular heart rate, abnormal lung sounds, rapid or irregular breathing, abnormal appearance of veins in the neck, swelling of legs or abdomen, and abnormal skin color. Diagnostic blood tests, x-rays, echocardiogram, electrocardiogram, cardiac catheterization, or coronary angiogram may also be performed.

How Is Pulmonary Edema Treated?

Treatment of pulmonary edema varies depending on the nature and severity of symptoms. Common treatments include the use of supplemental oxygen, breathing assistance via mechanical ventilator, diuretic medications to reduce pressure caused by the accumulation of fluid in the lungs, narcotic medications to reduce shortness of breath and anxiety, medications to dilate blood vessels to relieve pressure on the heart, and/or medications to regulate blood pressure.

How Pulmonary Edema Can Be Prevented

Pulmonary edema is preventable through the maintenance of a healthy lifestyle and controlling certain health conditions. Hypertension and diabetes are two common causes of pulmonary edema and should be regulated through proper screening and healthcare. People at risk for pulmonary edema should follow the treatment plan prescribed by their doctor, including taking all prescription medications as directed. Following a diet that is low in salt and fat, quitting smoking, maintaining a healthy weight, getting regular exercise, and avoiding triggers such as allergens are important factors in limiting the development of pulmonary edema. Another common recommendation is to reduce or manage stress in order to limit the risk of heart problems.

References

1. "Diseases and Conditions: Pulmonary Edema," Mayo Clinic, July 24, 2014.

2. "Pulmonary Edema," Medline Plus, National Institutes of Health (NIH), February 24, 2016.

3. "Pulmonary Edema," WebMD, April 15, 2016.

Chapter 31

Pulmonary Embolism

What Is a Pulmonary Embolism?

A pulmonary embolism (PE) is a sudden blockage in a lung artery. It usually happens when a blood clot breaks loose and travels through the bloodstream to the lungs. PE is a serious condition that can cause:

- Permanent damage to the lungs

- Low oxygen levels in your blood

- Damage to other organs in your body from not getting enough oxygen

Pulmonary embolism can be life-threatening, especially if a clot is large, or if there are many clots.

What Causes Pulmonary Embolism

The cause is usually a blood clot in the leg, called a "deep vein thrombosis" (DVT), that breaks loose and travels through the bloodstream to the lung.

This chapter includes text excerpted from "Pulmonary Embolism," Medline-Plus, National Institutes of Health (NIH), October 14, 2016.

Who Is at Risk for Pulmonary Embolism?

Anyone can get a PE, but certain things can raise your risk of PE:

- **Having surgery,** especially joint replacement surgery
- **Certain medical conditions,** including:
  - Cancers
  - Heart diseases
  - Lung diseases
  - A broken hip or leg bone or other trauma
- **Hormone-based medicines,** such as birth control pills or hormone replacement therapy
- **Pregnancy and childbirth.** The risk is highest for about six weeks after childbirth.
- **Not moving for long periods,** such as being on bed rest, having a cast, or taking a long plane flight
- **Age.** Your risk increases as you get older, especially after age 40.
- **Family history and genetics.** Certain genetic changes that can increase your risk of blood clots and PE.
- **Obesity**

What Are the Symptoms of Pulmonary Embolism?

Half the people who have pulmonary embolism have no symptoms. If you do have symptoms, they can include shortness of breath, chest pain, or coughing up blood. Symptoms of a blood clot include warmth, swelling, pain, tenderness, and redness of the leg.

How Is Pulmonary Embolism Diagnosed?

It can be difficult to diagnose PE. To make a diagnosis, your health-care provider will:

- Take your medical history, including asking about your symptoms and risk factors for PE
- Do a physical exam

- Run some tests, including various imaging tests and possibly some blood tests

What Are the Treatments for Pulmonary Embolism?

If you have PE, you need medical treatment right away. The goal of treatment is to break up clots and help keep other clots from forming. Treatment options include medicines and procedures.

Medicines

- **Anticoagulants,** or blood thinners, keep blood clots from getting larger and stop new clots from forming. You might get them as an injection, a pill, or through an I.V. (intravenous). They can cause bleeding, especially if you are taking other medicines that also thin your blood, such as aspirin.

- **Thrombolytics** are medicines to dissolve blood clots. You may get them if you have large clots that cause severe symptoms or other serious complications. Thrombolytics can cause sudden bleeding, so they are used if your PE is serious and may be life-threatening.

Procedures

- **Catheter-assisted thrombus removal** uses a flexible tube to reach a blood clot in your lung. Your healthcare provider can insert a tool in the tube to break up the clot or to deliver medicine through the tube. Usually, you will get medicine to put you to sleep for this procedure.

- **A vena cava filter** may be used in some people who cannot take blood thinners. Your healthcare provider inserts a filter inside a large vein called the "vena cava." The filter catches blood clots before they travel to the lungs, which prevents pulmonary embolism. But the filter does not stop new blood clots from forming.

Can Pulmonary Embolism Be Prevented?

Preventing new blood clots can prevent PE. Prevention may include

- Continuing to take blood thinners. It is also important to get regular checkups with your provider, to make sure that the dosage of your medicines is working to prevent blood clots but not causing bleeding.

- Heart-healthy lifestyle changes, such as heart-healthy eating, exercise, and, if you smoke, quitting smoking

- Using compression stockings to prevent DVT

- Moving your legs when sitting for long periods of time (such as on long trips)

- Moving around as soon as possible after surgery or being confined to a bed

Chapter 32

Pulmonary Hypertension

Pulmonary hypertension occurs when the pressure in the blood vessels that carry blood from your heart to your lungs is higher than normal. One type of pulmonary hypertension is pulmonary arterial hypertension (PAH). Pulmonary hypertension can happen on its own or be caused by another disease or condition. In the United States, the most common cause of pulmonary hypertension is left heart disease. Other conditions that can cause pulmonary hypertension include sickle cell disease (SCD); pulmonary embolus (PE), which is a type of venous thromboembolism (VTE); and chronic obstructive pulmonary disease (COPD).

The increased pressure in the blood vessels of the lungs means that your heart has to work harder to pump blood into the lungs. This can cause symptoms, such as shortness of breath, chest pain, and light-headedness. If left untreated, the increased pressure can damage your heart. This may lead to serious or life-threatening complications, such as heart failure or arrhythmias, which are irregular heart rhythms.

Causes of Pulmonary Hypertension

Your genes or other medical conditions can cause pulmonary hypertension. Certain medical conditions can damage, change, or block the blood vessels of the pulmonary arteries. The cause of pulmonary hypertension is not always clear.

This chapter includes text excerpted from "Pulmonary Hypertension," National Heart, Lung, and Blood Institute (NHLBI), April 18, 2017.

To understand pulmonary hypertension, it is helpful to understand the flow of blood through the heart and lungs. The right side of your heart receives oxygen-poor blood from your body's tissues. The pulmonary arteries connect your right heart and lungs. The heart pumps blood through the pulmonary arteries to the lungs to become oxygen-rich blood. The force or pressure of the blood against the walls of the pulmonary arteries is called the "pulmonary pressure."

Genes

Gene mutations are found in some people who have a family history of PAH. Mutations are also found often in patients who do not have a family history.

Medical Conditions

Many medical conditions can cause pulmonary hypertension. Pulmonary arterial hypertension is caused by conditions that result in narrowing of the pulmonary arteries themselves, such as scleroderma or human immunodeficiency virus (HIV). Narrowed blood vessels can increase blood pressure in the lungs.

Medical conditions that can cause pulmonary hypertension include:

- **Blood clots** in the lungs, called "pulmonary embolism," a type of VTE

- **Chronic exposure to high altitude**

- **Chronic kidney failure**

- **Congenital heart defects** or congenital narrowing of the pulmonary arteries

- **Connective tissue diseases,** such as scleroderma

- **HIV**

- **Infection with parasites,** such as schistosomiasis or Echinococcus, which are tapeworms

- **Left heart diseases,** such as left heart failure, which may be caused by high blood pressure throughout your body or ischemic heart disease; and heart valve diseases, such as aortic stenosis and mitral valve disease

- **Liver diseases,** such as cirrhosis, that lead to higher-than-normal blood pressures in the liver

- **Lung diseases,** such as COPD, interstitial lung disease, or sleep apnea

- **Metabolic disorders,** such as thyroid disorders or Gaucher disease

- **Sarcoidosis**

- **SCD**

- **Tumors in the lungs**

Risk Factors of Pulmonary Hypertension

You may have an increased risk for pulmonary hypertension because of your age, environment, family history and genetics, lifestyle habits, medicines you are taking, other medical conditions, or sex.

Age

Your risk of pulmonary hypertension goes up as you get older, although it may occur at any age. The condition is typically diagnosed between ages 30 and 60.

Environment

You may be at an increased risk of pulmonary hypertension if you have or are exposed to the following:

- **Asbestos** or silica

- **Infection** caused by parasites, such as schistosomiasis or Echinococcus, which are tapeworms

Family History and Genetics

Certain genetic disorders, such as Down syndrome, congenital heart disease (CHD), and Gaucher disease, can increase your risk of developing pulmonary hypertension.

A family history of blood clots or pulmonary embolism also increases your risk of developing pulmonary hypertension.

Lifestyle Habits

Unhealthy lifestyle habits can increase the risk of pulmonary hypertension. These habits include:

- Illegal drugs, such as cocaine and amphetamines
- Smoking

Medicines

Some medicines may increase your risk of pulmonary hypertension, including:

- **Chemotherapy medicines** to treat cancer, such as dasatinib, mitomycin C, and cyclophosphamide

- **Selective serotonin reuptake inhibitors (SSRIs)** to treat depression and anxiety. SSRIs may cause PAH in newborns whose mothers have taken these medicines during pregnancy.

- **Weight-loss drugs,** such as fenfluramine and dexfenfluramine, which are no longer approved for weight loss in the United States

Other Medical Conditions

Certain medical conditions may increase your risk of developing pulmonary hypertension:

- **Blood clotting disorders,** such as blood clots in the lungs, a higher-than-normal platelet count in your blood, and conditions that make your blood more likely to clot, such as protein S and C deficiency, factor V Leiden thrombophilia, antithrombin III deficiency, and antiphospholipid syndrome

- **Chronic kidney disease**

- **Diseases that change the structure of the chest wall,** such as scoliosis

- **Infections,** such as hepatitis B or C

- **Liver disease,** such as cirrhosis

- **Surgical removal of the spleen**

- **Thyroid diseases**

Sex

Pulmonary hypertension is more common in women than in men. Pulmonary hypertension with certain types of heart failure is also more common in women.

Screening and Prevention of Pulmonary Hypertension

To screen for pulmonary hypertension, your doctor will determine whether you have any known risk factors and may have you undergo screening tests. Screening is not usually performed unless you have known risk factors, such as scleroderma. Your doctor may recommend prevention strategies to help you lower your risk of developing pulmonary hypertension.

Tests to Screen

Based on your symptoms or risk factors, your doctor may recommend the following tests to screen for changes in the heart or lungs that may be related to pulmonary hypertension.

- **Echocardiography (Echo)** to look at your heart's function and structure and estimate pulmonary artery pressure

- **Electrocardiography (ECG or EKG)** to look for signs of changes in your heart or abnormal rhythms in your heart's electrical activity

- **Pulmonary function tests** to look for changes in lung function for conditions, such as systemic sclerosis, COPD, or interstitial lung diseases

Based on the results of these screening tests, your doctor may do follow-up tests to see whether you have higher-than-normal pressures in the pulmonary arteries. These other tests can help diagnose pulmonary hypertension.

Prevention Strategies

To help prevent pulmonary hypertension, your doctor may recommend controlling certain medical conditions, avoiding certain medicines or illegal drugs, and protecting yourself against environmental hazards that are risk factors.

Signs, Symptoms, and Complications of Pulmonary Hypertension

Signs and symptoms of pulmonary hypertension are sometimes hard to recognize, because they are similar to those of other medical conditions. People may have symptoms for years before being diagnosed with pulmonary hypertension. These symptoms may get worse over time and could eventually lead to serious complications, such as right heart failure.

Signs and Symptoms

Signs and symptoms of pulmonary hypertension may include the following:

- **Chest pain**
- **Cough** that is dry or may produce blood
- **Fatigue**
- **Hoarseness**
- **Light-headedness,** fainting, or dizziness
- **Nausea and vomiting**
- **Shortness of breath,** first with physical activity and then without it as the disease gets worse
- **Swelling** of your abdomen, legs, or feet caused by fluid buildup
- **Weakness**
- **Wheezing**

Complications

Complications of pulmonary hypertension may include the following:

- **Anemia**
- **Arrhythmias** and bundle branch blocks of the heart
- **Blood clots** in the pulmonary arteries
- **Bleeding in the lungs,** which may be life-threatening
- **Heart failure,** especially right ventricular failure
- **Liver damage** from increased pressure in the right heart
- **Pericardial effusion,** which is a collection of fluid in the sac-like structure around the heart
- **Pregnancy complications** that can be life-threatening for the mother and baby

Diagnosis of Pulmonary Hypertension

To diagnose pulmonary hypertension, your doctor may ask you questions about your medical history and do a physical exam. Your doctor may also test you for pulmonary hypertension based on your signs and symptoms and risk factors. A diagnosis of pulmonary hypertension will be made if tests show higher-than-normal pressure in the pulmonary arteries.

Confirming High Pressures in the Pulmonary Arteries

Normal pressure in the pulmonary arteries is between 11 and 20 millimeters of mercury (mm Hg) when measured by cardiac catheterization. Your doctor may perform the following tests to confirm high pressures in the pulmonary arteries.

- **Cardiac catheterization** to provide a definite diagnosis of pulmonary hypertension. A diagnosis of pulmonary hypertension is made if the pulmonary artery pressure is 25 mm Hg or greater while at rest.

- **Echocardiography** to estimate pulmonary artery pressure. An estimated pulmonary artery pressure of 35 to 40 mm Hg or greater on echocardiography suggests pulmonary hypertension. A diagnosis of pulmonary hypertension may be made when enough changes are seen on an echocardiogram. If the echocardiogram suggests pulmonary hypertension, then right heart catheterization may be the next step.

Medical History and Physical Exam

Your doctor may ask you about any signs and symptoms you have been experiencing and any risk factors, such as other medical conditions you have.

Your doctor will also perform a physical exam to look for signs that may help diagnose your condition. As part of this exam, your doctor may do the following:

- Check whether the oxygen levels in your blood are low. This may be done by pulse oximetry, in which a probe is placed on your finger to check your oxygen levels.

- Feel your liver to see if it is larger than normal

- Listen to your heart to see if there are changes in how it sounds, and also to find out if your heartbeat is faster than normal or irregular or if you have a new heart murmur

- Listen to your lungs for sounds that could be caused by heart failure or interstitial lung disease

- Look at the veins in your neck to see if they are larger than normal

- Look for swelling in your abdomen and legs that may be caused by fluid buildup

- Measure your blood pressure

Diagnostic Test

Your doctor may order blood tests and imaging tests to help diagnose pulmonary hypertension.

- **Blood tests** to look for increased risk of blood clots, stress on the heart, or anemia.

- **Cardiac Magnetic resonance imaging (MRI)** to get detailed pictures of the structure and functioning of the heart and surrounding blood vessels.

- **Chest x-ray** to look at the size and shape of the heart and surrounding blood vessels, including the pulmonary arteries.

- **Echocardiogram (echo)** to look for signs of pulmonary hypertension and also study the heart's structure and functioning. If the echocardiogram suggests pulmonary hypertension, then right heart catheterization may be the next step.

- **Electrocardiogram (ECG or EKG)** to look for signs of changes in your heart or abnormal rhythms in your heart's electrical activity caused by pulmonary hypertension. You may still have pulmonary hypertension if you have a normal ECG.

Tests for Other Medical Conditions

Your doctor may order additional tests to see whether another condition or medicine may be causing your pulmonary hypertension. Doctors can use this information to develop your treatment plan.

Treatment of Pulmonary Hypertension

If you are diagnosed with pulmonary hypertension, your doctor will determine your treatment plan based on the cause of disease, if it is known. Your doctor may recommend healthy lifestyle changes, medicines, or other treatments aimed at keeping your symptoms from getting worse, increasing your ability to exercise, improving heart function, and ensuring a better quality of life. There is no cure for pulmonary hypertension unless chronic blood clots in the lungs are the cause.

Healthy Lifestyle Changes

Depending on the cause of your pulmonary hypertension, your doctor may recommend healthy lifestyle changes.

- **Heart-healthy eating,** which includes eating less salt, to lower blood pressure or cholesterol if high levels of these contributed to the cause of your pulmonary hypertension. Eating less salt will help control your body fluids and may improve heart function.

- **Physical activity** as recommended and supervised by your doctor

- **Physical rehabilitation** to improve your ability to exercise and also boost your quality of life

Medicines

Medicines to treat pulmonary hypertension may include:

- **Anticoagulation or blood thinners** to prevent blood clots in people whose pulmonary hypertension is caused by chronic blood clots in the lungs. These thinners also can help some people who have PAH, heart failure, or other risk factors for blood clots.

- **Digitalis, or digoxin** to control the rate at which blood is pumped throughout the body.

- **Vasodilator therapy** to relax blood vessels and lower blood pressure in the pulmonary artery most affected in people who have PAH. This includes calcium channel blockers, such as nifedipine and diltiazem, as well as newer groups of medicines called "endothelin receptor antagonists" (ERAs) and "phosphodiesterase type 5 inhibitors" (PDE 5).

375

Procedures and Therapies

Your doctor may recommend a procedure, surgery, or therapy to treat pulmonary hypertension.

- **Oxygen therapy** if oxygen levels in the blood are too low.

- **Balloon atrial septostomy** to decrease pressure in the right heart chambers and improve the output of the left heart and oxygenation of the blood. In this procedure, a small hole is made in the wall between the right and left atria to allow blood to flow from the right to the left atrium.

- **Balloon pulmonary angioplasty** to lower the blood pressure in your pulmonary artery and improve heart function in people who cannot have a pulmonary endarterectomy.

- **Pulmonary endarterectomy** surgery to remove blood clots from the inside of the blood vessels of the lungs.

Treatments for Other Conditions

Your doctor may recommend medicines or procedures to treat the condition that is causing your pulmonary hypertension.

- Blood pressure medicines, such as angiotensin-converting enzymes inhibitors, beta-blockers, or calcium channel blockers when left heart disease is the cause

- Blood transfusions or hydroxyurea to treat SCD

- Heart valve repair

- Iron supplements to increase blood iron levels and improve anemia

Living with Pulmonary Hypertension

After you are diagnosed with pulmonary hypertension, it is important to follow your treatment plan, get regular care, and learn how to monitor your condition. Taking these steps can slow down the progression of the disease and may improve your condition. Your specific treatment plan will depend on the cause of your pulmonary hypertension, as well as how advanced it is.

Receive Routine Follow-Up Care

Your follow-up care may include recommendations such as these:

- **Participate in support groups, counseling, and education efforts** that can help you manage the activities of daily living, experience a successful pregnancy, and generally improve the quality of your life.

- **Get the recommended vaccines,** which often include a vaccine for pneumococcus and influenza, or flu shot every year at the start of flu season.

Monitor Your Condition

Talk to your doctor about new or concerning symptoms. People who have pulmonary hypertension may need regular tests. Your doctor may recommend the following to monitor your condition and treatment response:

- **Six-minute walk test** to monitor your ability to exercise

- **Blood tests** to check hemoglobin, iron, and electrolyte levels; kidney, liver, and thyroid function; your blood's ability to clot; and signs of stress on the heart

- **Cardiac catheterization**

- **Cardiac MRI** to monitor your heart's size and how well it is working

- **Chest x-ray**

- **Echocardiography** to monitor your heart's size and how well it is working, and measure the pressure in your right heart chambers

- **Electrocardiogram** to check for irregular heartbeats

- **Pulmonary function** tests to check for any change in your lung function

If your pulmonary hypertension is severe or does not respond to treatment, your doctor may talk to you about a lung transplant or a heart and lung transplant.

Prevent Complications over Your Lifetime

To help prevent some of the complications of pulmonary hypertension, your doctor may recommend the following.

- Make heart-healthy lifestyle changes, such as heart-healthy eating if your pulmonary hypertension is due to heart failure from ischemic heart disease or high blood pressure.

- Engage in regular physical activity. Before starting any exercise program, ask your doctor about what level of physical activity is right for you.

- Avoid high altitudes when possible and discuss with your doctor any plans for air travel or visits to places at high altitude.

- Talk to your doctor if you are planning to get pregnant, as there is an increased risk of pregnancy complications.

- Treat other medical conditions, such as COPD, heart conditions, and sleep apnea.

Learn the Warning Signs of Serious Complications and Have a Plan

Even with treatment, pulmonary hypertension may lead to serious complications, such as heart failure and arrhythmias. Know the signs and symptoms of pulmonary hypertension and how to recognize the possible complications.

If you are taking a blood thinner, this will increase your risk of bleeding. If you experience any abnormal bleeding, such as blood in your stool, black stool, or coughing up blood, contact your doctor right away. If you fall while taking a blood thinner, you are at higher risk for bleeding inside your head. Let your doctor know if you have fallen while taking a blood thinner.

Some treatments for pulmonary hypertension must be given through a long-term intravenous (IV) line. Call your doctor right away if you have any signs of infection. Signs of infection include redness, swelling, or yellow discharge where the IV is inserted; a fever of 100.3°F or higher; and chills.

Chapter 33

Cystic Fibrosis

Cystic fibrosis (CF) is a genetic condition that affects a protein in the body. People who have CF have a faulty protein that affects the body's cells, tissues, and the glands that make mucus and sweat.

Mucus is normally slippery and protects the linings of the airways, digestive tract, and other organs and tissues. People who have CF make thick, sticky mucus that can build up and lead to blockages, damage, or infections in the affected organs. Inflammation also causes damage to organs such as the lungs and pancreas.

Some people who have CF have few or no signs or symptoms, while others experience severe symptoms or life-threatening complications. Symptoms of CF depend on which organs are affected and the severity of the condition. The most serious and common complications of CF are problems with the lungs, also known as "pulmonary" or "respiratory problems," which may include serious lung infections. People who have CF often also have problems maintaining good nutrition, because they have a hard time absorbing the nutrients from food. This is a problem that can delay growth.

Your doctor may recommend treatments to improve lung function and manage other complications. Early treatment can improve your quality of life (QOL) and help you live longer.

Causes of Cystic Fibrosis

Cystic fibrosis is an inherited disease caused by mutations in a gene called the "*cystic fibrosis transmembrane conductance regulator*"

This chapter includes text excerpted from "Cystic Fibrosis," National Heart, Lung, and Blood Institute (NHLBI), March 13, 2019.

(*CFTR*) gene. The *CFTR* gene provides instructions for the CFTR protein. The CFTR protein is located in every organ of the body that makes mucus, including the lungs, liver, pancreas, and intestines, as well as sweat glands. The CFTR protein has also been found in other cells in the body, such as cells of the heart and the immune system. The mutations in the *CFTR* gene cause the CFTR protein to not work properly. This causes thick, sticky mucus and blockages in the lungs and digestive system.

Normally, mucus coats tiny hair-like structures called "cilia" in the airways of your lungs, which sweep the mucus particles up to the nose and mouth where your body can get rid of them. In people who have cystic fibrosis, this process does not work properly.

What Gene Mutations Cause Cystic Fibrosis

There are almost 2,000 known disease-causing mutations of the *CFTR* gene. Different mutations have different effects on how the CFTR protein is made and how it works. In the most common gene mutation, part of the *CFTR* gene is missing, resulting in a protein that does not work properly.

How Is Cystic Fibrosis Inherited?

Every person inherits two *CFTR* genes, one gene from each parent. Children who inherit a *CFTR* gene with a mutation from both parents will have cystic fibrosis. When a mutated *CFTR* gene is inherited from only one parent and a normal *CFTR* gene is inherited from the other, the person will be a cystic fibrosis carrier. CF carriers are generally healthy, but they can pass the mutated *CFTR* gene on to their children.

Figure 33.1 shows how two parents who are both CF carriers can pass a *CFTR* gene mutation on to their children.

Risk Factors of Cystic Fibrosis

A person may have an increased risk for CF because of her or his family history and genetics, and race or ethnicity.

Family History and Genetics

A person is at higher risk for having CF if one or both parents is a carrier of a mutated *CFTR* gene or has CF. A person is also at higher risk if a sibling, half-sibling, or first cousin has CF. More than 10 million Americans are carriers of a *CFTR* gene mutation, yet many of them do not know it.

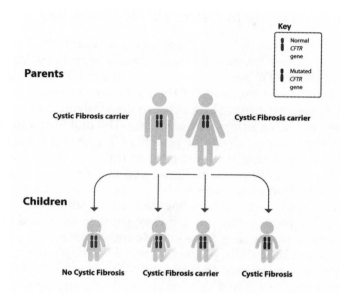

Figure 33.1. *Inheritance Pattern for Cystic Fibrosis*

This figure shows how CFTR genes are inherited. A person inherits 2 copies of the CFTR gene, 1 from each parent. If each parent has a normal CFTR gene and a mutated CFTR gene, each child has a 25 percent chance of inheriting 2 normal genes, a 50 percent chance of inheriting 1 normal gene and 1 gene with a mutation and being a cystic fibrosis (CF) carrier, and a 25 percent chance of inheriting 2 genes with mutations and having cystic fibrosis.

Race or Ethnicity

Cystic fibrosis is most common in people of northern European ancestry and less common in Hispanics and African Americans. It is relatively uncommon in Asian Americans.

Screening and Prevention of Cystic Fibrosis

Genetic testing may be performed to look for carriers, as well as to screen relatives of people who have CF. Genetic testing may also be used as prenatal screening tool to look for a mutated *CFTR* gene. All newborns in the United States are now screened for CF. Since universal screening for CF began relatively recently, there are still young people and adults who have not been screened.

Carrier Screening to Detect CFTR Mutations

Genetic testing can tell you if you carry a mutation of the *CFTR* gene. This is called "carrier testing." People who have inherited a mutation of the *CFTR* gene from one parent are CF carriers. People who have inherited a mutation of the *CFTR* gene from both parents will have CF. Genetic testing looks at your deoxyribonucleic acid (DNA) from a blood or saliva sample, or cells from the inside of your cheek.

The standard test to check for possible CF carriers looks for 23 of the most common disease-causing gene mutations. If you have a positive test, there is a 99 percent chance you are a carrier. However, if you have a negative test, there is still a small chance that you could carry a *CFTR* mutation that did not show up on the test.

Siblings of a person who has CF may want to be tested for cystic fibrosis whether or not they have symptoms. Other relatives, such as first cousins and half-siblings, may be tested if they have symptoms, or if the family is concerned that the individual may have CF. After a positive screening test, the diagnosis should be confirmed with further testing.

Prenatal Screening

Couples who are planning to have children may want to be tested to see if they are CF carriers. Genetic testing, such as the carrier screening described above, may be done before or during pregnancy. Often, the mother is tested first. However, if you are already pregnant, you and your partner may choose to be tested at the same time. If the father has a family history of CF, he may be tested first. Similar to standard genetic testing, prenatal screening uses a sample of blood, saliva, or cells from the inside of your cheek to check your deoxyribonucleic acid.

If one partner is a carrier for CF gene mutation, then the next step is to test the partner if this has not been done. If both parents are CF carriers, then prenatal diagnostic testing may be performed to see whether your unborn baby has CF or is a carrier.

Newborn Screening

When a child has CF, it is very important to diagnose it early to help prevent complications. Newborn screening for CF is performed during a baby's first two to three days of life. A few drops of blood from a heel prick are placed on a special card and analyzed in labs.

The type of newborn screening that is performed varies from state to state. Every state and the District of Columbia begins with a blood test to check for levels of a chemical made by the pancreas called "immunoreactive trypsinogen" (IRT). In people who have CF, IRT tends to be high. However, most babies with high levels of IRT do not have cystic fibrosis. IRT may also be high if the baby is premature, had a stressful delivery, or is a carrier of cystic fibrosis.

Some states test only IRT for CF newborn screening. Other states test IRT and also perform DNA testing. In states that test both IRT and DNA, if IRT is high, then the hospital will test the baby's DNA for some of the gene mutations that cause CF. After a positive screening test, the diagnosis should be confirmed with further testing.

Prevention Strategies

There is no way to prevent whether or not you have CF. Couples who are planning to have children and know that they are at risk of having a child with CF may want to meet with a genetic counselor. A genetic counselor can answer questions about the risk and explain the choices that are available.

Signs, Symptoms, and Complications of Cystic Fibrosis

Symptoms of CF depend on which organs are affected and the severity of the condition. Most patients who have CF have noticeable symptoms. Some patients have few or no signs or symptoms, while others experience severe symptoms or life-threatening complications. Symptoms may also change over time. The most common complications of CF affects the lungs and pancreas.

Signs and Symptoms

Cystic fibrosis most commonly affects the lungs. Some people who have CF may have wheezing and a cough that may produce mucus or blood.

Other signs and symptoms depend on the organs affected and may include:

- **Blockage of the intestine** in a baby soon after birth

- **Clubbing of fingers and toes** due to less oxygen getting to the hands and feet

- **Fever,** which may include night sweats

- **Gastrointestinal symptoms,** such as severe abdominal pain, chronic diarrhea, or constipation

- **Jaundice,** or yellow skin, for an abnormally long time after birth

- **Low body mass index (BMI)** or being underweight

- **Muscle and joint pain**

- **Delayed growth or puberty**

- **Salty skin** and saltier than normal sweat

- **Sinus infections**

Complications

Cystic fibrosis affects many parts and systems of the body. Complications will depend on the affected organs and the severity of the disease. People who have CF produce thick, sticky mucus that causes problems in the lungs and digestive system. The buildup of mucus in the lungs makes it easy for bacteria to grow and often leads to serious lung infections. People who have CF often have problems with nutrition, too, because their pancreas does not work properly.

Possible complications of CF include:

- **Allergic bronchopulmonary aspergillosis (ABPA),** which is an allergic reaction in the lungs to the fungus *Aspergillus*

- **Bronchiectasis,** a widening of the airways in the lungs caused by chronic inflammation or obstruction of the airways. This is a common complication of cystic fibrosis.

- **Cancers of the digestive tract,** including the esophagus, stomach, small bowel, large bowel, liver, and pancreas

- **Collapsed lung,** called "pneumothorax," resulting in the air in the space between your lung and chest wall

- **Diabetes** due to damage to the pancreas. The pancreas is where insulin is made.

- **Fertility problems**

- **Gastrointestinal complications,** such as distal intestinal obstruction syndrome (DIOS), in which your intestine becomes blocked by very thick intestinal contents. Another possible complication is rectal prolapse, in which part of the rectum sticks out through the anus.

- **Heart failure** because of lung damage

- **Hemoptysis**

- **Kidney problems** due to diabetes and some antibiotics, or kidney stones

- **Liver disease** or failure caused by blockage of the bile ducts in the liver, which leads to bile damaging your liver. This may lead to cirrhosis and a need for a liver transplant.

- **Lung infections** that may come back or be difficult to treat

- **Malnutrition** because the pancreas may not make enough enzymes to help digest and absorb nutrients from food

- **Mental-health problems,** such as depression and anxiety

- **Muscle and bone complications,** including low bone density and osteoporosis, joint pain and arthritis, and muscle pains

- **Pancreatitis** and low levels of pancreatic enzymes leading to nutritional deficiencies, including low levels of vitamins A, D, E, and K

- **Pulmonary exacerbations,** which are episodes of worsening cough, shortness of breath, and mucus production caused by airway inflammation and blockage from an increase in bacteria in your airways and lungs. These episodes may also cause fatigue, loss of appetite, and weight loss.

- **Salt loss syndrome**, in which your body quickly loses salt, or sodium and chloride, causing electrolyte and other imbalances

- **Urinary incontinence,** or loss of bladder control

Diagnosis of Cystic Fibrosis

Your doctor may diagnose CF based on your signs and symptoms and results from certain tests, such as genetic and sweat tests that are done to confirm screening tests.

Diagnostic Tests and Procedures

To diagnose CF, your doctor may recommend some of the following tests and procedures:

- **Genetic testing** to detect mutated *CFTR* genes. This test can confirm a positive CF screening test and sweat test. If genetic testing is done as part of newborn or other screening, it may not be repeated during the newborn stage.

- **Prenatal diagnostic tests** to diagnose CF in an unborn baby, using mutated *CFTR* genes. This is done with procedures that take either a sample of amniotic fluid, the liquid in the sac surrounding your unborn baby, or tissue from the placenta. Cells from these samples are checked for gene mutations. Infants with positive prenatal testing for CF will be further tested after birth to confirm the diagnosis of cystic fibrosis.

- **Sweat test** for high sweat chloride to see if you have high levels of chloride in your sweat. The sweat test is the standard test for diagnosing CF. It may be used if you have symptoms that may indicate CF, or to confirm a positive diagnosis from a screening of your newborn baby. A normal sweat chloride test alone does not mean you do not have CF. Lower levels of chloride may indicate the need for further testing to diagnose or rule out cystic fibrosis.

Table 33.1. Sweat Chloride Test Results

Chloride Level, mmol/L	Result
60 or greater	Cystic fibrosis diagnosis
30 to 59	Unclear diagnosis; further testing needed
Less than 30	Cystic fibrosis likely

The table shows how much chloride in a person's sweat sample must be present in order to determine whether the diagnosis for CF is positive, unclear, or unlikely. A chloride level of 60 millimoles per liter (mmol/L) or greater indicates CF. A chloride level of 30 to 59 mmol/L indicates a diagnosis of CF is unclear, and that further testing is needed. A chloride level of less than 30 mmol/L indicates a diagnosis of CF is unlikely.

How Is a Sweat Chloride Test Performed?

The sweat test detects a higher amount of chloride—a component of salt that is made of sodium and chloride—in the sweat of people who have CF. In order to make sweat for this test, a colorless, odorless chemical and a little electrical stimulation are applied to a small area of an arm or leg. The sweat is collected and sent to a hospital lab for testing.

Treatment of Cystic Fibrosis

While there is not yet a cure for CF, advances in treatment are helping people live longer, healthier lives. After early diagnosis, the goal is the proactive treatment to slow down lung disease as much as possible. You or your child will work with CF specialists. In newborns with a positive screening result, treatment may begin while the diagnosis is being confirmed. Treatment for CF is focused on airway clearance, medicines to prevent and fight infections, and surgery, if needed.

Your Healthcare Team

Your healthcare team will likely include CF specialist. This is a doctor who is familiar with the complex nature of CF. Your doctor may work with a medical team that specializes in CF, often at major medical centers. The United States has more than 100 CF Care Centers, with medical teams that include:

- Doctors specializing in the lungs, diabetes, and the digestive system
- Genetic counselors
- Nurses
- Nutritionists and dietitians
- Pharmacists
- Physical therapists
- Psychologists
- Respiratory therapists
- Social workers

Airway Clearance Techniques

Airway clearance techniques help loosen lung mucus so it can be cleared, reducing infections and improving breathing. The techniques include special ways of breathing and coughing, devices used by mouth and therapy vests that use vibrations to loosen mucus, and chest physical therapy. These techniques are often used along with medicines, such as bronchodilators and mucus thinners.

Medicines

Medicines to treat CF include those used to maintain and improve lung function, fight infections, clear mucus and help breathing, and work on the faulty CFTR protein. Your doctor may prescribe some of the following medicines to treat CF:

- **Antibiotics** to prevent or treat lung infections and improve lung function. Your doctor may prescribe oral, inhaled, or intravenous (IV) antibiotics.

- **Anti-inflammatory medicines,** such as ibuprofen or corticosteroids, to reduce inflammation. Inflammation causes many of the changes in CF, such as lung disease. Ibuprofen is especially beneficial for children, but side effects can include kidney and stomach problems. Corticosteroids can cause bone thinning and increased blood sugar and blood pressure.

- **Bronchodilators** to relax and open airways. These treatments are taken by inhaling them.

- **Mucus thinners** to make it easier to clear the mucus from your airways. These treatments are taken by inhaling them.

- **CFTR modulators** that help improve the function of the faulty CFTR protein. They improve lung function and help with weight gain. Examples include ivacaftor and lumacaftor.

Surgery

Surgery may be an option for people with advanced conditions.

Chapter 34

Traumatic Lung Disorders

Chapter Contents

Section 34.1

Acute Respiratory Distress Syndrome

This section includes text excerpted from "ARDS," National
Heart, Lung, and Blood Institute (NHLBI), May 18, 2014.
Reviewed August 2019.

Acute respiratory distress syndrome (ARDS) is a lung condition
that leads to low oxygen levels in the blood. ARDS can be life threatening because your body's organs need oxygen-rich blood to work well.
People who develop ARDS often are very ill with another disease or
have major injuries. They might already be in the hospital when they
develop ARDS.

To understand ARDS, it helps to understand how the lungs work.
When you breathe, air passes through your nose and mouth into your
windpipe. The air then travels to your lungs' air sacs. These sacs are
called "alveoli." Small blood vessels called "capillaries" run through
the walls of the air sacs. Oxygen passes from the air sacs into the
capillaries and then into the bloodstream. Blood carries the oxygen to
all parts of the body, including the body's organs.

In ARDS, infections, injuries, or other conditions cause fluid to build
up in the air sacs. This prevents the lungs from filling with air and
moving enough oxygen into the bloodstream. As a result, the body's
organs (such as the kidneys and brain) do not get the oxygen they need.
Without oxygen, the organs may not work well or at all.

People who develop ARDS often are in the hospital for other serious
health problems. Rarely, people who are not hospitalized have health
problems that lead to ARDS, such as severe pneumonia.

If you have trouble breathing, call your doctor right away. If you
have severe shortness of breath, call 911.

More people are surviving ARDS now than in the past. One likely
reason for this is that treatment and care for the condition have
improved. Survival rates for ARDS vary depending on age, the underlying cause of ARDS, associated illnesses, and other factors. Some people
who survive recover completely. Others may have lasting damage to
their lungs and other health problems. Researchers continue to look
for new and better ways to treat ARDS.

Other names of ARDS include:

- Acute lung injury

- Adult respiratory distress syndrome

- Increased-permeability pulmonary edema
- Noncardiac pulmonary edema

In the past, ARDS was called "stiff lung," "shock lung," and "wet lung."

Causes of Acute Respiratory Distress Syndrome

Many conditions or factors can directly or indirectly injure the lungs and lead to ARDS. Some common ones are:

- Sepsis. This is a condition in which bacteria infect the bloodstream.
- Pneumonia. This is an infection in the lungs.
- Severe bleeding caused by an injury to the body
- An injury to the chest or head, such as a severe blow
- Breathing in harmful fumes or smoke
- Inhaling vomited stomach contents from the mouth

It is not clear why some very sick or seriously injured people develop ARDS and others do not. Researchers are trying to find out why ARDS develops and how to prevent it.

Risk Factors of Acute Respiratory Distress Syndrome

People at risk for ARDS have a condition or illness that can directly or indirectly injure their lungs.

Direct Lung Injury

Conditions that can directly injure the lungs include:

- Pneumonia. This is an infection in the lungs.
- Breathing in harmful fumes or smoke
- Inhaling vomited stomach contents from the mouth
- Using a ventilator. This is a machine that helps people breathe; rarely, it can injure the lungs.
- Nearly drowning

Indirect Lung Injury

Conditions that can indirectly injure the lungs include:

- Sepsis. This is a condition in which bacteria infect the bloodstream.

- Severe bleeding caused by an injury to the body or having many blood transfusions

- An injury to the chest or head, such as a severe blow

- Pancreatitis. This is a condition in which the pancreas becomes irritated or infected. The pancreas is a gland that releases enzymes and hormones.

- Fat embolism. This is a condition in which fat blocks an artery. A physical injury, such as a broken bone, can lead to a fat embolism.

- Drug reaction

Signs, Symptoms, and Complications of Acute Respiratory Distress Syndrome

The first signs and symptoms of ARDS are feeling like you cannot get enough air into your lungs, rapid breathing, and a low blood oxygen level.

Other signs and symptoms depend on the cause of ARDS. They may occur before ARDS develops. For example, if pneumonia is causing ARDS, you may have a cough and fever before you feel short of breath.

Sometimes people who have ARDS develop signs and symptoms, such as low blood pressure, confusion, and extreme tiredness. This may mean that the body's organs, such as the kidneys and heart, are not getting enough oxygen-rich blood.

People who develop ARDS often are in the hospital for other serious health problems. Rarely, people who are not hospitalized have health problems that lead to ARDS, such as severe pneumonia.

If you have trouble breathing, call your doctor right away. If you have severe shortness of breath, call 911.

Complications from Acute Respiratory Distress Syndrome

If you have ARDS, you can develop other medical problems while in the hospital.

The most common problems are:

- **Infections.** Being in the hospital and lying down for a long time can put you at risk for infections, such as pneumonia. Being on a ventilator also puts you at higher risk for infections.

- **A pneumothorax (collapsed lung).** This is a condition in which air or gas collects in the space around the lungs. This can cause one or both lungs to collapse. The air pressure from a ventilator can cause this condition.

- **Lung scarring.** ARDS causes the lungs to become stiff (scarred). It also makes it hard for the lungs to expand and fill with air. Being on a ventilator also can cause lung scarring.

- **Blood clots.** Lying down for long periods can cause blood clots to form in your body. A blood clot that forms in a vein deep in your body is called a "deep vein thrombosis" (DVT). This type of blood clot can break off, travel through the bloodstream to the lungs, and block blood flow. This condition is called "pulmonary embolism."

Diagnosis of Acute Respiratory Distress Syndrome

Your doctor will diagnose ARDS based on your medical history, a physical exam, and test results.

Medical History

- Your doctor will ask whether you have or have recently had conditions that could lead to ARDS.

- Your doctor also will ask whether you have heart problems, such as heart failure. Heart failure can cause fluid to build up in your lungs.

Physical Exam

- Acute respiratory distress syndrome may cause abnormal breathing sounds, such as crackling. Your doctor will listen to your lungs with a stethoscope to hear these sounds.

- She or he also will listen to your heart and look for signs of extra fluid in other parts of your body. Extra fluid may mean you have heart or kidney problems.

- Your doctor will look for a bluish color on your skin and lips. A bluish color means your blood has a low level of oxygen. This is a possible sign of ARDS.

Diagnostic Tests

You may have ARDS or another condition that causes similar symptoms. To find out, your doctor may recommend one or more of the following tests.

Initial Tests

The first tests done are:

- **An arterial blood gas test.** This blood test measures the oxygen level in your blood using a sample of blood taken from an artery. A low blood oxygen level might be a sign of ARDS.

- **Chest x-ray.** This test creates pictures of the structures in your chest, such as your heart, lungs, and blood vessels. A chest x-ray can show whether you have extra fluid in your lungs.

- **Blood tests,** such as a complete blood count, blood chemistries, and blood cultures. These tests help find the cause of ARDS, such as an infection.

- **A sputum culture.** This test is used to study the spit you have coughed up from your lungs. A sputum culture can help find the cause of an infection.

Other Tests

Other tests used to diagnose ARDS include:

- **Chest computed tomography scan, or chest CT scan.** This test uses a computer to create detailed pictures of your lungs. A chest CT scan may show lung problems, such as fluid in the lungs, signs of pneumonia, or a tumor.

- **Heart tests that look for signs of heart failure.** Heart failure is a condition in which the heart cannot pump enough blood to meet the body's needs. This condition can cause fluid to build up in your lungs.

Treatment of Acute Respiratory Distress Syndrome

Acute respiratory distress syndrome is treated in a hospital's intensive care unit. Current treatment approaches focus on improving blood oxygen levels and providing supportive care. Doctors also will try to pinpoint and treat the underlying cause of the condition.

Oxygen Therapy

One of the main goals of treating ARDS is to provide oxygen to your lungs and other organs (such as your brain and kidneys). Your organs need oxygen to work properly. Oxygen usually is given through nasal prongs or a mask that fits over your mouth and nose. However, if your oxygen level does not rise or it is still hard for you to breathe, your doctor will give you oxygen through a breathing tube. She or he will insert the flexible tube through your mouth or nose and into your windpipe.

Before inserting the tube, your doctor will squirt or spray a liquid medicine into your throat (and possibly your nose) to make it numb. Your doctor also will give you medicine through an intravenous (IV) line in your bloodstream to make you sleepy and relaxed. The breathing tube will be connected to a machine that supports breathing (a ventilator). The ventilator will fill your lungs with oxygen-rich air. Your doctor will adjust the ventilator as needed to help your lungs get the right amount of oxygen. This also will help prevent injury to your lungs from the pressure of the ventilator.

You will use the breathing tube and ventilator until you can breathe on your own. If you need a ventilator for more than a few days, your doctor may do a tracheotomy. This procedure involves making a small cut in your neck to create an opening to the windpipe. The opening is called a "tracheostomy." Your doctor will place the breathing tube directly into the windpipe. The tube is then connected to the ventilator.

Supportive Care

Supportive care refers to treatments that help relieve symptoms, prevent complications, or improve quality of life. Supportive approaches used to treat ARDS include:

- Medicines to help you relax, relieve discomfort, and treat pain

- Ongoing monitoring of heart and lung function (including blood pressure and gas exchange)

- **Nutritional support.** People who have ARDS often suffer from malnutrition. Thus, extra nutrition may be given through a feeding tube.

- **Treatment for infections.** People who have ARDS are at higher risk for infections, such as pneumonia. Being on a ventilator also increases the risk of infections. Doctors use antibiotics to treat pneumonia and other infections.

- **Prevention of blood clots.** Lying down for long periods can cause blood clots to form in the deep veins of your body. These clots can travel to your lungs and block blood flow (a condition called "pulmonary embolism"). Blood-thinning medicines and other treatments, such as compression stocking (stockings that create gentle pressure up the leg), are used to prevent blood clots.

- **Prevention of intestinal bleeding.** People who receive long-term support from a ventilator are at increased risk of bleeding in the intestines. Medicines can reduce this risk.

- **Fluids.** You may be given fluids to improve blood flow through your body and to provide nutrition. Your doctor will make sure you get the right amount of fluids. Fluids usually are given through an IV line inserted into one of your blood vessels.

Section 34.2

Atelectasis

This section includes text excerpted from "Atelectasis," National Heart, Lung, and Blood Institute (NHLBI), September 18, 2018.

Atelectasis can happen when there is an airway blockage, when pressure outside the lung keeps it from expanding, or when there is not enough surfactant for the lung to expand normally. When your lungs do not fully expand and fill with air, they may not be able to deliver enough oxygen to your blood.

Atelectasis can happen at any age and for different reasons. For example, newborns whose lungs are not fully developed may have atelectasis due to respiratory distress syndrome. Atelectasis can also happen when a tumor, excess mucus, or a piece of food blocks an airway, or because of pneumothorax or pleural effusion.

You may be at higher risk of atelectasis if you smoke or have other conditions, including obesity, sleep apnea, or lung diseases such as asthma, chronic obstructive pulmonary disease (COPD), or cystic fibrosis (CF). You are also at higher risk if you recently had surgery.

The medicines used to make you sleep during surgery can affect the way your lungs work, or the procedure itself can make it painful to breathe deeply. To help prevent atelectasis during and after surgery, your medical team may ask you to stop smoking and give you breathing exercises, medicines, or a breathing device such as a Continuous positive airway pressure (CPAP) machine.

Atelectasis may not cause signs or symptoms if it affects only a small area of lung. If it affects a larger area of the lung, it can cause fever, shallow breathing, wheezing, or coughing. The most common test used to diagnose atelectasis is a chest x-ray. Bronchoscopy or imaging tests can confirm a diagnosis.

Atelectasis treatment can include breathing or coughing exercises, inhaled medicines, breathing devices, or surgery. Atelectasis usually gets better with time or treatment. However, if it is undiagnosed or untreated, serious complications can occur, including fluid buildup, pneumonia, and respiratory failure.

Section 34.3

Inhalation Injuries to the Lungs

This section includes text excerpted from "Inhalation Injuries," MedlinePlus, National Institutes of Health (NIH), August 16, 2016.

Inhalation injuries are acute injuries to your respiratory system and lungs. They can happen if you breathe in toxic substances, such as smoke (from fires), chemicals, particle pollution, and gases. Inhalation injuries can also be caused by extreme heat; these are a type of thermal injuries. Over half of deaths from fires are due to inhalation injuries.

Symptoms of inhalation injuries can depend on what you breathed in. But they often include:

- Coughing and phlegm

- A scratchy throat

- Irritated sinuses

- Shortness of breath

- Chest pain or tightness

- Headaches

- Stinging eyes

- A runny nose

If you have a chronic heart or lung problem, an inhalation injury can make it worse.

To make a diagnosis, your healthcare provider may use a scope to look at your airways and check for damage. Other possible tests include imaging tests of the lungs, blood tests, and lung function tests.

If you have an inhalation injury, your healthcare provider will make sure that your airway is not blocked. Treatment is with oxygen therapy, and in some cases, medicines. Some patients need to use a ventilator to breathe. Most people get better, but some people have permanent lung or breathing problems. Smokers and people who had a severe injury are at a greater risk of having permanent problems.

You can take steps to try to prevent inhalation injuries:

- At home, practice fire safety, which includes preventing fires and having a plan in case there is a fire

- If there is smoke from a wildfire nearby or lots of particulate pollution in the air, try to limit your time outdoors. Keep your indoor air as clean as possible by keeping windows closed and using an air filter. If you have asthma, another lung disease, or heart disease, follow your healthcare provider's advice about your medicines and respiratory management plan.

- If you are working with chemicals or gases, handle them safely and use protective equipment

Chapter 35

Lung Cancer

What Is Lung Cancer?

Cancer is a disease in which cells in the body grow out of control. When cancer starts in the lungs, it is called "lung cancer."

Lung cancer begins in the lungs and may spread to lymph nodes or other organs in the body, such as the brain. Cancer from other organs also may spread to the lungs. When cancer cells spread from one organ to another, they are called "metastases."

Lung cancers usually are grouped into two main types called "small cell" and "nonsmall cell." These types of lung cancer grow differently and are treated differently. Nonsmall cell lung cancer is more common than small cell lung cancer.

What Are the Risk Factors of Lung Cancer?

Research has found several risk factors that may increase your chances of getting lung cancer.

Smoking

Cigarette smoking is the number 1 risk factor for lung cancer. In the United States, cigarette smoking is linked to about 80 to 90 percent of lung cancer deaths. Using other tobacco products, such as cigars or

---

This chapter includes text excerpted from "What Is Lung Cancer," Centers for Disease Control and Prevention (CDC), July 19, 2018.

pipes also increases the risk for lung cancer. Tobacco smoke is a toxic mix of more than 7,000 chemicals. Many are poisons. At least 70 are known to cause cancer in people or animals.

People who smoke cigarettes are 15 to 30 times more likely to get lung cancer or die from lung cancer than people who do not smoke. Even smoking a few cigarettes a day or smoking occasionally increases the risk of lung cancer. The more years a person smokes and the more cigarettes smoked each day, the more risk goes up.

People who quit smoking have a lower risk of lung cancer than if they had continued to smoke, but their risk is higher than the risk for people who never smoked. Quitting smoking at any age can lower the risk of lung cancer.

Cigarette smoking can cause cancer almost anywhere in the body. Cigarette smoking causes cancer of the mouth and throat, esophagus, stomach, colon, rectum, liver, pancreas, voicebox (larynx), trachea, bronchus, kidney and renal pelvis, urinary bladder, and cervix, and causes acute myeloid leukemia.

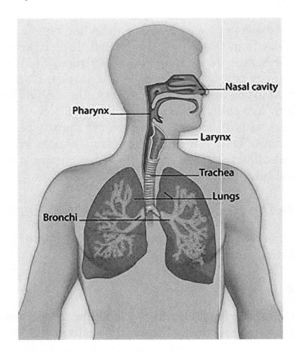

Figure 35.1. *Lung Diagram*

This illustration of the respiratory system shows the lungs, bronchi, trachea, larynx, pharynx, and nasal cavity.

Secondhand Smoke

Secondhand smoke and the harmful chemicals in it are known causes of sudden infant death syndrome (SIDS), respiratory infections, ear infections, and asthma attacks in infants and children. They are also known causes of heart disease, stroke, and lung cancer in adult nonsmokers.

Smoke from other people's cigarettes, pipes, or cigars (secondhand smoke) also causes lung cancer. When a person breathes in secondhand smoke, it is like she or he is smoking. In the United States, 2 out of 5 adults who do not smoke and half of the children are exposed to secondhand smoke, and about 7,300 people who never smoked die from lung cancer due to secondhand smoke every year.

Radon

Radon is a naturally occurring gas that comes from rocks and dirt and can get trapped in houses and buildings. It cannot be seen, tasted, or smelled. According to the U.S. Environmental Protection Agency (EPA), radon causes about 20,000 cases of lung cancer each year, making it the second leading cause of lung cancer. Nearly 1 out of every 15 homes in the United States is thought to have high radon levels. The EPA recommends testing homes for radon and using proven ways to lower high radon levels.

Other Substances

Examples of substances found at some workplaces that increase risk include asbestos, arsenic, diesel exhaust, and some forms of silica and chromium. For many of these substances, the risk of getting lung cancer is even higher for those who smoke.

Personal or Family History of Lung Cancer

If you are a lung cancer survivor, there is a risk that you may develop another lung cancer, especially if you smoke. Your risk of lung cancer may be higher if your parents, brothers or sisters, or children have had lung cancer. This could be true because they also smoke, or they live or work in the same place where they are exposed to radon and other substances that can cause lung cancer.

Radiation Therapy to the Chest

Cancer survivors who had radiation therapy (RT) to the chest are at higher risk of lung cancer.

Diet

Scientists are studying many different foods and dietary supplements to see whether they change the risk of getting lung cancer. There is much we still need to know. It is known that smokers who take beta-carotene supplements have increased risk of lung cancer.

Also, arsenic in drinking water (primarily from private wells) can increase the risk of lung cancer.

What Are the Symptoms of Lung Cancer?

Different people have different symptoms for lung cancer. Some people have symptoms related to the lungs. Some people whose lung cancer has spread to other parts of the body (metastasized) have symptoms specific to that part of the body. Some people just have general symptoms of not feeling well. Most people with lung cancer do not have symptoms until the cancer is advanced. Lung cancer symptoms may include:

- Coughing that gets worse or does not go away

- Chest pain

- Shortness of breath

- Wheezing

- Coughing up blood

- Feeling very tired all the time

- Weight loss with no known cause

Other changes that can sometimes occur with lung cancer may include repeated bouts of pneumonia and swollen or enlarged lymph nodes (glands) inside the chest in the area between the lungs.

These symptoms can happen with other illnesses, too. If you have some of these symptoms, talk to your doctor, who can help find the cause.

What Can You Do to Reduce Your Risk of Lung Cancer?

You can help lower your risk of lung cancer in the following ways:

- **Do not smoke.** Cigarette smoking causes about 80 to 90 percent of lung cancer deaths in the United States. The most important thing you can do to prevent lung cancer is to not start smoking or to quit if you smoke.

- **Avoid secondhand smoke.** Smoke from other people's cigarettes, cigars, or pipes is called "secondhand smoke." Make your home and car smoke-free.

- **Get your home tested for radon.** The EPA recommends that all homes be tested for radon.

- **Be careful at work.** Health and safety guidelines in the workplace can help workers avoid carcinogens—things that can cause cancer.

Who Should Be Screened for Lung Cancer?

Screening means testing for a disease when there are no symptoms or history of that disease. Doctors recommend a screening test to find a disease early, when treatment may work better.

The only recommended screening test for lung cancer is low-dose computed tomography (also called a "low-dose CT scan," or LDCT). In this test, an x-ray machine scans the body and uses low doses of radiation to make detailed pictures of the lungs.

Who Should Be Screened?

The U.S. Preventive Services Task Force (USPSTF) recommends yearly lung cancer screening with LDCT for people who:

- Have a history of heavy smoking

- Smoke now or have quit within the past 15 years

- Are between 55 and 80 years old

Heavy smoking means a smoking history of 30 pack years or more. A pack year is smoking an average of 1 pack of cigarettes per day for 1 year. For example, a person could have a 30 pack-year history by smoking 1 pack a day for 30 years or 2 packs a day for 15 years.

Risks of Screening

Lung cancer screening has at least three risks:

- A lung cancer screening test can suggest that a person has lung cancer when no cancer is present. This is called a "false-positive

403

result." False-positive results can lead to follow-up tests and surgeries that are not needed and may have more risks.

- A lung cancer screening test can find cases of cancer that may never have caused a problem for the patient. This is called "overdiagnosis." Overdiagnosis can lead to treatment that is not needed.

- Radiation from repeated LDCT tests can cause cancer in otherwise healthy people.

That is why lung cancer screening is recommended only for adults who have no symptoms but who are at high risk for developing the disease because of their smoking history and age. If you are thinking about getting screened, talk to your doctor. If lung cancer screening is right for you, your doctor can refer you to a high-quality screening facility.

The best way to reduce your risk of lung cancer is to not smoke and to avoid secondhand smoke. Lung cancer screening is not a substitute for quitting smoking.

When Should Screening Stop?

The Task Force recommends that yearly lung cancer screening stop when the person being screened:

- Turns 81 years old

- Has not smoked in 15 years

- Develops a health problem that makes her or him unwilling or unable to have surgery if lung cancer is found

How Is Lung Cancer Diagnosed and Treated?
Types of Lung Cancer

The two main types of lung cancer are small cell lung cancer and nonsmall cell lung cancer. These categories refer to what the cancer cells look like under a microscope. Nonsmall cell lung cancer is more common than small cell lung cancer.

Staging

If lung cancer is diagnosed, other tests are done to find out how far it has spread through the lungs, lymph nodes, and the rest of the body.

This process is called "staging." The type and stage of lung cancer tells doctors what kind of treatment you need.

Types of Treatment

Lung cancer is treated in several ways, depending on the type of lung cancer and how far it has spread. People with nonsmall cell lung cancer can be treated with surgery, chemotherapy, radiation therapy, targeted therapy, or a combination of these treatments. People with small cell lung cancer are usually treated with radiation therapy and chemotherapy.

- **Surgery.** An operation where doctors cut out cancer tissue.

- **Chemotherapy.** Using special medicines to shrink or kill the cancer. The drugs can be pills you take or medicines given in your veins, or sometimes both.

- **Radiation therapy.** Using high-energy rays (similar to x-rays) to kill the cancer.

- **Targeted therapy.** Using drugs to block the growth and spread of cancer cells. The drugs can be pills you take or medicines given in your veins.

Doctors from different specialties often work together to treat lung cancer. Pulmonologists are doctors who are experts in diseases of the lungs. Surgeons are doctors who perform operations. Thoracic surgeons specialize in chest, heart, and lung surgery. Medical oncologists are doctors who treat cancer with medicines. Radiation oncologists are doctors who treat cancers with radiation.

Complementary and Alternative Medicine

Complementary and alternative medicine are medicines and health practices that are not standard cancer treatments.

- **Complementary medicine** is used in addition to standard treatments. Examples include acupuncture, dietary supplements, massage therapy, hypnosis, and meditation.

- **Alternative medicine** is used instead of standard treatments. Examples include special diets, megadose vitamins, herbal preparations, special teas, and magnet therapy.

Many kinds of complementary and alternative medicine have not been tested scientifically and may not be safe. Talk to your doctor about the risks and benefits before you start any kind of complementary or alternative medicine.

Which Treatment Is Right for Me?

Choosing the treatment that is right for you may be hard. Talk to your cancer doctor about the treatment options available for your type and stage of cancer. Your doctor can explain the risks and benefits of each treatment and their side effects. Side effects are how your body reacts to drugs or other treatments.

Sometimes people get an opinion from more than one cancer doctor. This is called a "second opinion." Getting a second opinion may help you choose the treatment that is right for you.

Living with Lung Cancer

When you have been diagnosed with cancer, you are considered a cancer survivor from that moment throughout the rest of your life.

Finding lung cancer earlier and making new treatments available are helping more lung cancer survivors live longer. It is important to get the treatment you need when you need it. You deserve timely and appropriate care for your lung cancer and its symptoms (including pain), as well as any side effects of treatment. Molecular testing (also called "tumor" or "biomarker testing") may help you make decisions about treatment.

Talk with your healthcare provider about how a survivorship care plan can help you coordinate your follow-up care to support your physical and emotional health.

Take steps to stay healthy. This can lower your risk of getting cancer again or having the cancer come back.

Some cancer survivors may blame themselves or feel that others blame them for having cancer. Lung cancer survivors may have these feelings of blame or stigma. You may find it helpful to talk about your experiences and feelings with a social worker or mental-health professional. You may also find it helpful to share your story with other cancer survivors or listen to their stories.

Chapter 36

Hypoventilation Syndrome

Chapter Contents

Section 36.1

Congenital Central Hypoventilation Syndrome

This section includes text excerpted from "Congenital Central
Hypoventilation Syndrome," Genetics Home Reference (GHR),
National Institutes of Health (NIH), September 2008.
Reviewed August 2019.

Congenital central hypoventilation syndrome (CCHS) is a disorder
that affects breathing. People with this disorder take shallow breaths
(hypoventilate), especially during sleep, resulting in a shortage of
oxygen and a buildup of carbon dioxide in the blood. Ordinarily, the
part of the nervous system that controls involuntary body processes
(autonomic nervous system) would react to such an imbalance by stimulating the individual to breathe more deeply or wake up. This reaction
is impaired in people with CCHS, and they must be supported with
a machine to help them breathe (mechanical ventilation) or a device
that stimulates a normal breathing pattern (diaphragm pacemaker).
Some affected individuals need this support 24 hours a day, while
others need it only at night.

Symptoms of CCHS usually become apparent shortly after birth.
Affected infants hypoventilate upon falling asleep and exhibit a bluish
appearance of the skin or lips (cyanosis). Cyanosis is caused by lack
of oxygen in the blood. In some milder cases, CCHS may be diagnosed
later in life. In addition to the breathing problem, people with this
disorder may have difficulty regulating their heart rate and blood pressure, for example in response to exercise or changes in body position.
They may have abnormalities in the nerves that control the digestive
tract (Hirschsprung disease), resulting in severe constipation, intestinal blockage, and enlargement of the colon. They are also at increased
risk of developing certain tumors of the nervous system called "neuro-
blastomas," "ganglioneuromas," and "ganglioneuroblastomas." Some
affected individuals develop learning difficulties or other neurological
problems, which may be worsened by oxygen deprivation if treatment
to support their breathing is not completely effective.

Individuals with CCHS usually have eye abnormalities, including
a decreased response of the pupils to light. They also have decreased
perception of pain, low body temperature, and occasional episodes of
profuse sweating.

People with CCHS, especially children, may have a characteristic
appearance with a short, wide, somewhat flattened face often described

as "box-shaped." Life expectancy and the extent of any cognitive disabilities depend on the severity of the disorder, timing of the diagnosis, and the success of treatment.

Frequency of Congenital Central Hypoventilation Syndrome

Congenital central hypoventilation syndrome is a relatively rare disorder. Approximately 1,000 individuals with this condition have been identified. Researchers believe that some cases of sudden infant death syndrome (SIDS) or sudden unexplained death in children may be caused by undiagnosed CCHS.

Causes of Congenital Central Hypoventilation Syndrome

Mutations in the *PHOX2B* gene cause CCHS. The *PHOX2B* gene provides instructions for making a protein that acts early in development to help promote the formation of nerve cells (neurons) and regulate the process by which the neurons mature to carry out specific functions (differentiation). The protein is active in the neural crest, which is a group of cells in the early embryo that give rise to many tissues and organs. Neural crest cells migrate to form parts of the autonomic nervous system, many tissues in the face and skull, and other tissue and cell types.

Mutations are believed to interfere with the *PHOX2B* protein's role in promoting neuron formation and differentiation, especially in the autonomic nervous system, resulting in the problems regulating breathing and other body functions that occur in CCHS.

Inheritance Pattern for Congenital Central Hypoventilation Syndrome

This condition is inherited in an autosomal dominant pattern, which means one copy of the altered gene in each cell is sufficient to cause the disorder.

More than 90 percent of cases of CCHS result from new mutations in the *PHOX2B* gene. These cases occur in people with no history of the disorder in their family. Occasionally an affected person inherits the mutation from one affected parent. The number of such cases has been increasing as better treatment has allowed more affected individuals to live into adulthood.

About 5 to 10 percent of affected individuals inherit the mutation from a seemingly unaffected parent with somatic mosaicism. Somatic mosaicism means that some of the body's cells have a *PHOX2B* gene mutation, and others do not. A parent with mosaicism for a *PHOX2B* gene mutation may not show any signs or symptoms of CCHS.

Section 36.2

Obesity Hypoventilation Syndrome

This section includes text excerpted from "Obesity Hypoventilation Syndrome," National Heart, Lung, and Blood Institute (NHLBI), August 24, 2018.

It is not clear why obesity hypoventilation syndrome (OHS) affects some people who have obesity and not others. Extra fat on your neck or chest or across your abdomen can make it difficult to breathe deeply and may produce hormones that affect your body's breathing patterns. You may also have a problem with the way your brain controls your breathing. Most people who have OHS, also have sleep apnea.

You can help prevent this condition by maintaining a healthy weight. If you have been diagnosed with obesity, your doctor may screen you for OHS by measuring your blood oxygen or carbon dioxide levels.

If you have OHS, you may feel sluggish or sleepy during the day, have headaches, or feel out of breath. You or a loved one may notice you often snore loudly, choke or gasp, or have trouble breathing at night. Your symptoms may get worse over time. Complications of OHS include pulmonary hypertension; right heart failure, also known as "cor pulmonale;" and secondary erythrocytosis.

To diagnose OHS, your doctor will perform a physical exam to measure your weight and height, calculate your body mass index (BMI), and measure your waist and neck circumference. Your doctor may perform other tests, such as pulmonary function tests, sleep studies, a chest x-ray, or an arterial blood gas or serum bicarbonate test. Other blood tests may help rule out other causes or be used to plan your treatment. You may be diagnosed at the hospital if you have trouble breathing and go to the emergency room with respiratory failure. You may be diagnosed with tests routinely performed before surgery.

If you are diagnosed with OHS, your doctor may recommend healthy lifestyle changes, such as aiming for a healthy weight and being physically active. You may also need a continuous positive airway pressure (CPAP) machine or other breathing device to help keep your airways open and increase blood oxygen levels. Other treatments may include weight loss surgery, medicines, or a tracheostomy.

To prevent complications, use your CPAP device as instructed and continue with your doctor's recommended healthy lifestyle changes. Tell your doctor about new signs and symptoms, such as swelling around your ankles, chest pain, lightheadedness, or wheezing. Talk to your doctor if you will be flying or need surgery, as these situations can increase your risk for serious complications.

Chapter 37

Lymphangioleiomyomatosis

Lymphangioleiomyomatosis (LAM) is a rare lung disease that mostly affects women of childbearing age. In people with LAM, abnormal muscle-like cells begin to grow out of control in certain organs or tissues, especially the lungs, lymph nodes, and kidneys. Over time, these LAM cells can destroy the normal lung tissue. As a result, air cannot move freely in and out of the lungs. In some cases, this means the lungs cannot supply enough oxygen to the body's other organs.

There are two types of LAM. LAM that occurs sporadically is called "sporadic LAM." When LAM occurs in association with a rare disease called "tuberous sclerosis complex" (TSC), it is called "TSC-LAM." Doctors may diagnose LAM with imaging tests such as high-resolution computed tomography (CT) scans and blood tests for vascular endothelial growth factor D (VEGF-D). Other tests and procedures may be needed to diagnose LAM.

Doctors treat LAM with sirolimus (rapamycin), a medicine that stabilizes lung function, treats an abnormal fluid buildup in the lung called "chylothorax," and improves overall quality of life (QOL). They may also prescribe other medicines or therapies to control other symptoms or complications.

Lymphangioleiomyomatosis has no cure. It is important to get routine follow-up care because the disease tends to worsen over time. How quickly the disease worsens varies. More than half of women

---

This chapter includes text excerpted from "LAM," National Heart, Lung, and Blood Institute (NHLBI), October 30, 2015. Reviewed August 2019.

who have LAM will develop a serious condition called "pneumothorax," or "collapsed lung," that requires immediate treatment. Over time, LAM may cause permanent damage to the lungs and cause potentially fatal respiratory failure. Lung transplant is a treatment option for some women whose lungs have been severely damaged by LAM.

Causes of Lymphangioleiomyomatosis

Researchers do not know the exact cause of LAM or why it mainly affects women, but they believe genes and the female hormone estrogen play a role.

Genes

People with LAM or TSC-LAM have abnormal *TSC1* or *TSC2* genes. These genes are known to cause another rare genetic disease called "tuberous sclerosis complex" (TSC).

Abnormal *TSC* genes make proteins that cannot control cell growth and cell movement in the body. As a result, abnormal muscle-like cells begin to grow out of control in certain organs or tissues, such as the lungs, kidney, and lymph nodes. These abnormal cell growths cause the signs, symptoms, and complications of LAM.

Estrogen Hormone

Estrogen is thought to play a role in LAM because the condition:

- Primarily affects women

- Worsens in a pattern that matches up with a women's menstrual cycle, during pregnancy, and after using medicines such as birth control that contain estrogen

- Has been known to stop worsening in some women who have entered menopause

Risk Factors of Lymphangioleiomyomatosis

Lymphangioleiomyomatosis is a rare disease that mostly affects women of childbearing age. LAM can occur in older women as well, although this is less common. Women with tuberous sclerosis complex (TSC) have an increased risk of developing TSC-LAM.

In rare cases, LAM has been reported in men.

Signs, Symptoms, and Complications of Lymphangioleiomyomatosis

The uncontrolled growth of LAM cells and their effect on nearby body tissues causes the signs, symptoms, and complications of LAM. Symptoms tend to start when women are between the ages of 20 and 40.

Usually, TSC-LAM is milder than sporadic LAM and may not cause symptoms affecting the lungs. However, the severity of the disease varies from patient to patient and it is still possible for some women with sporadic LAM to also have mild disease without symptoms and some women with TSC-LAM to have more severe disease with worse symptoms and complications.

Signs

Signs of LAM are:

- Lung cysts detected by chest imaging tests
- Increased VEGF-D levels in the blood. VEGF-D is a vascular growth factor involved in tumor spread.
- Reduced lung function
- Reduced oxygen levels in the blood

Symptoms

The most common symptoms are:

- Chest pain or aches that may worsen when you breathe in
- Fatigue that may affect your overall QOL
- Frequent cough that may occur with bloody phlegm
- Shortness of breath that at first may occur only during high-energy activities but over time may happen after simple activities such as dressing and showering
- Wheezing or a whistling sound when you breathe

Complications

Possible complications of LAM include any of the following:

- **Angiomyolipomas and other tumors.** Many women who have LAM get tumors in their kidneys, called "angiomyolipomas."

415

Women who have LAM also may develop large tumors in the lymph node or growths in other organs such as the liver.

- **Blood in the urine.** This may occur in women who have kidney tumors.

- **Enlarged lymph nodes.** These usually occur in the abdomen or the chest. Very rarely, enlarged lymph nodes may occur in locations where they can be felt, such as the neck or under the arms.

- **Pleural effusions.** This condition can occur if bodily fluids collect in the space between the lung and the chest wall. Often the fluid contains a milky substance called "chylothorax." The excess fluid in the chest may cause shortness of breath because the lung has less room to expand.

- **Pneumothorax or collapsed lung.** This potentially life-threatening condition occurs when air leaks out of the lung and into the space between the lung and chest wall, an area called the "pleural space." In LAM, a pneumothorax can occur if lung cysts rupture through the lining of a lung. Air that collects in the space between the lung and chest wall must be removed to reinflate the lung. A collapsed lung can cause pain and shortness of breath. Sometimes one lung will collapse repeatedly. Pneumothorax usually requires urgent medical care and treatment.

- **Swelling or the buildup of fluid.** This can happen in the abdomen, pelvic area, legs, ankles, or feet. Pain may also occur with the swelling.

When a person has LAM, abnormal muscle-like cells begin to grow out of control in certain organs or tissues, especially the lungs, lymph nodes, and kidneys. Over time, these LAM cells can destroy the normal lung tissue. As a result, air no longer moves freely in and out of the lungs. In some cases, this means the lungs cannot supply enough oxygen to the body's other organs.

Diagnosis of Lymphangioleiomyomatosis

Methods for diagnosing LAM have improved, making it possible to diagnose the disease at an early stage. LAM is diagnosed based on your medical history and the results from diagnostic lung function tests, imaging tests such as high-resolution CT scans, VEGF-D blood tests, or other procedures. To help diagnose your condition, you may want to see a pulmonologist, a doctor who specializes in lung diseases and conditions, who has experience providing care to patients with LAM.

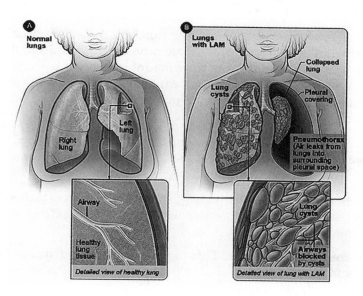

Figure 37.1. *Normal Lungs and Lungs with Lymphangioleiomyomatosis*

Figure A shows the location of the lungs and airways in the body. The inset image shows a cross-section of a healthy lung. Figure B shows a view of the lungs with LAM and a collapsed lung (pneumothorax). The inset image shows a cross-section of a lung with LAM.

Medical History

Your doctor will ask you about your medical history to see if you have signs and symptoms related to LAM. Your doctor may ask how long you have had symptoms and whether they have become worse over time.

Many women may not know they have it because many of LAM's signs and symptoms are the same as those of other diseases, such as asthma, emphysema, and bronchitis. But, your doctor will want to rule out those other conditions before making a final diagnosis.

Diagnostic Tests and Procedures

Your doctor may recommend tests to show how well your lungs are working and what your lung tissue looks like. These tests can show whether your lungs are delivering enough oxygen to your blood. You also may have tests to check for complications of LAM.

Lung Function Tests

- **Lung function tests.** For lung function tests, you breathe through a mouthpiece into a machine called a "spirometer." The spirometer measures the amount of air you breathe in and out. Other lung function tests can show how much air your lungs can hold and how well your lungs deliver oxygen to your blood.

- **Arterial blood gas tests.** Your doctor may take a blood sample from an artery in your wrist to measure your blood oxygen levels and to determine if you need oxygen therapy.

- **Pulse oximetry.** For this test, a small sensor is attached to your finger or ear. The sensor uses light to estimate how much oxygen is in your blood.

- **Six-minute walk test.** This test measures the distance you can walk in six minutes. It can help determine if you need oxygen therapy while exercising.

Imaging Tests

- **Chest x-ray.** A chest x-ray creates a picture of the structures in your chest, such as your heart and lungs. The test can show a collapsed lung or fluid in your chest. In the early stages of LAM, your chest x-rays may look normal. As the disease gets worse, the x-rays may detect cysts in your lungs and assess how cysts change over time.

- **High-resolution CT (HRCT) scan.** The most useful imaging test for diagnosing LAM is a high-resolution CT scan of the chest. This test creates a computer-generated picture of your lungs. The picture shows more detail than the pictures from a chest x-ray. An HRCT scan can show cysts, excess fluid, a collapsed lung, and enlarged lymph nodes. The test also can show how much normal lung tissue has been replaced by the LAM cysts. HRCT scans of your abdomen and pelvis can show whether you have growths in your kidneys, other abdominal organs, or lymph nodes.

Blood Tests for VEGF-D

Your doctor may take a blood sample from a vein in your arm to measure VEGF-D levels. The VEGF-D blood tests test may help confirm the diagnosis of LAM in patients whose HRCT scans show lung cysts that suggest a patient has LAM.

VEGF-D levels of 800 pg/mL (picograms per milliliter) or more can help your doctor confirm that you have LAM. Because you may still have LAM if your levels are less than 800 pg/mL, your doctor may have you undergo other diagnostic procedures that look for LAM cells.

Procedures That Look for LAM Cells

If lung function, imaging, or blood VEGF-D tests cannot diagnose LAM, your doctor may recommend one of the following procedures to collect tissue samples that can be used to detect LAM cells.

- **Video-assisted thoracoscopic surgery (VATS).** In this procedure, your doctor inserts a small, lighted tube into little cuts made in your chest wall. This lets him or her look inside your chest and snip out a few small pieces of lung tissue. VATS is done in a hospital. The procedure is not major surgery, but it does require general anesthesia to make you sleep during the procedure.

- **Open lung biopsy.** In this procedure, your doctor removes a few small pieces of lung tissue through a cut made in your chest wall between your ribs. An open lung biopsy is done in a hospital. You will be given medicine to make you sleep during the procedure. Open lung biopsies are rarely done anymore because the recovery time is much longer than the recovery time from VATS.

- **Transbronchial biopsy.** In this procedure, your doctor inserts a long, narrow, flexible, lighted tube down your windpipe and into your lungs. He or she then snips out bits of lung tissue using a tiny device. This procedure usually is done in a hospital. Your mouth and throat are numbed to prevent pain. Because only a small amount of tissue is collected, it is possible that this test will not provide enough information.

- **Other biopsies.** Your doctor also can diagnose LAM using the results from other tissue biopsies, such as biopsies of lymph nodes or abdominal or pelvic lesions.

Other Tests

If your chest imaging tests show that you have pleural effusions, your doctor may order a pleural fluid analysis. For this test, a fluid sample is taken from the pleural space, which is a thin space between two layers of tissue that line the lungs and chest cavity. Doctors use a procedure called "thoracentesis" to collect the fluid sample. The fluid is studied for the milky substance called "chylothorax."

If you are diagnosed with sporadic LAM, your doctor may advise you to have a CT scan or magnetic resonance imaging (MRI) scan of your head. These tests can help screen for underlying tuberous sclerosis complex (TSC), a condition that can also cause kidney growths and lung cysts. If a woman who has cysts in her lungs is found to have TSC, the doctor will diagnose TSC-associated LAM or TSC–LAM.

Treatment of Lymphangioleiomyomatosis

While there is no cure for LAM, doctors treat LAM with sirolimus (rapamycin), a medicine that stabilizes lung function, treats an abnormal fluid buildup in the lung called "chylothorax," and improves overall QOL. They may also prescribe other medicines or therapies to control other symptoms or complications.

You may want to see a pulmonologist doctor who specializes in lung diseases and conditions, especially LAM, to help treat your condition.

Medicines

Your doctor may prescribe sirolimus (rapamycin) to treat your condition, or bronchodilators or oxygen therapy to help you breathe better. Lung function tests can sometimes show whether these medicines are likely to help you.

- **Sirolimus (rapamycin).** Studies have shown that sirolimus helps regulate the abnormal growth and movement of LAM cells. Sirolimus stabilizes lung function and improves QOL, shrinks abnormal kidney and lymph node growths, and reduces abnormal fluid in the lung called "chylothorax." The latest clinical guidelines recommend sirolimus for people with LAM if they have abnormal or declining lung function or in some patients with LAM who have pleural effusions containing chylothorax. Sirolimus may also reduce the size of angiomyolipomas and, therefore, may be a treatment option before procedures that remove or shrink kidney tumors.

Sirolimus does have side effects, some of which can be serious. If you have LAM, talk with your doctor about the benefits and risks of this medicine, and whether it is an option for you.

- **Bronchodilators**. If you are having trouble breathing or are wheezing, your doctor may prescribe bronchodilators. These medicines relax the muscles around the airways. This helps the airways open up, making it easier for you to breathe.

- **Oxygen therapy**. If the level of oxygen in your blood is low, your doctor may suggest oxygen therapy. Oxygen usually is given through nasal prongs or a mask. At first, you may need oxygen only while exercising. It also may help to use it while sleeping. Over time, you may need full-time oxygen therapy.

The latest clinical guidelines, which are based on currently available clinical data, do not recommend the following medicines to treat LAM:

- **Doxycycline**, an antibiotic that did not show a clinical benefit when used to treat LAM.

- **Hormone therapies** including certain medicines—progestins, gonadotrophin-releasing hormone (GnRH) agonists, selective estrogen receptor modulators (SERMs) such as tamoxifen—or surgical procedures. While these therapies had previously been used to treat LAM, newer analyses suggest they do not produce clinical benefit in all patients with LAM. If you are taking any of these hormone medicines, talk to your doctor to see if you need to discontinue their use.

Procedures That Remove Air or Fluid from the Chest or Abdomen

Several procedures can remove excess air or fluid from your chest or abdomen. Removing fluid from your chest by thoracentesis or from your abdomen by paracentesis may help relieve discomfort and shortness of breath.

Your doctor often can remove the fluid with a needle and syringe. If large amounts of fluid build up in your chest, your doctor may have to insert a tube into your chest to remove the fluid.

Removing air from your chest may relieve shortness of breath and chest pain caused by a pneumothorax, or collapsed lung. Your doctor usually can remove the air with a tube. The tube is inserted into your chest between your side ribs. Often, the tube is attached to a suction device. If this procedure does not work, or if your lungs repeatedly collapse, you may need surgery.

If fluid or air often leak into your chest, your doctor may recommend a procedure called "pleurodesis" to prevent repeat episodes. Your doctor may inject a chemical at the site of the leakage. The chemical fuses your lung and chest wall together, which removes the space for leakage.

Your doctor may do this procedure at your bedside in the hospital. You will be given medicine to prevent pain. The procedure also can be done in an operating room using video-assisted thoracoscopy. In this case, you will be given medicine to make you sleep during the procedure.

Procedures That Remove or Shrink Kidney Tumors

Kidney tumors, or angiomyolipomas, often do not cause symptoms, but sometimes they can cause ongoing pain or bleeding. If this happens, you may need surgery to remove some of them. If bleeding is not too severe, a radiologist often can block the blood vessels feeding the kidney tumors. This may cause them to shrink.

Lung Transplant

Some patients who have severe lung damage due to advanced LAM may be eligible for lung transplants. While lung transplants can improve lung function and QOL for eligible patients, they have a high risk of complications, including infections and rejection of the transplanted lung by the body.

Studies suggest that more than three-quarters of women with LAM who receive a lung transplant survive for at least three years. In a few cases, doctors have found LAM cells in the newly transplanted lungs. However, the LAM cells generally do not stop the transplanted lung from working.

Living with Lymphangioleiomyomatosis

Not long ago, doctors thought women who had LAM would not live more than 10 years after diagnosis. With earlier diagnosis and newer treatment, patients with LAM are living longer, with some living more than 20 years after diagnosis.

For your follow-up care, you may want to see a pulmonologist, a doctor who specializes in lung diseases and conditions, and who has experience providing care to patients with LAM. Your doctor will monitor your condition to see if it is stable or getting worse and causing serious complications. Also, your doctor may recommend other medical care, including vaccines, lifestyle changes, and pregnancy and birth control planning.

Monitor Your Condition

If you have LAM, it is important for you to have routine follow-up care so your doctor can monitor your condition to see if it is stable or worsening. LAM has no cure, and the disease tends to worsen over time. How quickly the disease worsens varies between patients.

In the early stages of LAM, you usually can do your normal daily activities. These may include attending school, going to work, and doing common physical activities such as walking upstairs. In the later stages of LAM, you may find it harder to be active and you may need oxygen therapy.

Serious and possibly life-threatening complications can occur if you have LAM. More than half of women who have LAM develop pneumothorax, or collapsed lung. LAM may cause death from respiratory failure.

Lung Transplant is a treatment option for patients whose lungs have been damaged by LAM.

Receive Other Medical Care

In addition to monitoring your condition, your doctor may recommend emotional support to improve your QOL, vaccines to prevent lung infections, lifestyle changes to improve your overall health and avoid some complications, tests or medicines to care for your bones, and pregnancy and birth control options.

Emotional Support

Living with LAM may cause fear, anxiety, depression, and stress. Your doctor can evaluate how your condition is affecting your activity level and mental health. To improve your QOL, your doctor may recommend medicines to treat pain, fatigue, or mental-health concerns or serious depression that you may have.

Other steps you can take that may help include:

- Seeking support from family and friends to help relieve stress and anxiety. Let your loved ones know how you feel and what they can do to help you.

- Talking with your doctors or a professional counselor about how you feel

- Joining a patient support group to help you adjust to living with LAM

Vaccines for Lung Health

Take steps to care for your lungs. For example, talk with your doctor about getting a pneumococcal pneumonia vaccine and a yearly influenza or flu shot.

Lifestyle Changes

If you have LAM, taking good care of your health is important. Your doctor may recommend you adopt the following healthy lifestyle changes, many of which are also heart-healthy.

- Make healthy eating choices.

- Be physically active.

- Get plenty of rest.

- Quit smoking. Talk to your doctor about programs and products that can help you quit smoking. If you have trouble quitting smoking on your own, consider joining a support group. Many hospitals, workplaces, and community groups offer classes to help people quit smoking. Ask your family members and friends to support you in your efforts to quit.

Also, check with your doctor before traveling by air or traveling to areas where medical attention is not readily available. Also, talk to your doctor before traveling to places where the amount of oxygen in the air is low.

Care for Your Bones

Some women who have LAM may be at risk for osteoporosis if they have undergone permanent hormonal therapy such as oophorectomy or are receiving certain hormone therapy medicines. This is in part because many hormone therapies affect estrogen, and estrogen is important for keeping bones strong. While newer clinical guidelines do not recommend hormone therapies for the treatment of LAM, your doctor may order tests to measure your bone density if you have previously had an oophorectomy or are still on hormone therapies for other conditions. If you have lost bone density, your doctor may prescribe medicines or calcium and vitamin D supplements to prevent more bone loss.

Pregnancy and Birth Control Planning

Because hormone changes during pregnancy can worsen LAM, it is important to talk to your pulmonologist and obstetrician before you get pregnant.

Most doctors do not recommend birth control pills containing estrogen to women who have LAM because estrogen is thought to contribute to or worsen LAM. If you have LAM, talk to your doctors about birth-control options.

Chapter 38

Neuromuscular and Kidney Diseases That Impact Lung Function

Chapter Contents

Section 38.1

Amyotrophic Lateral Sclerosis

This section includes text excerpted from "Amyotrophic Lateral
Sclerosis (ALS) Fact Sheet," National Institute of Neurological
Disorders and Stroke (NINDS), May 14, 2019.

Amyotrophic lateral sclerosis (ALS) is a group of rare neurological diseases that mainly involve the nerve cells (neurons) responsible for controlling voluntary muscle movement. Voluntary muscles produce movements such as chewing, walking, and talking. The disease is progressive, meaning the symptoms get worse over time. As of now, there is no cure for ALS and no effective treatment to halt or reverse, the progression of the disease.

Amyotrophic lateral sclerosis belongs to a wider group of disorders known as "motor neuron diseases," which are caused by gradual deterioration (degeneration) and death of motor neurons. Motor neurons are nerve cells that extend from the brain to the spinal cord and to muscles throughout the body. These motor neurons initiate and provide vital communication links between the brain and the voluntary muscles.

Messages from motor neurons in the brain (called "upper motor neurons") are transmitted to motor neurons in the spinal cord and to motor nuclei of brain (called "lower motor neurons") and from the spinal cord and motor nuclei of the brain to a particular muscle or muscles.

In ALS, both the upper motor neurons and the lower motor neurons degenerate or die, and stop sending messages to the muscles. Unable to function, the muscles gradually weaken, start to twitch (called "fasciculations"), and waste away (atrophy). Eventually, the brain loses its ability to initiate and control voluntary movements.

Early symptoms of ALS usually include muscle weakness or stiffness. Gradually all muscles under voluntary control are affected, and individuals lose their strength and the ability to speak, eat, move, and even breathe.

Most people with ALS die from respiratory failure, usually within 3 to 5 years from when the symptoms first appear. However, about 10 percent of people with ALS survive for 10 or more years.

Who Gets Amyotrophic Lateral Sclerosis

In 2016 the Centers for Disease Control and Prevention (CDC) estimated that between 14,000 to 15,000 Americans have ALS. ALS is a common neuromuscular disease worldwide. It affects people of all races and ethnic backgrounds.

There are several potential risk factors for ALS including:

- **Age.** Although the disease can strike at any age, symptoms most commonly develop between the ages of 55 and 75.

- **Gender.** Men are slightly more likely than women to develop ALS. However, as we age, the difference between men and women disappears.

- **Race and ethnicity.** Most likely to develop the disease are Caucasians and non-Hispanics.

Some studies suggest that military veterans are about 1.5 to 2 times more likely to develop ALS. Although the reason for this is unclear, possible risk factors for veterans include exposure to lead, pesticides, and other environmental toxins. ALS is recognized as a service-connected disease by the U.S. Department of Veterans Affairs (VA).

Sporadic Amyotrophic Lateral Sclerosis

The majority of ALS cases (90% or more) are considered sporadic. This means the disease seems to occur at random with no clearly associated risk factors and no family history of the disease. Although family members of people with sporadic ALS are at an increased risk for the disease, the overall risk is very low and most will not develop amyotrophic lateral sclerosis.

Familial Amyotrophic Lateral Sclerosis

About 5 to 10 percent of all ALS cases are familial, which means that an individual inherits the disease from her or his parents. The familial form of ALS usually only requires one parent to carry the gene responsible for the disease. Mutations in more than a dozen genes have been found to cause familial ALS. About 25 to 40 percent of all familial cases (and a small percentage of sporadic cases) are caused by a defect in a gene known as *"chromosome 9 open reading frame 72,"* or *C9ORF72*. Interestingly, the same mutation can be associated with atrophy of frontal-temporal lobes of the brain causing frontal-temporal lobe dementia (FTD). Some individuals carrying this mutation may show signs of both motor neuron and dementia symptoms (ALS-FTD). Another 12 to 20 percent of familial cases result from mutations in the gene that provides instructions for the production of the enzyme copper-zinc superoxide dismutase 1 (*SOD1*).

What Are the Symptoms of Amyotrophic Lateral Sclerosis?

The onset of ALS can be so subtle that the symptoms are overlooked but gradually these symptoms develop into more obvious weakness or atrophy that may cause a physician to suspect ALS. Some of the early symptoms include:

- Fasciculations (muscle twitches) in the arm, leg, shoulder, or tongue

- Muscle cramps

- Tight and stiff muscles (spasticity)

- Muscle weakness affecting an arm, a leg, neck or diaphragm

- Slurred and nasal speech

- Difficulty chewing or swallowing

For many individuals, the first sign of ALS may appear in the hand or arm as they experience difficulty with simple tasks such as buttoning a shirt, writing, or turning a key in a lock. In other cases, symptoms initially affect one of the legs, and people experience awkwardness when walking or running or they notice that they are tripping or stumbling more often.

When symptoms begin in the arms or legs, it is referred to as "limb onset" ALS. Other individuals first notice speech or swallowing problems, termed "bulbar onset" ALS. Regardless of where the symptoms first appear, muscle weakness and atrophy spread to other parts of the body as the disease progresses. Individuals may develop problems with moving, swallowing (dysphagia), speaking or forming words (dysarthria), and breathing (dyspnea).

Although the sequence of emerging symptoms and the rate of disease progression vary from person to person, eventually individuals will not be able to stand or walk, get in or out of bed on their own, or use their hands and arms. Individuals with ALS usually have difficulty swallowing and chewing food, which makes it hard to eat normally and increases the risk of choking. They also burn calories at a faster rate than most people without ALS. Due to these factors, people with ALS tend to lose weight rapidly and can become malnourished.

Because people with ALS usually retain their ability to perform higher mental processes, such as reasoning, remembering, understanding, and problem solving, they are aware of their progressive loss of function and may become anxious and depressed. A small percentage of individuals may experience problems with language or decision-making, and there is growing evidence that some may even develop a form of dementia over time.

Individuals with ALS will have difficulty breathing as the muscles of the respiratory system weaken. They eventually lose the ability to breathe on their own and must depend on a ventilator. Affected individuals also face an increased risk of pneumonia during later stages of the disease. Besides muscle cramps that may cause discomfort, some individuals with ALS may develop painful neuropathy (nerve disease or damage).

How Is Amyotrophic Lateral Sclerosis Diagnosed?

No one test can provide a definitive diagnosis of ALS. ALS is primarily diagnosed based on detailed history of the symptoms and signs observed by a physician during physical examination along with a series of tests to rule out other mimicking diseases. However, the presence of upper and lower motor neuron symptoms strongly suggests the presence of the disease.

Physicians will review an individual's full medical history and conduct a neurologic examination at regular intervals to assess whether symptoms such as muscle weakness, atrophy of muscles, and spasticity are getting progressively worse.

Amyotrophic lateral sclerosis symptoms in the early stages of the disease can be similar to those of a wide variety of other, more treatable diseases or disorders. Appropriate tests can exclude the possibility of other conditions.

Muscle and Imaging Tests

Electromyography (EMG), a special recording technique that detects electrical activity of muscle fibers, can help diagnose ALS. Another common test is a nerve conduction study (NCS), which measures electrical activity of the nerves and muscles by assessing the nerve's ability to send a signal along the nerve or to the muscle. Specific abnormalities in the NCS and EMG may suggest, for example, that the individual has a form of peripheral neuropathy (damage to peripheral nerves outside of the brain and spinal cord) or myopathy (muscle disease) rather than ALS.

A physician may also order a magnetic resonance imaging (MRI) test, a noninvasive procedure that uses a magnetic field and radio waves to produce detailed images of the brain and spinal cord. Standard MRI scans are generally normal in people with ALS. However, they can reveal other problems that may be causing the symptoms, such as a spinal cord tumor, a herniated disk in the neck that compresses the spinal cord, syringomyelia (a cyst in the spinal cord), or cervical spondylosis (abnormal wear affecting the spine in the neck).

Laboratory Tests

Based on the person's symptoms, test results, and findings from the examination, a physician may order tests on blood and urine samples to eliminate the possibility of other diseases.

Tests for Other Diseases and Disorders

Infectious diseases such as human immunodeficiency virus (HIV), human T-cell leukemia virus (HTLV), polio, and West Nile virus can, in some cases, cause ALS-like symptoms. Neurological disorders such as multiple sclerosis (MS), post-polio syndrome (PPS), multifocal motor neuropathy, and spinal and bulbar muscular atrophy (Kennedy disease) also can mimic certain features of the disease and should be considered by physicians attempting to make a diagnosis. Fasciculations and muscle cramps also occur in benign conditions.

Because of the prognosis carried by this diagnosis and the variety of diseases or disorders that can resemble ALS in the early stages of the disease, individuals may wish to obtain a second neurological opinion.

What Causes Amyotrophic Lateral Sclerosis

The cause of ALS is not known, and scientists do not yet know why ALS strikes some people and not others. However, evidence from scientific studies suggests that both genetics and environment play a role in the development of ALS.

Genetics

An important step toward determining ALS risk factors was made in 1993 when scientists supported by the National Institute of Neurological Disorders and Stroke (NINDS) discovered that mutations in the *SOD1* gene were associated with some cases of familial ALS. Although it is still not clear how mutations in the *SOD1* gene lead to motor neuron degeneration, there is increasing evidence that the gene playing a role in producing mutant SOD1 protein can become toxic.

Since then, more than a dozen additional genetic mutations have been identified, many through NINDS-supported research, and each of these gene discoveries is providing new insights into possible mechanisms of amyotrophic lateral sclerosis.

The discovery of certain genetic mutations involved in ALS suggests that changes in the processing of ribonucleic acid (RNA) molecules may lead to ALS-related motor neuron degeneration. RNA molecules are one of the major macromolecules in the cell involved in directing the synthesis of specific proteins as well as gene regulation and activity.

Other gene mutations indicate defects in the natural process in which malfunctioning proteins are broken down and used to build new ones, known as "protein recycling." Still others point to possible defects in the structure and shape of motor neurons, as well as increased susceptibility to environmental toxins. Overall, it is becoming increasingly clear that a number of cellular defects can lead to motor neuron degeneration in amyotrophic lateral sclerosis.

In 2011 another important discovery was made when scientists found that a defect in the *C9ORF72* gene is not only present in a significant subset of individuals with ALS but also in some people with a type of frontotemporal dementia (FTD). This observation provides evidence for genetic ties between these two neurodegenerative disorders. Most researchers now believe ALS and some forms of FTD are related disorders.

Environmental Factors

In searching for the cause of ALS, researchers are also studying the impact of environmental factors. Researchers are investigating a number of possible causes such as exposure to toxic or infectious agents, viruses, physical trauma, diet, and behavioral and occupational factors.

For example, researchers have suggested that exposure to toxins during warfare, or strenuous physical activity, are possible reasons for why some veterans and athletes may be at increased risk of developing amyotrophic lateral sclerosis.

Although there has been no consistent association between any environmental factor and the risk of developing ALS, future research may show that some factors are involved in the development or progression of the disease.

How Is Amyotrophic Lateral Sclerosis Treated?

No cure has yet been found for ALS. However, there are treatments available that can help control symptoms, prevent unnecessary complications, and make living with the disease easier.

Supportive care is best provided by multidisciplinary teams of healthcare professionals such as physicians; pharmacists; physical, occupational, and speech therapists; nutritionists; social workers; respiratory therapists and clinical psychologists; and home care and hospice nurses. These teams can design an individualized treatment plan and provide special equipment aimed at keeping people as mobile, comfortable, and independent as possible.

Medication

The U.S. Food and Drug Administration (FDA) has approved the drugs riluzole (Rilutek) and edaravone (Radicava) to treat ALS. Riluzole is believed to reduce damage to motor neurons by decreasing levels of glutamate, which transports messages between nerve cells and motor neurons. Clinical trials in people with ALS showed that riluzole prolongs survival by a few months, particularly in the bulbar form of the disease, but does not reverse the damage already done to motor neurons. Edaravone has been shown to slow the decline in clinical assessment of daily functioning in persons with ALS.

Physicians can also prescribe medications to help manage symptoms of ALS, including muscle cramps, stiffness, excess saliva and phlegm, and the pseudobulbar affect (involuntary or uncontrollable episodes of crying and/or laughing, or other emotional displays). Drugs also are available to help individuals with pain, depression, sleep disturbances, and constipation. Pharmacists can give advice on the proper use of medications and monitor a person's prescriptions to avoid risks of drug interactions.

Physical Therapy

Physical therapy and special equipment can enhance an individual's independence and safety throughout the course of ALS. Gentle, low-impact aerobic exercise such as walking, swimming, and stationary bicycling can strengthen unaffected muscles, improve cardiovascular health, and help people fight fatigue and depression. Range of motion and stretching exercises can help prevent painful spasticity and shortening (contracture) of muscles.

Physical therapists can recommend exercises that provide these benefits without overworking muscles. Occupational therapists can suggest devices such as ramps, braces, walkers, and wheelchairs that help individuals conserve energy and remain mobile.

Speech Therapy

People with ALS who have difficulty speaking may benefit from working with a speech therapist, who can teach adaptive strategies to speak louder and more clearly. As ALS progresses, speech therapists can help people maintain the ability to communicate. They can recommend aids such as computer-based speech synthesizers that use eye-tracking technology and can help people develop ways for responding to yes-or-no questions with their eyes or by other nonverbal means.

Some people with ALS may choose to use voice banking while they are still able to speak as a process of storing their own voice for future use in computer-based speech synthesizers. These methods and devices help people communicate when they can no longer speak or produce vocal sounds.

Nutritional Support

Nutritional support is an important part of the care of people with ALS. It has been shown that individuals with ALS will get weaker if they lose weight. Nutritionists can teach individuals and caregivers how to plan and prepare small meals throughout the day that provide enough calories, fiber, and fluid and how to avoid foods that are difficult to swallow. People may begin using suction devices to remove excess fluids or saliva and prevent choking. When individuals can no longer get enough nourishment from eating, doctors may advise inserting a feeding tube into the stomach. The use of a feeding tube also reduces the risk of choking and pneumonia that can result from inhaling liquids into the lungs.

Breathing Support

As the muscles responsible for breathing start to weaken, people may experience shortness of breath during physical activity and difficulty breathing at night or when lying down. Doctors may test an individual's breathing to determine when to recommend a treatment called "noninvasive ventilation" (NIV). NIV refers to breathing support that is usually delivered through a mask over the nose and/or mouth.

Initially, NIV may only be necessary at night. When muscles are no longer able to maintain normal oxygen and carbon dioxide levels, NIV may be used full-time. NIV improves the quality of life (QOL) and prolongs survival for many people with amyotrophic lateral sclerosis.

Because the muscles that control breathing become weak, individuals with ALS may also have trouble generating a strong cough. There are several techniques to help people increase forceful coughing, including mechanical cough assist devices and breath stacking. In breath stacking, a person takes a series of small breaths without exhaling until the lungs are full, briefly holds the breath, and then expels the air with a cough.

As the disease progresses and muscles weaken further, individuals may consider forms of mechanical ventilation (respirators) in which a machine inflates and deflates the lungs. Doctors may place a breathing tube through the mouth or may surgically create a hole at the front of the neck and insert a tube leading to the windpipe (tracheostomy). The tube is connected to a respirator.

Individuals with ALS and their families often consider several factors when deciding whether and when to use ventilation support. These devices differ in their effect on a person's QOL and in cost. Although ventilation support can ease problems with breathing and prolong survival, it does not affect the progression of ALS. People may choose to be fully informed about these considerations and the long-term effects of life without movement before they make decisions about ventilation support.

Section 38.2

Goodpasture Syndrome

This section includes text excerpted from "Goodpasture Syndrome," National Institute of Diabetes and Digestive and Kidney Diseases (NIDDK), May 2012. Reviewed August 2019.

What Is Goodpasture Syndrome?

Goodpasture syndrome is a pulmonary-renal syndrome, which is a group of acute illnesses involving the kidneys and lungs. Goodpasture syndrome includes all of the following conditions:

- Glomerulonephritis—inflammation of the glomeruli, which are tiny clusters of looping blood vessels in the kidneys that help filter wastes and extra water from the blood

- The presence of anti-glomerular basement membrane (GBM) antibodies; the GBM is part of the glomeruli and is composed of collagen and other proteins

- Bleeding in the lungs

In Goodpasture syndrome, immune cells produce antibodies against a specific region of collagen. The antibodies attack the collagen in the lungs and kidneys.

Ernest Goodpasture first described the syndrome during the influenza pandemic of 1919 when he reported on a patient who died from bleeding in the lungs and kidney failure. Diagnostic tools to confirm Goodpasture syndrome were not available at that time, so it is not known whether the patient had true Goodpasture syndrome or vasculitis. Vasculitis is an autoimmune condition—a disorder in which the body's immune system attacks the body's own cells and organs—that involves inflammation in the blood vessels and can cause similar lung and kidney problems.

Goodpasture syndrome is sometimes called "anti-GBM disease." However, the anti-GBM disease is only one cause of pulmonary-renal syndromes, including Goodpasture syndrome.

Goodpasture syndrome is fatal unless quickly diagnosed and treated.

What Causes Goodpasture Syndrome

The causes of Goodpasture syndrome are not fully understood. People who smoke or use hair dyes appear to be at increased risk for this condition. Exposure to hydrocarbon fumes, metallic dust, and certain drugs, such as cocaine, may also raise a person's risk. Genetics may also play a part, as a small number of cases have been reported in more than one family member.

What Are the Symptoms of Goodpasture Syndrome?

The symptoms of Goodpasture syndrome may initially include fatigue, nausea, vomiting, and weakness. The lungs are usually affected before or at the same time as the kidneys, and symptoms can include shortness of breath and coughing, sometimes with blood. The progression from initial symptoms to the lungs being affected may be very rapid. Symptoms that occur when the kidneys are affected include blood in the urine or foamy urine, swelling in the legs, and high blood pressure.

How Is Goodpasture Syndrome Diagnosed?

A healthcare provider may order the following tests to diagnose Goodpasture syndrome:

- **Urinalysis.** Urinalysis is testing of a urine sample. The urine sample is collected in a special container in a healthcare provider's office or commercial facility and can be tested in the same location or sent to a lab for analysis. For the test, a nurse or technician places a strip of chemically treated paper, called a "dipstick," into the urine. Patches on the dipstick change color when protein or blood are present in urine. A high number of red blood cells and high levels of protein in the urine indicate kidney damage.

- **Blood test.** A blood test involves drawing blood at a healthcare provider's office or commercial facility and sending the sample to a lab for analysis. The blood test can show the presence of anti-GBM antibodies.

- **Chest x-ray.** An x-ray of the chest is performed in a healthcare provider's office, outpatient center, or hospital by an x-ray technician, and the images are interpreted by a radiologist—a doctor who specializes in medical imaging. Abnormalities in the lungs, if present, can be seen on the x-ray.

438

- **Biopsy.** A biopsy is a procedure that involves taking a piece of kidney tissue for examination with a microscope. The biopsy is performed by a healthcare provider in a hospital with light sedation and local anesthetic. The healthcare provider uses imaging techniques such as ultrasound or a computerized tomography scan to guide the biopsy needle into the kidney. The tissue is examined in a lab by a pathologist—a doctor who specializes in diagnosing diseases. The test can show crescent-shaped changes in the glomeruli and lines of antibodies attached to the GBM.

How Is Goodpasture Syndrome Treated?

Goodpasture syndrome is usually treated with

- **Immunosuppressive medications,** such as cyclophosphamide, to keep the immune system from making antibodies

- **Corticosteroid medications** to suppress the body's autoimmune response

- **Plasmapheresis**—a procedure that uses a machine to remove blood from the body, separate certain cells from the plasma, and return just the cells to the person's body; the anti-GBM antibodies remain in the plasma and are not returned to the person's body

Plasmapheresis is usually continued for several weeks, and immunosuppressive medications may be given for 6 to 12 months, depending on the response to therapy. In most cases, bleeding in the lungs stops and no permanent lung damage occurs. Damage to the kidneys, however, may be long-lasting. If the kidneys fail, blood-filtering treatments called "dialysis" or kidney transplantation may become necessary.

Section 38.3

Muscular Dystrophy

This section contains text excerpted from the following sources:
Text beginning with the heading "What Is Muscular Dystrophy?"
is excerpted from "Muscular Dystrophy," Centers for Disease
Control and Prevention (CDC), July 5, 2019; Text beginning with
the heading "What Causes Muscular Dystrophy" is excerpted from
"Muscular Dystrophy: Hope through Research," National Institute of
Neurological Disorders and Stroke (NINDS), May 7, 2019.

What Is Muscular Dystrophy?

Muscular dystrophies (MD) are a group of diseases caused by defects in a person's genes. Over time, this muscle weakness decreases mobility and makes the tasks of daily living difficult. There are many muscular dystrophies and the Centers for Disease Control and Prevention (CDC) studies the major types.

Different types of MD affect specific groups of muscles, have a specific age when signs and symptoms are first seen, vary in how severe they can be, and are caused by imperfections in different genes. MD can run in the family, or a person might be the first one in their family to have the condition.

Muscular dystrophy is rare, and there is not a lot of data on how many people are affected by the condition. Much of the information comes from outside the United States. Scientists at the CDC are working to estimate the number of people with each type of MD in the United States.

Types of Muscular Dystrophy

The major types of MD are:

- Duchenne/Becker (DMD/BMD)

- Myotonic (MMD)

- Limb-Girdle (LGMD)

- Facioscapulohumeral (FSH)

- Congenital (CMD) and myopathies

- Distal (DD)

- Oculopharyngeal (OPMD)

- Emery-Dreifuss (EDMD)

What Causes Muscular Dystrophy

All of the MD are inherited and involve a mutation in one of the thousands of genes that program proteins critical to muscle integrity. The body's cells do not work properly when a protein is altered or produced in insufficient quantity (or sometimes missing completely). Many cases of MD occur from spontaneous mutations that are not found in the genes of either parent, and this defect can be passed to the next generation.

Genes are like blueprints: they contain coded messages that determine a person's characteristics or traits. They are arranged along 23 rod-like pairs of chromosomes with one half of each pair being inherited from each parent. Each half of a chromosome pair is similar to the other, except for one pair, which determines the sex of the individual. Muscular dystrophies can be inherited in three ways:

- **Autosomal dominant inheritance** occurs when a child receives a normal gene from one parent and a defective gene from the other parent. Autosomal means the genetic mutation can occur on any of the 22 nonsex chromosomes in each of the body's cells. Dominant means only one parent is needed to pass along the abnormal gene in order to produce the disorder. In families where one parent carries a defective gene, each child has a 50 percent chance of inheriting the gene and, therefore, the disorder. Males and females are equally at risk and the severity of the disorder can differ from person to person.

- **Autosomal recessive inheritance** means that both parents must carry and pass on the faulty gene. The parents each have one defective gene but are not affected by the disorder. Children in these families have a 25 percent chance of inheriting both copies of the defective gene and a 50 percent chance of inheriting one gene and, therefore, becoming a carrier, able to pass along the defect to their children. Children of either sex can be affected by this pattern of inheritance.

- **X-linked (or sex-linked) recessive inheritance** occurs when a mother carries the affected gene on one of her two X chromosomes and passes it to her son (males always inherit an X chromosome from their mother and a Y chromosome from their father, while daughters inherit an X chromosome from each parent). Sons of carrier mothers have a 50 percent chance of inheriting the disorder. Daughters also have a 50 percent chance of inheriting the defective gene but usually are not affected, since the healthy X chromosome they receive from their father can offset the faulty one received from their mother. Affected fathers cannot pass an X-linked disorder to their sons but their daughters will be carriers of that disorder. Carrier females occasionally can exhibit milder symptoms of MD.

How Many People Have Muscular Dystrophy?

Muscular dystrophy occurs worldwide, affecting all races. Its incidence varies, as some forms are more common than others. Its most common form in children, Duchenne muscular dystrophy, affects approximately 1 in every 3,500 to 6,000 male births each year in the United States. Some types of MD are more prevalent in certain countries and regions of the world. Many muscular dystrophies are familial, meaning there is some family history of the disease. Duchenne cases often have no prior family history. This is likely due to the large size of the dystrophin gene that is implicated in the disorder, making it a target for spontaneous mutations.

How Does Muscular Dystrophy Affect Muscles?

Muscles are made up of thousands of muscle fibers. Each fiber is actually a number of individual cells that have joined together during development and are encased by an outer membrane. Muscle fibers that make up individual muscles are bound together by connective tissue.

Muscles are activated when an impulse, or signal, is sent from the brain through the spinal cord and peripheral nerves (nerves that connect the central nervous system to sensory organs and muscles) to the neuromuscular junction (the space between the nerve fiber and the muscle it activates). There, a release of the chemical acetylcholine triggers a series of events that cause the muscle to contract.

The muscle fiber membrane contains a group of proteins—called the "dystrophin-glycoprotein complex"—which prevents damage as muscle fibers contract and relax. When this protective membrane is damaged, muscle fibers begin to leak the protein creatine kinase (needed for the chemical reactions that produce energy for muscle contractions) and take on excess calcium, which causes further harm. Affected muscle fibers eventually die from this damage, leading to progressive muscle degeneration.

Although MD can affect several body tissues and organs, it most prominently affects the integrity of muscle fibers. The disease causes muscle degeneration, progressive weakness, fiber death, fiber branching and splitting, phagocytosis (in which muscle fiber material is broken down and destroyed by scavenger cells), and, in some cases, chronic or permanent shortening of tendons and muscles. Also, overall muscle strength and tendon reflexes are usually lessened or lost due to replacement of muscle by connective tissue and fat.

How Are the Muscular Dystrophies Diagnosed?

Both the individual's medical history and a complete family history should be thoroughly reviewed to determine if the muscle disease is secondary to a disease affecting other tissues or organs or is an inherited condition. It is also important to rule out any muscle weakness resulting from prior surgery, exposure to toxins, or current medications that may affect the person's functional status or rule out many acquired muscle diseases. Thorough clinical and neurological exams can rule out disorders of the central and/or peripheral nervous systems, identify any patterns of muscle weakness and atrophy, test reflex responses and coordination, and look for contractions.

Various laboratory tests may be used to confirm the diagnosis of MD.

Blood and Urine Tests

Blood and urine tests can detect defective genes and help identify specific neuromuscular disorders. For example:

- Creatine kinase is an enzyme that leaks out of damaged muscle. Elevated creatine kinase levels may indicate muscle damage, including some forms of MD, before physical symptoms become apparent. Levels are significantly increased in the early stages of Duchenne and Becker MD. Testing can also determine if a young woman is a carrier of the disorder.

- The level of serum aldolase, an enzyme involved in the breakdown of glucose, is measured to confirm a diagnosis of skeletal muscle disease. High levels of the enzyme, which is present in most body tissues, are noted in people with MD and some forms of myopathy.

- Myoglobin is measured when injury or disease in skeletal muscle is suspected. Myoglobin is an oxygen-binding protein found in cardiac and skeletal muscle cells. High blood levels of myoglobin are found in people with MD.

- Polymerase chain reaction (PCR) can detect some mutations in the dystrophin gene. Also known as "molecular diagnosis" or "genetic testing," PCR is a method for generating and analyzing multiple copies of a fragment of DNA.

- Serum electrophoresis is a test to determine quantities of various proteins in a person's DNA. A blood sample is placed on specially treated paper and exposed to an electric current. The charge forces the different proteins to form bands that indicate the relative proportion of each protein fragment.

Exercise Tests

Exercise tests can detect elevated rates of certain chemicals following exercise and are used to determine the nature of the MD or other muscle disorder. Some exercise tests can be performed bedside while others are done at clinics or other sites using sophisticated equipment. These tests also assess muscle strength. They are performed when the person is relaxed and in the proper position to allow technicians to measure muscle function against gravity and detect even slight muscle weakness. If weakness in respiratory muscles is suspected, respiratory capacity may be measured by having the person take a deep breath and count slowly while exhaling.

Diagnostic Imaging

Diagnostic imaging can help determine the specific nature of a disease or condition. One such type of imaging, called "magnetic resonance imaging" (MRI), is used to examine muscle quality, any atrophy or abnormalities in size, and fatty replacement of muscle tissue, as well as to monitor disease progression. MRI scanning equipment creates a strong magnetic field around the body. Radio waves are then passed through the body to trigger a resonance signal that can be detected at different angles within the body. A computer processes this resonance into either a three-dimensional picture or a two-dimensional "slice" of the tissue being scanned. MRI is a noninvasive, painless procedure. Other forms of diagnostic imaging for MD include phosphorus magnetic resonance spectroscopy, which measures cellular response to exercise and the amount of energy available to muscle fiber, and ultrasound imaging (also known as "sonography"), which uses high-frequency sound waves to obtain images inside the body. The sound wave echoes are recorded and displayed on a computer screen as a real-time visual image. Ultrasound may be used to measure muscle bulk. MRI scans of the brain may be useful in diagnosing certain forms of congenital muscular dystrophy where structural brain abnormalities are typically present.

Muscle Biopsies

Muscle biopsies are used for diagnostic purposes, and in research settings, to monitor the course of disease and treatment effectiveness. Using local or general anesthesia, a physician or surgeon can remove a small sample of muscle for analysis. The sample may be gathered either surgically, through a slit made in the skin, or by needle biopsy, in which a thin hollow needle is inserted through the skin and into the muscle. A small piece of muscle remains in the hollow needle when it is removed from the body. The muscle specimen is stained and examined to determine whether the person has muscle disease, nerve disease (neuropathy), inflammation, or another myopathy. Muscle biopsies can sometimes also assist in carrier testing. With the advent of accurate molecular techniques, muscle biopsy is less frequently needed to diagnose muscular dystrophies. Muscle biopsy is still necessary to make the diagnosis in most of the acquired muscle diseases.

Immunofluorescence

Immunofluorescence testing can detect specific proteins such as dystrophin within muscle fibers. Following biopsy, fluorescent markers are used to stain the sample that has the protein of interest.

Electron Microscopy

Electron microscopy can identify changes in subcellular components of muscle fibers. Electron microscopy can also identify changes that characterize cell death, mutations in muscle cell mitochondria, and an increase in connective tissue seen in muscle diseases such as MD. Changes in muscle fibers that are evident in a rare form of distal MD can be seen using an electron microscope.

Neurophysiology Studies

Neurophysiology studies can identify physical and/or chemical changes in the nervous system.

- **Nerve conduction velocity studies** measure the speed and strength with which an electrical signal travels along a nerve. A small surface electrode stimulates a nerve, and a recording electrode detects the resulting electrical signal either elsewhere on the same nerve or on a muscle controlled by that nerve. The response can be assessed to determine whether nerve damage is present.

- **Repetitive stimulation studies** involve electrically stimulating a motor nerve several times in a row to assess the function of the neuromuscular junction. The recording electrode is placed on a muscle controlled by the stimulated nerve, as is done for a routine motor nerve conduction study.

- **Electromyography (EMG)** can record muscle fiber and motor unit activity. A tiny needle containing an electrode is inserted through the skin into the muscle. The electrical activity detected in the muscle can be displayed on a monitor, and can also be heard when played through a speaker. Results may reveal electrical activity characteristic of MD or other neuromuscular disorders.

How Are the Muscular Dystrophies Treated?

There is no specific treatment that can stop or reverse the progression of any form of MD. All forms of MD are genetic and cannot be prevented at this time, aside from the use of prenatal screening interventions. However, available treatments are aimed at keeping the person independent for as long as possible and prevent complications that result from weakness, reduced mobility, and cardiac and respiratory difficulties. Treatment may involve a combination of approaches, including physical therapy, drug therapy, and surgery. The available treatments are sometimes quite effective and can have a significant impact on life expectancy and quality of life.

Assisted Ventilation

Assisted ventilation is often needed to treat respiratory muscle weakness that accompanies many forms of MD, especially in the later stages. Air that includes supplemental oxygen is fed through a flexible mask (or, in some cases, a tube inserted through the esophagus and into the lungs) to help the lungs inflate fully. Since respiratory difficulty may be most extreme at night, some individuals may need overnight ventilation. Many people prefer noninvasive ventilation, in which a mask worn over the face is connected by a tube to a machine that generates intermittent bursts of forced air that may include supplemental oxygen. Some people with Duchenne MD, especially those who are overweight, may develop obstructive sleep apnea and require nighttime ventilation. Individuals on a ventilator may also require the use of a gastric feeding tube.

Drug Therapy

Drug therapy may be prescribed to delay muscle degeneration. Corticosteroids such as prednisone can slow the rate of muscle deterioration in Duchenne MD and help children retain strength and prolong independent walking by as much as several years. However, these medicines have side effects such as weight gain, facial changes, loss of linear (height) growth, and bone fragility that can be especially troubling in children. Immunosuppressive drugs such as cyclosporine and azathioprine can delay some damage to dying muscle cells. Drugs that may provide short-term relief from myotonia (muscle spasms and weakness) include mexiletine; phenytoin; baclofen, which blocks signals sent from the spinal cord to contract the muscles; dantrolene, which interferes with the process of muscle contraction; and quinine. The Food and Drug Administration has granted accelerated approval of the drug Exondys 51 to treat individuals who have a confirmed mutation of the dystrophin gene amenable to exon 15 skipping. The accelerated approval means the drug can be administered to selected individuals who meet the rare disease criteria while the company works on additional trials to learn more about the effectiveness of the drug. Drugs for myotonia may not be effective in myotonic MD but work well for myotonia congenita, a genetic neuromuscular disorder characterized by the slow relaxation of the muscles. Respiratory infections may be treated with antibiotics.

Physical Therapy

Physical therapy can help prevent deformities, improve movement, and keep muscles as flexible and strong as possible. Options include passive stretching, postural correction, and exercise. A program is developed to meet the individual's needs. Therapy should begin as soon as possible following diagnosis, before there is joint or muscle tightness.

- Passive stretching can increase joint flexibility and prevent contractures that restrict movement and cause loss of function.

When done correctly, passive stretching is not painful. The therapist or other trained health professional slowly moves the joint as far as possible and maintain the position for about 30 seconds. The movement is repeated several times during the session. Passive stretching on children may be easier following a warm bath or shower.

- Regular, moderate exercise can help people with MD maintain range of motion and muscle strength, prevent muscle atrophy, and delay the development of contractures. Individuals with a weakened diaphragm can learn coughing and deep breathing exercises that are designed to keep the lungs fully expanded.

- Postural correction is used to counter the muscle weakness, contractures, and spinal irregularities that force individuals with MD into uncomfortable positions. When possible, individuals should sit upright, with feet at a 90-degree angle to the floor. Pillows and foam wedges can help keep the person upright, distribute weight evenly, and cause the legs to straighten. Armrests should be at the proper height to provide support and prevent leaning.

- Support aids such as wheelchairs, splints and braces, other orthopedic appliances, and overhead bed bars (trapezes) can help maintain mobility. Braces are used to help stretch muscles and provide support while keeping the person ambulatory. Spinal supports can help delay scoliosis. Night splints, when used in conjunction with passive stretching, can delay contractures. Orthotic devices such as standing frames and swivel walkers help people remain standing or walking for as long as possible, which promotes better circulation and improves calcium retention in bones.

- Repeated low-frequency bursts of electrical stimulation to the thigh muscles may produce a slight increase in strength in some boys with Duchenne MD, though this therapy has not been proven to be effective.

Occupational Therapy

Occupational therapy may help some people deal with progressive weakness and loss of mobility. Some individuals may need to learn new job skills or new ways to perform tasks while other persons may need to change jobs. Assistive technology may include modifications to home and workplace settings and the use of motorized wheelchairs, wheelchair accessories, and adaptive utensils.

Speech Therapy

Speech therapy may help individuals whose facial and throat muscles have weakened. Individuals can learn to use special communication devices, such as a computer with voice synthesizer

Dietary Changes

Dietary changes have not been shown to slow the progression of MD. Proper nutrition is essential, however, for overall health. Limited mobility or inactivity resulting from muscle weakness can contribute to obesity, dehydration, and constipation. A high-fiber, high-protein, low-calorie diet combined with recommended fluid intake may help. Feeding techniques can help people with MD who have a swallowing disorder and find it difficult to pass from or liquid from the mouth to the stomach.

What Is the Prognosis for Muscular Dystrophy?

The prognosis varies according to the type of MD and the speed of progression. Some types are mild and progress very slowly, allowing normal life expectancy, while others are more severe and result in functional disability and loss of ambulation. Life expectancy often depends on the degree of muscle weakness, as well as the presence and severity of respiratory and/or cardiac complications.

Section 38.4

Myasthenia Gravis

This section includes text excerpted from "Myasthenia Gravis
Fact Sheet," National Institute of Neurological Disorders
and Stroke (NINDS), May 2017.

Myasthenia gravis is a chronic autoimmune neuromuscular disease that causes weakness in the skeletal muscles, which are responsible for breathing and moving parts of the body, including the arms and legs.

The hallmark of myasthenia gravis is muscle weakness that worsens after periods of activity and improves after periods of rest. Certain muscles such as those that control eye and eyelid movement, facial expression, chewing, talking, and swallowing are often (but not always) involved in the disorder. The muscles that control breathing and neck and limb movements may also be affected.

There is no known cure but with available therapies most cases of myasthenia gravis are not as "grave" as the name implies. Available treatments can control symptoms and often allow people to have a relatively high QOL. Most individuals with the condition have a normal life expectancy.

What Causes Myasthenia Gravis

Myasthenia gravis is caused by an error in the transmission of nerve impulses to muscles. It occurs when normal communication between the nerve and muscle is interrupted at the neuromuscular junction—the place where nerve cells connect with the muscles they control.

Neurotransmitters are chemicals that neurons, or brain cells, use to communicate information. Normally when electrical signals or impulses travel down a motor nerve, the nerve endings release a neurotransmitter called "acetylcholine." Acetylcholine travels from the nerve ending and binds to acetylcholine receptors on the muscle. The binding of acetylcholine to its receptor activates the muscle and causes a muscle contraction.

In myasthenia gravis, antibodies (immune proteins) block, alter, or destroy the receptors for acetylcholine at the neuromuscular junction, which prevents the muscle from contracting. In most individuals with myasthenia gravis, this is caused by antibodies to the acetylcholine receptor itself. However, antibodies to other proteins, such as muscle-specific kinase (MuSK) protein, can also lead to impaired transmission at the neuromuscular junction.

These antibodies are produced by the body's own immune system. Myasthenia gravis is an autoimmune disease because the immune system—which normally protects the body from foreign organisms—mistakenly attacks itself.

The thymus is a gland that controls immune function and maybe associated with myasthenia gravis. Located in the chest behind the breast bone, the gland is largest in children. It grows gradually until puberty, and then gets smaller and is replaced by fat. Throughout childhood, the thymus plays an important role in the development of the immune system because it is responsible for producing T-lymphocytes or T cells, a specific type of white blood cell that protects the body from viruses and infections.

In many adults with myasthenia gravis, the thymus gland remains large. People with the disease typically have clusters of immune cells in their thymus gland similar to lymphoid hyperplasia—a condition that usually only happens in the spleen and lymph nodes during an active immune response. Some individuals with myasthenia gravis develop thymomas (tumors of the thymus gland). Thymomas are most often harmless, but they can become cancerous.

The thymus gland plays a role in myasthenia gravis, but its function is not fully understood. Scientists believe that the thymus gland may give incorrect instructions to developing immune cells, ultimately causing the immune system to attack its own cells and tissues and produce acetylcholine receptor antibodies—setting the stage for the attack on neuromuscular transmission.

What Are the Symptoms of Myasthenia Gravis?

Although myasthenia gravis may affect any skeletal muscle, muscles that control eye and eyelid movement, facial expression, and swallowing are most frequently affected. The onset of the disorder may be sudden and symptoms often are not immediately recognized as myasthenia gravis.

In most cases, the first noticeable symptom is weakness of the eye muscles. In others, difficulty swallowing and slurred speech may be the first signs. The degree of muscle weakness involved in myasthenia gravis varies greatly among individuals, ranging from a localized form limited to eye muscles (ocular myasthenia), to a severe or generalized form in which many muscles—sometimes including those that control breathing—are affected.

Symptoms may include:

- Drooping of one or both eyelids (ptosis)
- Blurred or double vision (diplopia) due to weakness of the muscles that control eye movements
- A change in facial expression
- Difficulty swallowing
- Shortness of breath
- Impaired speech (dysarthria)
- Weakness in the arms, hands, fingers, legs, and neck

Who Gets Myasthenia Gravis

Myasthenia gravis affects both men and women and occurs across all racial and ethnic groups. It most commonly impacts young adult women (under 40) and older men (over 60), but it can occur at any age, including childhood. Myasthenia gravis is not inherited nor is it contagious. Occasionally, the disease may occur in more than one member of the same family.

Although myasthenia gravis is rarely seen in infants, the fetus may acquire antibodies from a mother affected with myasthenia gravis—a condition called "neonatal myasthenia." Generally, neonatal myasthenia gravis is temporary and the child's symptoms usually disappear within two to three months after birth. Rarely, children of a healthy mother may develop congenital myasthenia. This is not an autoimmune disorder. It is caused by defective genes that produce abnormal proteins in the neuromuscular junction and can cause similar symptoms to myasthenia gravis.

How Is Myasthenia Gravis Diagnosed?

A doctor may perform or order several tests to confirm the diagnosis, including:

- **A physical and neurological examination.** A physician will first review an individual's medical history and conduct a physical examination. In a neurological examination, the physician will check muscle strength and tone, coordination, sense of touch, and look for impairment of eye movements.

- **An edrophonium test.** This test uses injections of edrophonium chloride to briefly relieve weakness in people with myasthenia gravis. The drug blocks the breakdown of acetylcholine and temporarily increases the levels of acetylcholine at the neuromuscular junction. It is usually used to test ocular muscle weakness.

- **A blood test.** Most individuals with myasthenia gravis have abnormally elevated levels of acetylcholine receptor antibodies. A second antibody—called the "anti-MuSK antibody"—has been found in about half of individuals with myasthenia gravis who do not have acetylcholine receptor antibodies. A blood test can also detect this antibody. However, in some individuals with myasthenia gravis, neither of these antibodies is present. These individuals are said to have seronegative (negative antibody) myasthenia.

- **Electrodiagnostics.** Diagnostic tests include repetitive nerve stimulation, which repeatedly stimulates a person's nerves with small pulses of electricity to tire specific muscles. Muscle fibers in myasthenia gravis, as well as other neuromuscular disorders, do not respond as well to repeated electrical stimulation compared to muscles from normal individuals. Single fiber electromyography (EMG), considered the most sensitive test for myasthenia gravis, detects impaired nerve-to-muscle transmission. EMG can be very helpful in diagnosing mild cases of myasthenia gravis when other tests fail to demonstrate abnormalities.

- **Diagnostic imaging.** Diagnostic imaging of the chest using computed tomography (CT) or magnetic resonance imaging (MRI) may identify the presence of a thymoma.

- **Pulmonary function testing.** Measuring breathing strength can help predict if respiration may fail and lead to a myasthenic crisis.

Because weakness is a common symptom of many other disorders, the diagnosis of myasthenia gravis is often missed or delayed (sometimes up to two years) in people who experience mild weakness or in those individuals whose weakness is restricted to only a few muscles.

What Is a Myasthenic Crisis?

A myasthenic crisis is a medical emergency that occurs when the muscles that control breathing weaken to the point where individuals require a ventilator to help them breathe.

Approximately 15 to 20 percent of people with myasthenia gravis experience at least one myasthenic crisis. This condition usually requires immediate medical attention and may be triggered by infection, stress, surgery, or an adverse reaction to medication. However, up to one-half of people may have no obvious cause for their myasthenic crisis. Certain medications have been shown to cause myasthenia gravis. However, sometimes these medications may still be used if it is more important to treat an underlying condition.

How Is Myasthenia Gravis Treated?

Myasthenia gravis can generally be controlled. There are several therapies available to help reduce and improve muscle weakness.

- **Thymectomy.** This operation to remove the thymus gland (which often is abnormal in individuals with myasthenia gravis) can reduce symptoms and may cure some people, possibly by rebalancing the immune system. A National Institute of Neurological Disorders and Stroke (NINDS)-funded study found that thymectomy is beneficial both for people with thymoma and those with no evidence of the tumors. The clinical trial followed 126 people with myasthenia gravis and no visible thymoma and found that the surgery reduced muscle weakness and the need for immunosuppressive drugs.

- **Anticholinesterase medications.** Medications to treat the disorder include anticholinesterase agents such as mestinon or pyridostigmine, which slow the breakdown of acetylcholine at the neuromuscular junction and thereby improve neuromuscular transmission and increase muscle strength.

- **Immunosuppressive drugs.** These drugs improve muscle strength by suppressing the production of abnormal antibodies. They include prednisone, azathioprine, mycophenolate mofetil, tacrolimus, and rituximab. The drugs can cause significant side effects and must be carefully monitored by a physician.

- **Plasmapheresis and intravenous immunoglobulin.** These therapies may be options in severe cases of myasthenia gravis. Individuals can have antibodies in their plasma (a liquid component in blood) that attack the neuromuscular junction. These treatments remove the destructive antibodies, although their effectiveness usually only lasts for a few weeks to months.

- **Plasmapheresis** is a procedure using a machine to remove harmful antibodies in plasma and replace them with good plasma or a plasma substitute.

- **Intravenous immunoglobulin** is a highly concentrated injection of antibodies pooled from many healthy donors that temporarily changes the way the immune system operates. It works by binding to the antibodies that cause myasthenia gravis and removing them from circulation.

What Is the Prognosis for Myasthenia Gravis?

With treatment, most individuals with myasthenia can significantly improve their muscle weakness and lead full lives. Sometimes the severe weakness of myasthenia gravis may cause respiratory failure, which requires immediate emergency medical care.

Some cases of myasthenia gravis may go into remission—either temporarily or permanently—and muscle weakness may disappear completely so that medications can be discontinued. Stable, long-lasting complete remissions are the goal of thymectomy and may occur in about 50 percent of individuals who undergo this procedure.

Part Five

Pediatric
Respiratory Disorders

Chapter 39

Asthma in Children

Asthma is a serious disease causing wheezing, difficulty breathing, and coughing. Over a lifetime, it can cause permanent lung damage. About 16 percent of Black children and 7 percent of White children have asthma. While it is not known what causes asthma, it is known how to prevent asthma attacks or at least make them less severe. Nowadays, children with asthma and their caregivers report fewer attacks, missed school days, and hospital visits. More children with asthma are learning to control their asthma using an asthma action plan. Still, more than half of children with asthma had one or more attacks in 2016. Every year, 1 in 6 children with asthma visits the Emergency Department with about 1 in 20 children with asthma hospitalized for asthma.

Doctors, nurses, and other healthcare providers are:

- Teaching children and parents to manage asthma by using a personalized action plan shared with school staff and other caregivers. Such a plan helps children use medicine properly and avoid asthma triggers such as tobacco smoke, pet dander, and air pollution.

- Working with community health workers, pharmacists, and others to ensure that children with asthma receive needed services

This chapter includes text excerpted from "Asthma in Children," Centers for Disease Control and Prevention (CDC), May 10, 2018.

- Working with children and parents to assess each child's asthma, prescribe appropriate medicines, and determine whether home health visits would help prevent attacks

Problem of Asthma in Children

Half of the children with asthma had 1 or more attacks in 2016. Asthma attacks are going down but, there are still too many.

- Attacks have gone down in children of all races and ethnicities from 2001 through 2016.

- About 50 percent of children with asthma had an attack in 2016.

- Asthma attacks occurred most frequently among children younger than age 5 in 2016.

- Emergency Department and urgent care center visits related to asthma attacks were highest among children ages 0 to 4 years and Non-Hispanic Black children.

Using medicine as prescribed can prevent asthma attacks.

- Inhaled corticosteroids and other control medicines can prevent asthma attacks.

- Rescue inhalers or nebulizers can give quick relief of symptoms

- But about half of children who are prescribed asthma control medicines do not use them regularly.

What Can Be Done to Prevent Asthma in Children
The Role of Federal Government

The federal government is:

- Working with state, territorial, private, and nongovernment partners to support medical management, asthma self-management education, and, for people at high risk, home visits to reduce triggers and help with asthma management

- Providing guidelines, tools such as asthma action plans, and educational messages to help children, their caregivers, and healthcare professionals better manage asthma

- Promoting policies and best practices to reduce exposure to indoor and outdoor asthma triggers such as tobacco smoke and air pollution

- Tracking asthma rates and assuring efficient and effective use of resources invested in asthma services

The Role of Healthcare Providers

The doctors, nurses, and other healthcare providers are:

- Teaching children and parents to manage asthma by using a personalized action plan shared with school staff and other caregivers. Such a plan helps children use medicine properly and avoid asthma triggers such as tobacco smoke, pet dander, and air pollution.
- Working with community health workers, pharmacists, and others to ensure that children with asthma receive needed services
- Working with children and parents to assess each child's asthma, prescribe appropriate medicines, and determine whether home health visits would help prevent attacks

The Role of Payers and Health Insurance Providers

Some payers and health insurance plans are:

- Reimbursing healthcare providers for the education of children with asthma, including development of their personalized asthma action plans
- Providing training and incentives for healthcare providers to practice guidelines-based medical management
- Taking actions to improve access to and proper use of asthma medications and devices
- Providing each child with asthma with the medical and community-based services needed to control her or his asthma

The Role of Children and Parents

Parents and children are:

- Learning about asthma, how to manage it, and how to recognize the warning signs of an asthma attack
- Taking steps to reduce asthma triggers such as tobacco smoke, mold, and pet dander in the home. If caregivers smoke, they should try to quit or at least never smoke around children.

461

- Making sure children use their asthma controller medicine as prescribed
- Communicating with schools, other family members, caregivers, and healthcare providers about the child's asthma action plan and about asthma symptoms

The Role of School

Schools are:

- Educating school nurses and other school staff about asthma and how to help children control it
- Carrying out asthma-friendly policies to help children follow their action plans, including stocking quick-relief medications, letting older children carry controller and rescue medicines, and helping children take part in school activities, such as exercising indoors when air quality is poor

Chapter 40

Bronchopulmonary Dysplasia

Bronchopulmonary dysplasia, or BPD, is a serious lung condition that affects newborns. BPD mostly affects premature newborns who need oxygen therapy, which is oxygen given through nasal prongs, a mask, or a breathing tube.

Most newborns who develop BPD are born more than 10 weeks before their due dates, weigh less than 2 pounds at birth, and have breathing problems. Infections that occur before or shortly after birth also can contribute to BPD.

Most babies who develop BPD are born with respiratory distress syndrome (RDS), a breathing disorder that mostly affects premature newborns. If premature newborns still require oxygen therapy by the time they reach 36 weeks gestation, they are diagnosed with BPD.

Some newborns may need long-term oxygen or breathing support from nasal continuous positive airway pressure (NCPAP) machines, ventilators, and medicines, such as bronchodilators. They may continue to have breathing problems throughout childhood and even into adulthood.

As children who have BPD grow, their parents can help reduce the risk of BPD complications. Parents can encourage healthy eating habits and good nutrition. They also can avoid cigarette smoke and other lung irritants.

This chapter includes text excerpted from "Bronchopulmonary Dysplasia," National Heart, Lung, and Blood Institute (NHLBI), June 29, 2019.

Causes of Bronchopulmonary Dysplasia

Bronchopulmonary dysplasia is a type of neonatal respiratory disease that develops as a result of a newborn's lungs not developing normally while the baby is growing in the womb or not developing fully if the baby was born premature. These babies' lungs are fragile and can be easily irritated or inflamed after birth. Ventilation, high levels of oxygen, or infections can also damage premature newborns' lungs.

Ventilation

Newborns who have breathing problems or cannot breathe on their own may need ventilator support. Ventilators are machines that use pressure to blow air into the airways and lungs.

Although ventilator support can help premature newborns survive, the machine's pressure might irritate and harm the babies' lungs. For this reason, doctors only recommend ventilator support when necessary.

High Levels of Oxygen

Newborns who have breathing problems might need oxygen therapy. This treatment helps the newborns' organs get enough oxygen to work well.

However, high levels of oxygen may inflame the lining of the lungs and injure the airways. Also, high levels of oxygen can slow lung development in premature newborns.

Infections

Infections may inflame the lungs. As a result, the airways narrow, which makes it harder for premature newborns to breathe. Lung infections also increase the babies' need for extra oxygen and breathing support.

Risk Factors of Bronchopulmonary Dysplasia

The more premature a newborn is and the lower his or her birth weight, the greater the risk of BPD. Most newborns who develop BPD are born more than 10 weeks before their due dates, weigh less than 2 pounds at birth, and have breathing problems. Infections that occur before or shortly after birth also can contribute to BPD.

The number of babies who have BPD is higher now than in the past. This is because of advances in care that help more premature newborns survive.

Many babies who develop BPD are born with serious respiratory distress syndrome (RDS). However, some babies who have mild RDS or do not have RDS also develop BPD. Studies show that genetic factors may also play a role in causing BPD, but more studies are needed.

Screening and Prevention of Bronchopulmonary Dysplasia

Taking steps to ensure a healthy pregnancy might prevent your newborn from being born before her or his lungs have fully developed. These steps include:

- Following a healthy eating plan
- Managing any medical conditions you have
- Not smoking and avoiding tobacco smoke, alcohol, and illegal drugs
- Preventing infections
- Seeing your doctor regularly during your pregnancy

Your doctor may give you injections of a corticosteroid medicine if she or he thinks you may give birth too early. This medicine can speed up the development of the lungs, brain, and kidneys in your baby and surfactant production. Usually, within about 24 hours of your taking this medicine, the baby's lungs start making enough surfactant. This will reduce the newborn's risk of respiratory distress syndrome, which can lead to BPD.

Signs, Symptoms, and Complications of Bronchopulmonary Dysplasia

Many babies who develop BPD are born with RDS. The first sign of BPD is when premature newborns—usually those born more than 10 weeks early—still need oxygen therapy by the time they reach 36 weeks gestation.

Newborns who have severe BPD may have trouble feeding, which can lead to delayed growth. These babies also may develop:

- **Pulmonary hypertension**, which is increased pressure in the pulmonary arteries. These arteries carry blood from the heart to the lungs to pick up oxygen.

- **Cor pulmonale**, which is failure of the right side of the heart. Ongoing high blood pressure in the pulmonary arteries and the lower right chamber of the heart causes this condition.

Diagnosis of Bronchopulmonary Dysplasia

Newborns who are born early—usually more than 10 weeks before their due dates—and still need oxygen therapy by the time they reach their original due dates are diagnosed with BPD.

Bronchopulmonary dysplasia can be mild, moderate, or severe. The diagnosis depends on how much extra oxygen a baby needs at the time of the original due date. It also depends on how long the baby needs oxygen therapy.

To help confirm a diagnosis of BPD, doctors may recommend tests, such as:

- **Chest x-ray** to show large areas of air and signs of inflammation or infection in the lung seen in severe cases of BPD. A chest x-ray also can detect problems, such as a collapsed lung, and show whether the lungs are not developing normally.

- **Blood tests** to see whether a newborn has enough oxygen in the blood. Blood tests also can help determine whether an infection is causing the newborn's breathing problems.

- **Echocardiography (echo)** to rule out heart defects or pulmonary hypertension as the cause of the newborn's breathing problems

Treatment of Bronchopulmonary Dysplasia

Treatment in the neonatal intensive care unit (NICU) is designed to limit stress on newborns and meet their basic needs of warmth, nutrition, and protection. Treatment of BPD usually includes breathing support with an NCPAP machine or a ventilator, other supportive treatments, and other procedures and treatments.

Once doctors diagnose BPD, some or all of the treatments used for RDS will continue in the NICU.

Breathing Support

Newborns who have BPD often need breathing support, or oxygen therapy, until their lungs start making enough surfactant. A mechanical ventilator usually was used. The ventilator was connected to a breathing tube that ran through the newborn's mouth or nose into the windpipe.

Nowadays, more and more newborns are receiving breathing support from NCPAP. NCPAP gently pushes air into the baby's lungs through prongs placed in the newborn's nostrils.

Other Supportive Treatments

Treatment in the NICU helps limit stress on babies and meet their basic needs of warmth, nutrition, and protection. Such treatment may include:

- Checking liquid intake to make sure that fluid does not build up in the baby's lungs

- Checking pulmonary artery pressure with echocardiography for moderate or severe BPD

- Checking the amount of oxygen in the blood using sensors on fingers or toes

- Giving fluids and nutrients through needles or tubes inserted into the newborn's veins. This helps prevent malnutrition and promotes growth. Nutrition is critical to the growth and development of the lungs. Later, babies may be given breast milk or newborn formula through feeding tubes that are passed through their noses or mouths and into their stomachs or intestines.

- Measuring blood pressure, heart rate, breathing, and temperature through sensors taped to the baby's body

- Using a radiant warmer or incubator to keep newborns warm and reduce the risk of hypothermia

- As BPD improves, babies are slowly weaned off NCPAP or ventilators until they can breathe on their own. These newborns will likely need oxygen therapy for some time.

Other Procedures and Treatments

Newborns who have BPD may spend several weeks or months in the hospital. This allows them to get the care they need, which may include:

Tracheostomy to provide long-term ventilator support. A tracheostomy is a surgically made hole. It goes through the front of the neck and into the trachea, or windpipe. Your child's doctor will put the breathing tube from the ventilator through the hole. A tracheostomy can allow your baby to interact more with you and the NICU staff, start talking and develop other skills.

Physical therapy to help strengthen your child's muscles and clear mucus out of the lungs.

Living with Bronchopulmonary Dysplasia

After your baby leaves the hospital, she or he will likely need follow-up care. It is important to follow your child's treatment plan and get regular care. It is also important to take care of your mental health as you care for your baby at home.

Receive Routine Follow-Up Care

Your child will likely continue on all or some of the treatments that were started at the hospital, including:

- Medicines, such as bronchodilators, steroids, and diuretics

- Oxygen therapy or breathing support from NCPAP or a ventilator

- Extra nutrition and calories, which may be given through a feeding tube

- Preventive treatment with a medicine called "palivizumab" for severe respiratory syncytial virus (RSV). This common virus leads to mild, cold-like symptoms in adults and older, healthy children. However, in newborns—especially those in high-risk groups—RSV can lead to severe breathing problems.

Your child also should have regular checkups with and timely vaccinations from a pediatrician, a doctor who specializes in treating children. If your child needs oxygen therapy or a ventilator at home, a pulmonary specialist might be involved in her or his care.

Ongoing Health Issues and Developmental Delays

Newborns who have BPD may have health problems even after they leave the hospital. These include:

- **Delayed growth** during their first two years. Children who survive borderline personality disorder (BPD) usually are smaller than other children of the same age.

- **Increased risk for infections,** such as colds and the flu. If these children develop respiratory infections, they may need to be treated in a hospital.

- **Lung problems** throughout childhood and even into adulthood. These problems can include underdeveloped lungs and asthma.

- **Need for ongoing oxygen therapy or breathing support** from nasal continuous positive airway pressure (NCPAP) or a ventilator. A pulmonary specialist may help with your child's long-term care and make treatment recommendations.

- **Trouble swallowing.** This may put them at risk for getting food stuck in their airways. This condition is called "aspiration," and it can cause infection. Children who have BPD may need help from a specialist to learn how to swallow correctly.

Babies who have very severe BPD also may develop other problems, such as:

- **Apnea.** This is a condition in which breathing stops for short periods.

- **Poor coordination and muscle tone**

- **Delayed speech and problems** with vision and hearing

- **Learning problems**

- **Gastroesophageal reflux disease (GERD).** This is a condition in which the stomach contents back up into the esophagus during or after a feeding. The esophagus is the passage leading from the mouth to the stomach. GERD may lead to aspiration.

The risk of these complications increases in newborns who are very small at birth.

Chapter 41

Childhood Interstitial Lung Disease

Childhood interstitial lung disease, or chILD, is a broad term for a group of rare lung diseases that can affect babies, children, and teens. These diseases have some similar symptoms, such as chronic cough, rapid breathing, and shortness of breath.

These diseases also harm the lungs in similar ways. For example, they damage the tissues that surround the lungs' alveoli and bronchial tubes (airways). Sometimes these diseases directly damage the air sacs and airways.

The various types of chILD can decrease lung function, reduce blood oxygen levels, and disturb the breathing process.

Researchers have only begun to study, define, and understand chILD in the last decade. As of now, they do not know how many children have chILD. They also do not know how many children have each type of chILD.

Diagnosing chILD and its specific diseases is hard because chILD is rare and complex. Also, chILD is a broad term for a group of diseases with similar symptoms—it is not a precise diagnosis.

Interstitial lung disease (ILD) also occurs in adults. However, the cause of ILD in adults may be different than the cause in children.

This chapter includes text excerpted from "Childhood Interstitial Lung Disease," National Heart, Lung, and Blood Institute (NHLBI), January 13, 2011. Reviewed August 2019.

Some types of chILD are similar to the adult forms of the disease. They may even have the same names as the adult forms, such as hypersensitivity pneumonitis, immunodeficiency-associated lung disease, and bronchiolitis obliterans.

However, research shows that the course and outcomes of these diseases often are very different for children than for adults.

Some ILDs only occur in children. They include:

- Lung growth abnormalities

- Neuroendocrine cell hyperplasia of infancy (NEHI)

- Pulmonary interstitial glycogenosis

- Developmental disorders, such as alveolar capillary dysplasia

Each form of chILD may differ in its severity and how it is treated. Thus, getting a correct diagnosis is vital for understanding and treating your child's illness.

You may want to consult a pediatric pulmonologist. This is a doctor who specializes in diagnosing and treating children who have lung diseases and conditions. This doctor's training and experience can help her or him diagnose chILD.

The outlook for children who have chILD also depends on the specific type of disease they have. Some diseases are very severe and lead to early death. Others are chronic (long-term) diseases that parents and the child's medical team must work together to manage.

At this time, chILD has no cure. However, some children who have certain diseases, such as neuroendocrine hyperplasia of infancy (NEHI), may slowly improve over time.

Researchers are now starting to learn more about the causes of chILD. They Are also trying to find distinct patterns and traits for the various forms of chILD.

Types of Childhood Interstitial Lung Disease

The broad term "childhood interstitial lung disease" (chILD) refers to a group of rare lung diseases that can affect babies, children, and teens. Some of these diseases are more common in certain age groups.

Diseases more common in infancy include:

- Surfactant dysfunction mutations

- Developmental disorders, such as alveolar capillary dysplasia

- Lung growth abnormalities

- Neuroendocrine cell hyperplasia of infancy (NEHI)
- Pulmonary interstitial glycogenosis (PIG)

Diseases more common in children older than two years of age and teens include:

- Idiopathic interstitial pneumonias:
  - Nonspecific interstitial pneumonia (NSIP)
  - Cryptogenic organizing pneumonia (COP)
  - Acute interstitial pneumonia
  - Desquamative interstitial pneumonia
  - Lymphocytic interstitial pneumonia (LIP)
- Other primary disorders:
  - Alveolar hemorrhage syndromes
  - Aspiration syndromes
  - Hypersensitivity pneumonitis
  - Infectious or postinfectious disease (bronchiolitis obliterans)
  - Eosinophilic pneumonia
  - Pulmonary alveolar proteinosis
  - Pulmonary infiltrates with eosinophilia
  - Pulmonary lymphatic disorders (lymphangiomatosis, lymphangiectasis)
  - Pulmonary vascular disorders (haemangiomatosis)
- ILD associated with systemic disease processes:
  - Connective tissue diseases
  - Histiocytosis
  - Malignancy-related lung disease
  - Sarcoidosis
  - Storage diseases
- Disorders of the compromised immune system:
  - Opportunistic infection

- Disorders related to therapeutic intervention

- Lung and bone marrow transplant-associated lung diseases

- Diffuse alveolar damage of unknown cause

The various types of chILD can affect many parts of the lungs, including the alveoli (air sacs), bronchial tubes (airways), and capillaries. (Capillaries are the tiny blood vessels that surround the air sacs.) The structures of the lung that chILD may affect are shown in the illustration below.

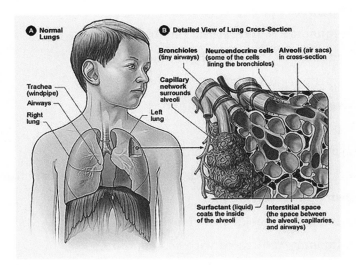

Figure 41.1. *Normal Lungs and Lung Structures*

Figure A shows the location of the lungs and airways in the body. Figure B is a detailed view of the lung structures that childhood interstitial lung disease may affect, such as the bronchioles, neuroendocrine cells, alveoli, capillary network, surfactant, and interstitial space.

Causes of Childhood Interstitial Lung Disease

Researchers do not yet know all of the causes of childhood interstitial lung disease (chILD). Many times, these diseases have no clear cause.

Some conditions and factors that may cause or lead to chILD include:

- **Inherited conditions**, such as surfactant disorders. Surfactant is a liquid that coats the inside of the lungs. It helps with breathing and may help protect the lungs from bacterial and viral infections.

- **Birth defects** that cause problems with the structure or function of the lungs

- **Aspiration.** This term refers to inhaling substances—such as food, liquid, or vomit—into the lungs. Inhaling these substances can injure the lungs. Aspiration may occur in children who have swallowing problems or gastroesophageal reflux disease (GERD). GERD occurs if acid from the stomach backs up into the throat.

- **Immune system disorders.** The immune system protects the body against bacteria, viruses, and toxins. Children who have immune system disorders are not able to fight illness and disease as well as children who have healthy immune systems.

- **Exposure to irritant substances in the environment**, such as molds and chemicals

- **Some cancer treatments**, such as radiation and chemotherapy

- **Systemic or autoimmune diseases**, such as collagen vascular disease or inflammatory bowel disease. Systemic diseases are diseases that involve many of the body's organs. Autoimmune diseases occur if the body's immune system mistakenly attacks the body's tissues and cells.

- **Transplants**, such as a bone marrow transplant or a lung

Risk Factors of Childhood Interstitial Lung Disease

Childhood interstitial lung disease is rare. Most children are not at risk for chILD. However, some factors increase the risk of developing chILD. These risk factors include:

- Having a family history of interstitial lung disease or chILD

- Having an inherited surfactant disorder or a family history of this type of disorder. Surfactant is a liquid that coats the inside of the lungs. It helps with breathing and may help protect the lungs from bacterial and viral infections.

- Having problems with aspiration. This term "aspiration" refers to inhaling substances—such as food, liquid, or vomit—into the lungs.

- Having an immune system disorder. The immune system protects the body against bacteria, viruses, and toxins. Children who have immune system disorders are not able to fight illness and disease as well as children who have healthy immune systems.

- Being exposed to substances in the environment that can irritate the lungs, such as molds and chemicals

- Having a systemic or autoimmune disease, such as collagen vascular disease or inflammatory bowel disease. Systemic diseases are diseases that involve many of the body's organs. Autoimmune diseases occur if the body's immune system mistakenly attacks the body's tissues and cells.

- Undergoing some cancer treatments, such as radiation and chemotherapy

- Having a bone marrow transplant or a lung transplant

Certain types of chILD are more common in infants and young children, while others can occur in children of any age.

The risk of death seems to be higher for children who have chILD and pulmonary hypertension, developmental or growth disorders, bone marrow transplants, or certain surfactant problems.

Signs, Symptoms, and Complications of Childhood Interstitial Lung Disease

Childhood interstitial lung disease (chILD) has many signs and symptoms because the disease has many forms. Signs and symptoms may include:

- Fast breathing, which also is called "tachypnea"

- Labored breathing, which also is called "respiratory distress"

- Low oxygen levels in the blood, which also is called "hypoxemia"

- Recurrent coughing, wheezing, or crackling sounds in the chest

- Shortness of breath during exercise (in older children) or while eating (in infants), which also is called "dyspnea"

- Poor growth or failure to gain weight

- Recurrent pneumonia or bronchiolitis

If your child has any of these signs and symptoms, contact her or his doctor. The doctor may refer you to a pediatric pulmonologist. This is a doctor who specializes in diagnosing and treating children who have lung diseases and conditions.

Diagnosis of Childhood Interstitial Lung Disease

Doctors diagnose chILD based on a child's medical and family histories and the results from tests and procedures. To diagnose chILD, doctors may first need to rule out other diseases as the cause of a child's symptoms.

Early diagnosis of chILD may help doctors stop or even reverse lung function problems. Often though, doctors find chILD hard to diagnose because:

- There are many types of the disease and a range of underlying causes

- The disease's signs and symptoms are the same as those for many other diseases

- The disease may coexist with other diseases

Going to a pediatric pulmonologist who has experience with chILD is helpful. A pediatric pulmonologist is a doctor who specializes in diagnosing and treating children who have lung diseases and conditions.

Medical and Family Histories

Your child's medical history can help her or his doctor diagnose chILD. The doctor may ask whether your child:

- Has severe breathing problems that occur often

- Has had severe lung infections

- Had serious lung problems as a newborn

- Has been exposed to possible lung irritants in the environment, such as birds, molds, dusts, or chemicals

- Has ever had radiation or chemotherapy treatment

- Has an autoimmune disease, certain birth defects, or other medical conditions. (Autoimmune diseases occur if the body's immune system mistakenly attacks the body's tissues and cells.)

The doctor also may ask how old your child was when symptoms began, and whether other family members have or have had severe lung diseases. If they have, your child may have an inherited form of chILD.

Diagnostic Tests and Procedures

No single test can diagnose the many types of chILD. Thus, your child's doctor may recommend one or more of the following tests. For some of these tests, infants and young children may be given medicine to help them relax or sleep.

- **Chest x-ray.** This painless test creates pictures of the structures inside your child's chest, such as the heart, lungs, and blood vessels. A chest x-ray can help rule out other lung diseases as the cause of your child's symptoms.

- **High-resolution CT scan (HRCT).** An HRCT scan uses x-rays to create detailed pictures of your child's lungs. This test can show the location, extent, and severity of lung disease.

- **Lung function tests.** These tests measure how much air your child can breathe in and out, how fast she or he can breathe air out, and how well your child's lungs deliver oxygen to the blood. Lung function tests can assess the severity of lung disease. Infants and young children may need to have these tests at a center that has special equipment for children.

- **Bronchoalveolar lavage.** For this procedure, the doctor injects a small amount of saline (saltwater) through a tube inserted in the child's lungs. The fluid helps bring up cells from the tissues around the air sacs. The doctor can then look at these cells under a microscope. This procedure can help detect an infection, lung injury, bleeding, aspiration, or an airway problem.

- Various tests to rule out conditions, such as asthma, cystic fibrosis, acid reflux, heart disease, neuromuscular disease, and immune deficiency

- Various tests for systemic diseases linked to chILD. Systemic diseases are diseases that involve many of the body's organs

- Blood tests to check for inherited (genetic) diseases and disorders

If these tests do not provide enough information, your child's doctor may recommend a lung biopsy. A lung biopsy is the most reliable way to diagnose chILD and the specific disease involved.

A lung biopsy is a surgical procedure that is done in a hospital. Before the biopsy, your child will receive medicine to make her or him sleep. During the biopsy, the doctor will take small samples of lung tissue from several places in your child's lungs. This often is done using video-assisted thoracoscopy. For this procedure, the doctor inserts a small tube with a light and camera (endoscope) into your child's chest through small cuts between the ribs. The endoscope provides a video image of the lungs and allows the doctor to collect tissue samples. After the biopsy, the doctor will look at these samples under a microscope.

Treatment of Childhood Interstitial Lung Disease

Childhood interstitial lung disease is rare, and little research has been done on how to treat it. At this time, chILD has no cure. However, some children who have certain diseases, such as neuroendocrine cell hyperplasia of infancy, may slowly improve over time.

Current treatment approaches include supportive therapy, medicines, and, in the most serious cases, lung transplants.

Supportive Therapy

Supportive therapy refers to treatments that help relieve symptoms or improve quality of life. Supportive approaches used to relieve common chILD symptoms include:

- **Oxygen therapy.** If your child's blood oxygen level is low, she or he may need oxygen therapy. This treatment can improve breathing, support growth, and reduce strain on the heart.

- **Bronchodilators.** These medications relax the muscles around your child's airways, which helps open the airways and makes breathing easier.

- **Breathing devices.** Children who have severe disease may need ventilators or other devices to help them breathe easier.

- **Extra nutrition.** This treatment can help improve your child's growth and help her or him gain weight. Close monitoring of growth is especially important.

- **Techniques and devices to help relieve lung congestion.** These may include chest physical therapy (CPT) or wearing a vest that helps move mucus (a sticky substance) to the upper airways so it can be coughed up. CPT may involve pounding the chest and back over and over with your hands or a device to loosen mucus in the lungs so that your child can cough it up.

- **Supervised pulmonary rehabilitation (PR).** PR is a broad program that helps improve the well-being of people who have chronic (ongoing) breathing problems.

Medicines

Corticosteroids are a common treatment for many children who have chILD. These medicines help reduce lung inflammation. Other medicines can help treat specific types or causes of chILD. For example, antimicrobial medicines can treat a lung infection. Acid-blocking medicines can prevent acid reflux, which can lead to aspiration.

Lung Transplant

A lung transplant may be an option for children who have severe chILD if other treatments have not worked. As of now, lung transplants are the only effective treatment for some types of chILD that have a high risk of death, such as alveolar capillary dysplasia and certain surfactant dysfunction mutations.

Early diagnosis of these diseases gives children the chance to receive lung transplants. So far, the chILD does not appear to come back in patients' transplanted lungs.

Living with Childhood Interstitial Lung Disease

Caring for a child who has chILD can be challenging. However, you can take steps to help your child manage her or his disease.

Make sure your child gets ongoing care and seek support to help you, your child, and your other family members cope with the effects of chILD on daily life.

Ongoing Care

Work with your child's healthcare team to manage your child's symptoms and keep her or him as healthy as possible.

This team may include doctors, nurses, dietitians, social workers, physical therapists, and home health aides. Each of these specialists may have services that can help you and your child cope with her or his lung disease.

You also can take other steps to help manage your child's care. For example:

- Give your child all of her or his prescribed medicines. Make sure to take your child to all follow-up medical visits.

- Work with your child's healthcare team to ensure that your child is getting good nutrition. Your child's healthcare team also can suggest physical activities that meet your child's needs.

- Ask your child's doctor about warning signs of worsening lung disease and when to seek emergency medical care. Agree on a plan of action if these warning signs occur.

- Keep complete records of your child's care and any instructions you receive. This information can help you manage care at home and inform various doctors about your child's medical history and status.

Many children who have chILD need oxygen therapy to help them breathe easier. Portable oxygen units can make it easier for your child to move around and do many daily activities.

If your child's doctor prescribes oxygen therapy, work with a home equipment provider to make sure you have the supplies and equipment you need. Trained personnel will show you how to use the equipment correctly and safely.

Ongoing Support

Your child may need support to help other people in her or his life understand the special needs related to chILD. For example, you may want to talk with your child's teachers about your child's illness. You can work with the teachers to decide how to meet your child's special school-related needs.

You also may want to alert relatives, caregivers, friends, and parents of friends about your child's illness. Let them know about your child's usual care and any signs or symptoms that require emergency care.

Taking care of yourself also is important. Managing your child's disease and ongoing care can be stressful. You and your family members may feel sad, guilty, or overwhelmed.

Social workers and mental-health providers can help you cope with your feelings and provide support. They also can connect you with family support groups. Taking part in a support group can show you how other people have coped with chILD.

Chapter 42

Croup

What Is Croup?

Croup is an inflammation of the vocal cords (larynx) and windpipe (trachea). It causes difficulty breathing, a barking cough, and a hoarse voice. It is also known with the names "spasmodic croup" as well as "viral croup."

What Causes Croup

The cause is usually a virus, often parainfluenza virus. Other causes include:

- Allergies
- Reflux

What Are the Symptoms of Croup?

Croup often starts out such as a cold. But then the vocal cords and windpipe become swollen, causing the hoarseness and the cough. There may also be a fever and high-pitched noisy sounds when breathing.

The symptoms are usually worse at night, and last for about three to five days. Croup is more common in the fall and winter.

This chapter includes text excerpted from "Croup," MedlinePlus, National Institutes of Health (NIH), December 31, 2016.

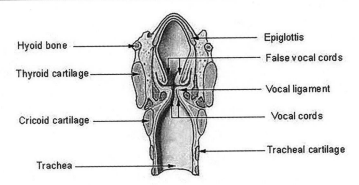

Figure 42.1. *Larynx* (Source: "Larynx and Trachea—SEER Training," Surveillance, Epidemiology, and End Results Program (SEER), National Cancer Institute (NCI).)

The larynx plays an essential role in human speech. During sound production, the vocal cords close together and vibrate as air expelled from the lungs passes between them.

Who Are at Risk of Croup?

Children between the ages of six months and three years have the highest risk of getting croup. They may also have more severe symptoms.

How Is Croup Treated?

Most cases of viral croup are mild and can be treated at home. Rarely, croup can become serious and interfere with your child's breathing. If you are worried about your child's breathing, call your healthcare provider right away.

Managing Recurrent Croup in Children*

Presently children who experience recurring croup symptoms receive a variety of treatments. This is because it is not clear which treatment may be best. Some children are given inhaled steroids (similar to what children with asthma use). Others are carefully watched and cautioned to avoid potential triggers (certain foods, environmental allergens, etc.), and should episodes of croup recur they are treated with a short course of oral steroids.

*Text excerpted from "Management of Recurrent Croup," ClinicalTrials. gov, National Institutes of Health (NIH), November 13, 2017.

Chapter 43

Human Metapneumovirus

Human metapneumovirus (HMPV) can cause upper and lower respiratory disease in people of all ages, especially among young children, older adults, and people with weakened immune systems. Discovered in 2001, HMPV is in the paramyxovirus family along with respiratory syncytial virus (RSV). Broader use of molecular diagnostic testing has increased identification and awareness of HMPV as an important cause of upper and lower respiratory infection.

Symptoms of Human Metapneumovirus

Symptoms commonly associated with HMPV include cough, fever, nasal congestion, and shortness of breath. Clinical symptoms of HMPV infection may progress to bronchitis or pneumonia and are similar to other viruses that cause upper and lower respiratory infections. The estimated incubation period is three to six days, and the median duration of illness can vary depending upon severity but is similar to other respiratory infections caused by viruses.

This chapter includes text excerpted from "Human Metapneumovirus (HMPV) Clinical Features," Centers for Disease Control and Prevention (CDC), May 14, 2019.

Surveillance and Seasonality of Human Metapneumovirus

Surveillance data from the Centers for Disease Control and Prevention's (CDC) National Respiratory and Enteric Virus Surveillance System (NREVSS) shows HMPV to be most active during late winter and spring in temperate climates.

Transmission of Human Metapneumovirus

Human metapneumovirus is most likely spread from an infected person to others through

- Secretions from coughing and sneezing

- Close personal contact, such as touching or shaking hands

- Touching objects or surfaces that have the viruses on them then touching the mouth, nose, or eyes

In the United States, HMPV circulates in distinct annual seasons. HMPV circulation begins in winter and lasts until or through spring. HMPV, RSV, and influenza can circulate simultaneously during the respiratory virus season.

Prevention and Treatment of Human Metapneumovirus

As of now, there is no specific antiviral therapy to treat HMPV and no vaccine to prevent HMPV. Medical care is supportive. However, you can help prevent the spread of HMPV and other respiratory viruses by following these steps:

- Wash your hands often with soap and water for at least 20 seconds

- Avoid touching your eyes, nose, or mouth with unwashed hands

- Avoid close contact with people who are sick

Patients who have cold-like symptoms should:

- Cover their mouth and nose when coughing and sneezing

- Wash their hands frequently and correctly (with soap and water for at least 20 seconds)

- Avoid sharing their cups and eating utensils with others

- Refrain from kissing others

- Stay at home when they are sick

In addition, cleaning possible contaminated surfaces (such as door-knobs and shared toys) may potentially help stop the spread of HMPV.

Since HMPV is a recently recognized respiratory virus, healthcare professionals may not routinely consider or test for HMPV. However, healthcare professionals should consider HMPV testing during winter and spring, especially when HMPV is commonly circulating.

Laboratory Diagnosis of Human Metapneumovirus

Infection with HMPV can be confirmed usually by:

- Direct detection of viral genome by polymerase chain reaction assays

- Direct detection of viral antigens in respiratory secretions using immunofluorescence or enzyme immunoassay

Chapter 44

Pulmonary Sequestration

Pulmonary sequestration is a rare congenital (present from birth) malformation where nonfunctioning lung tissue is separated from the rest of the lung and supplied with blood from an unusual source, often an artery from systemic circulation. Pulmonary sequestrations may be defined as "intralobular" or "extralobular," depending on their location. Symptoms may include a chronic or recurrent cough, respiratory distress or lung infection. Treatment depends on the location and may involve surgery.

Symptoms of Pulmonary Sequestration

Typical symptoms seen in infants with extralobular pulmonary sequestration include cough, respiratory problems, feeding difficulties, or congestive heart failure, although many infants have no symptoms. Chronic infections are not common. Extralobular pulmonary sequestration is commonly associated with other birth defects, including diaphragmatic hernia and other lung malformations, such as congenital cystic adenomatoid malformation and bronchogenic cysts, pectus excavatum, pericardial problems, and duplication cysts. This type of sequestration accounts for 25 percent of all sequestrations.

Intralobular pulmonary sequestration is characterized by recurrent infections, hemoptysis, or pleural effusion. A chronic or recurrent

This chapter includes text excerpted from "Pulmonary Sequestration," Genetic and Rare Diseases Information Center (GARD), National Center for Advancing Translational Sciences (NCATS), August 15, 2016.

cough is common. A chest radiograph may reveal a solid or fluid (cystic) lesion in the lower lobe, more often on the left side. Intralobular pulmonary sequestration is often diagnosed later than extralobular pulmonary sequestration, in childhood or adulthood. It accounts for 75 percent of all sequestrations and affects males and females in equal numbers. Intralobular pulmonary sequestration is not commonly associated with other congenital anomalies.

Causes of Pulmonary Sequestration

Pulmonary sequestration appears to result from abnormal budding of the primitive foregut. The tissue in this accessory lung bud migrates with the developing lung, but does not communicate with it. It receives its blood supply from vessels that connect to the aorta or one of its side branches. The arterial supply is derived in most cases from the thoracic aorta (75%) or the abdominal aorta (20%). In some cases (15%), two different arteries supply the blood.

If the accessory lung bud develops early in embryonic development, the pulmonary sequestration occurs among the normal lung tissue, where it is encased within the pleural sac. This results in intralobular pulmonary sequestration. Venous drainage of intralobular pulmonary sequestration is usually through the pulmonary circulation. If the accessory lung bud develops later, extralobular pulmonary sequestration results. This type of pulmonary sequestration is separated from the normal lung tissue by its own visceral pleura and can occur above, within, or below the diaphragm. Venous drainage is usually through systemic circulation.

Inheritance Pattern of Pulmonary Sequestration

While the vast majority of pulmonary sequestration cases occur in isolation (without any family history), rare familial cases have been reported. Therefore, a genetic component cannot be ruled out.

Treatment of Pulmonary Sequestration

Due to the risk of infection and bleeding, intralobar pulmonary sequestrations are usually removed, either by segmentectomy (removal of part of the lung) or lobectomy (removal of the full lobe). Angiography along with computed tomography (CT) scan (with or without contrast) and magnetic resonance imaging (MRI) are generally used to visualize the origins of the blood supply before surgery is performed.

Traditional treatment of extralobular pulmonary sequestration involves surgical removal via mini-thoracotomy for patients that are experiencing symptoms. Less invasive surgery techniques may include thoracoscopic surgery and coil embolization.

Chapter 45

Respiratory Distress Syndrome of the Newborn

Respiratory distress syndrome (RDS) is a common breathing disorder that affects newborns. RDS occurs most often in babies born preterm, affecting nearly all newborns who are born before 28 weeks of pregnancy. Less often, RDS can affect full-term newborns.

Respiratory distress syndrome is more common in premature newborns because their lungs are not able to make enough surfactant. Surfactant is a foamy substance that keeps the lungs fully expanded so that newborns can breathe in air once they are born.

Without enough surfactant, the lungs collapse and the newborn has to work hard to breathe. She or he might not be able to breathe in enough oxygen to support the body's organs. Most babies who develop RDS show signs of breathing problems and a lack of oxygen at birth or within the first few hours that follow. The lack of oxygen can damage the baby's brain and other organs if not treated promptly. RDS may change over time to become bronchopulmonary dysplasia (BPD). This is another breathing disorder that may affect babies, especially premature babies.

Respiratory distress syndrome usually develops in the first 24 hours after birth. If premature newborns still have breathing problems by the time they reach 36 weeks gestation, they may be diagnosed with

This chapter includes text excerpted from "Respiratory Distress Syndrome," National Heart, Lung, and Blood Institute (NHLBI), April 9, 2019.

BPD. Some of the life-saving treatments used for RDS may contribute to BPD. Some newborns who have RDS recover and never get BPD.

Due to better treatments and medical advances, most newborns who have RDS survive. However, these babies may need extra medical care after going home. Some babies have complications from RDS or its treatments. Serious complications may include chronic breathing problems, such as asthma and BPD; impaired vision; and movement, learning, or behavior problems.

Causes of Respiratory Distress Syndrome

Respiratory distress syndrome is a type of neonatal respiratory disease that is caused most often by a lack of surfactant in the lungs. A fetus's lungs start making surfactant during the third trimester of pregnancy, or weeks 26 through labor and delivery. Surfactant coats the insides of the air sacs, or alveoli in the lungs. This helps keep the lungs open so breathing can occur after birth. To understand respiratory distress syndrome, it helps to learn about how the lungs work.

Without enough surfactant, the lungs may collapse when the newborn exhales. The newborn then has to work harder to breathe. She or he might not be able to get enough oxygen to support the body's organs.

Some full-term newborns develop RDS because they have faulty genes that affect how their bodies make surfactant.

Risk Factors of Respiratory Distress Syndrome

Certain factors may increase the risk that your newborn will have RDS. These factors include:

- Infection
- Premature delivery. The earlier your baby is born, the greater her or his risk for RDS. Most cases of RDS occur in babies born before 28 weeks of pregnancy.
- Problems with your baby's lung development
- Stress during your baby's delivery, especially if you lose a lot of blood
- You having diabetes

Your baby also is at greater risk for RDS if you require an emergency cesarean delivery before your baby is full term. You may need an emergency cesarean delivery because of a condition, such as a detached placenta, that puts you or your newborn at risk.

Planned cesarean deliveries that occur before a baby's lungs have fully matured can also increase your baby's risk for RDS. Your doctor can do tests before delivery that show whether it is likely that your baby's lungs are fully developed. These tests determine the age of the fetus or lung maturity.

Screening and Prevention of Respiratory Distress Syndrome

Taking steps to ensure a healthy pregnancy might prevent your newborn from being born before her or his lungs have fully developed. These steps include:

- Following a healthy eating plan
- Managing any medical conditions you have
- Not smoking and avoiding tobacco smoke, alcohol, and illegal drugs
- Preventing infections
- Seeing your doctor regularly during your pregnancy

Your doctor may give you injections of a corticosteroid medicine if she or he thinks you may give birth too early. This medicine can speed up development of the lungs, brain, and kidneys in your baby and surfactant production. Usually, within about 24 hours of your taking this medicine, the baby's lungs start making enough surfactant.

Treatment with corticosteroids can reduce your baby's risk for RDS. If the baby does develop RDS, it may not be as serious.

Signs, Symptoms, and Complications of Respiratory Distress Syndrome

Signs and symptoms of RDS usually happen at birth or within the first few hours that follow. Depending on the severity of a newborn's RDS, she or he may develop other medical problems.

Signs and Symptoms

Signs and symptoms of RDS include:

- Grunting sounds

- Rapid, shallow breathing

- Sharp pulling inward of the muscles between the ribs when breathing

- Widening of the nostrils, or flaring, with each breath

The newborn also may have pauses in breathing that last for a few seconds. This condition is called "apnea."

Complications

Many babies who are born with RDS develop BPD. If babies born with RDS still require oxygen therapy by the time they reach their original due dates, they are diagnosed with BPD.

Depending on the severity of a newborn's RDS, she or he may develop other medical problems.

- **Bleeding in the brain,** which can delay cognitive development or cause intellectual disabilities or cerebral palsy

- **Blood and blood vessel complications.** Newborns who have RDS may develop sepsis. This infection can be life-threatening.

- **Bowel disease** called "necrotizing enterocolitis"

- **Impaired vision, including blindness**

- **Kidney failure**

- **Lung complications.** These may include atelectasis; leakage of air from the lungs into the chest cavity called "pneumothorax," a type of pleural disorder; and bleeding in the lung, or hemorrhage. Some of the life-saving treatments used for RDS may cause bronchopulmonary dysplasia.

- **Patent ductus arteriosus,** a type of congenital heart defect. The ductus arteriosus connects pulmonary arteries to the aorta. If it remains open, it can strain the heart and increase blood pressure in the lung arteries.

Diagnosis of Respiratory Distress Syndrome

Respiratory distress syndrome is common in premature newborns. Thus, doctors usually recognize and begin treating the disorder as soon as babies are born.

Doctors also do several tests to rule out other conditions that could be causing a newborn's breathing problems. The tests also can confirm that the doctors have diagnosed the condition correctly.

The tests include:

- **Chest x-ray** to show whether a newborn has signs of RDS. A chest x-ray also can detect problems, such as a collapsed lung, that may require urgent treatment.

- **Blood tests** to see whether a newborn has enough oxygen in the blood. Blood tests also can help find out whether an infection is causing the newborn's breathing problems.

- **Echocardiography (echo)** to rule out heart defects as the cause of the newborn's breathing problems

Treatment of Respiratory Distress Syndrome

Treatment for RDS usually begins as soon as a newborn is born, sometimes in the delivery room. Treatments for RDS include surfactant replacement therapy, breathing support from a ventilator or nasal continuous positive airway pressure (NCPAP) machine, or other supportive treatments.

Most newborns who show signs of RDS are quickly moved to a neonatal intensive care unit (NICU). There they receive around-the-clock treatment from healthcare professionals who specialize in treating premature newborns.

Surfactant Replacement Therapy

Surfactant helps keep the lungs open so that a newborn can breathe in air once she or he is born. Babies who have RDS get surfactant until their lungs are able to start making the substance on their own. Surfactant is usually given through a breathing tube. The tube allows the surfactant to go directly into the baby's lungs.

Once the surfactant is given, the breathing tube is connected to a ventilator, or the baby may get breathing support from NCPAP.

Surfactant often is given right after birth in the delivery room to try to prevent or treat RDS. It also may be given several times in the days that follow, until the baby is able to breathe better.

Some women are given medicines called "corticosteroids" during pregnancy. These medicines can speed up surfactant production and lung development in a fetus. Even if you had these medicines, your newborn may still need surfactant replacement therapy after birth.

Breathing Support

Newborns who have RDS often need breathing support, or oxygen therapy, until their lungs start making enough surfactant. Until recently, a mechanical ventilator usually was used. The ventilator was connected to a breathing tube that ran through the newborn's mouth or nose into the windpipe.

More and more newborns are receiving breathing support from NCPAP. NCPAP gently pushes air into the baby's lungs through prongs placed in the newborn's nostrils.

Other Supportive Treatments

Treatment in the NICU helps limit stress on babies and meet their basic needs of warmth, nutrition, and protection. Such treatment may include:

- **Checking liquid intake** to make sure that fluid does not build up in the baby's lungs

- **Checking the amount of oxygen in the blood** using sensors on fingers or toes

- **Giving fluids and nutrients** through needles or tubes inserted into the newborns' veins. This helps prevent malnutrition and promotes growth. Nutrition is critical to the growth and development of the lungs. Later, babies may be given breast milk or newborn formula through feeding tubes that are passed through their noses or mouths and into their throats.

- **Measuring blood pressure, heart rate, breathing, and temperature** through sensors taped to the baby's body

- **Using a radiant warmer or incubator** to keep newborns warm and reduce the risk of hypothermia

Living with Respiratory Distress Syndrome

After your baby leaves the hospital, she or he will likely need follow-up care. It is important to follow your child's treatment plan and get regular care. It is also important to take care of your mental health as you care for your baby at home.

Receive Routine Follow-Up Care

Your baby may need special care after leaving the neonatal intensive care unit (NICU), including:

- Special hearing and eye exams
- Speech or physical therapy
- Specialty care for other medical problems caused by premature birth

Talk to your child's doctor about ongoing care for your newborn and any other medical concerns you have.

Ongoing Health Issues and Developmental Delays

Newborns who have RDS may have health problems even after they leave the hospital. These include:

- **Delayed growth during their first two years.** Children who survive RDS usually are smaller than other children of the same age.

- **Increased risk for infections, such as colds and the flu.** If these children develop respiratory infections, they may need to be treated in a hospital.

- **Lung problems throughout childhood and even into adulthood.** These problems can include underdeveloped lungs and asthma.

- **Need for ongoing oxygen therapy or breathing support from nasal Continuous Positive Airway Pressure (nCPAP) or a ventilator.** A pulmonary specialist may help with your child's long-term care and make treatment recommendations.

- **Trouble swallowing.** This may put them at risk for getting food stuck in their airways. This condition is called "aspiration," and it can cause infection. Children who have RDS may need help from a specialist to learn how to swallow correctly.

- **Apnea,** a condition in which breathing stops for short periods

- **Poor coordination and muscle tone**

- **Delayed speech and problems with vision and hearing**

- **Learning problems**

- **Gastroesophageal reflux disease (GERD),** a condition in which the stomach contents back up into the esophagus during or after a feeding. The esophagus is the passage leading from the mouth to the stomach. GERD may lead to aspiration.

The risk of these complications increases in newborns who are very small at birth.

Prevent and Treat Complications over Your Child's Lifetime

You can take steps to help manage your child's RDS and help her or him recover.

- **Try to prevent infection.** Wash your hands often, and discourage visits from family and friends who are sick. Keep your baby away from large day care centers and crowds to avoid colds, the flu, and other infections.

- **Do not smoke in your home.** Keep your baby away from substances that could irritate the lungs, such as cigarette smoke.

- **Get recommended childhood vaccines.**

- **Treat complications of RDS.** Your doctor may give your child antibiotics for infections. Treatment for patent ductus arteriosus, a possible complication of RDS, includes medicines, catheter procedures, or surgery.

- **Call your child's doctor if you see any signs of respiratory infection.** These may include irritability, fever, stuffy nose, cough, changes in breathing patterns, and wheezing.

Take Care of Your Mental Health

Caring for a premature newborn can be challenging. You may experience:

- Emotional distress, including feelings of guilt, anger, and depression

- Anxiety about your baby's future

- A feeling of a lack of control over the situation

- Financial stress

- Problems relating to your baby while she or he is in the NICU

- Fatigue

- Frustration that you cannot breastfeed your newborn right away. You can pump and store your breast milk for later use.

  You can take steps to help yourself during this difficult time.

- **Ask questions about your newborn's condition** and what is involved in daily care. This will help you feel more confident about your ability to care for your baby at home.

- **Learn as much as you can** about what happens in the NICU. You can help your baby during her or his stay there and begin to bond with the baby before she or he comes home.

- **Seek out support from family, friends, and hospital staff.** Ask the case manager or social worker at the hospital what you will need after your baby leaves the hospital. The doctors and nurses can assist with questions about your newborn's care. Also, you may want to ask whether your community has a support group for parents of premature newborns.

- **Visit your baby in the NICU as much as possible.** Spend time talking to your baby and holding and touching her or him.

Chapter 46

Respiratory Syncytial Virus

Respiratory syncytial virus, or RSV, is a common respiratory virus that usually causes mild, cold-like symptoms. Most people recover in a week or two, but RSV can be serious, especially for infants and older adults. In fact, RSV is the most common cause of bronchiolitis (inflammation of the small airways in the lung) and pneumonia (infection of the lungs) in children younger than one year of age in the United States. It is also a significant cause of respiratory illness in older adults.

Respiratory Syncytial Virus in Infants and Young Children

Respiratory syncytial virus can be dangerous for some infants and young children. Each year in the United States, an estimated 57,000 children younger than 5 years old are hospitalized due to RSV infection. Those at greatest risk for severe illness from RSV include:

- Premature infants

- Very young infants, especially those six months and younger

- Children younger than two years old with chronic lung disease

- Children younger than two years old with chronic heart disease

---

This chapter includes text excerpted from "Respiratory Syncytial Virus Infection (RSV)," Centers for Disease Control and Prevention (CDC), June 26, 2018.

- Children with weakened immune systems
- Children who have neuromuscular disorders, including those who have difficulty swallowing or clearing mucus secretions

Severe Respiratory Syncytial Virus Infection

Virtually all children get an RSV infection by the time they are two years old. Most of the time RSV will cause a mild, cold-like illness, but it can also cause severe illness, such as:

- Bronchiolitis (inflammation of the small airways in the lung)
- Pneumonia (infection of the lungs)

1 to 2 out of every 100 children younger than 6 months of age with RSV infection may need to be hospitalized. Those who are hospitalized may require oxygen, intubation, and/or mechanical ventilation (help with breathing). Most improve with this type of supportive care and are discharged in a few days.

Early Symptoms of Respiratory Syncytial Virus

Respiratory syncytial virus may not be severe when it first starts. However, it can become more severe a few days into the illness. Early symptoms of RSV may include:

- Runny nose
- Decrease in appetite
- Cough, which may progress to wheezing

Respiratory Syncytial Virus in Very Young Infants

Infants who get an RSV infection almost always show symptoms. This is different from adults who can sometimes get RSV infections and not have symptoms. In very young infants (less than six months old), the only symptoms of RSV infection may be:

- Irritability
- Decreased activity
- Decreased appetite
- Apnea (pauses while breathing)
- Fever, which may not always occur with RSV infections

What You Should Do If You or Your Loved One Is at High Risk for Severe Respiratory Syncytial Virus Disease

Respiratory syncytial virus season occurs each year in most regions of the U.S. during fall, winter, and spring. If you have contact with an infant or young child or an older adult, you should take extra care to keep them healthy by doing the following:

- **Wash your hands often.** Wash your hands often with soap and water for 20 seconds, and help young children do the same. If soap and water are not available, use an alcohol-based hand sanitizer. Washing your hands will help protect you from germs.

- **Keep your hands off your face.** Avoid touching your eyes, nose, and mouth with unwashed hands. Germs spread this way.

- **Avoid close contact with sick people.** Avoid close contact, such as kissing, and sharing cups or eating utensils with people who have cold-like symptoms.

- **Cover your coughs and sneezes.** Cover your mouth and nose with a tissue or your upper shirt sleeve when coughing or sneezing. Throw the tissue in the trash afterward.

- **Clean and disinfect surfaces.** Clean and disinfect surfaces and objects that people frequently touch, such as toys and doorknobs. When people infected with RSV touch surfaces and objects, they can leave behind germs. Also, when they cough or sneeze, droplets containing germs can land on surfaces and objects.

- **Stay home when you are sick.** If possible, stay home from work, school, and public areas when you are sick. This will help protect others from catching your illness.

Symptoms and Care
Respiratory Syncytial Virus Symptoms

Symptoms of RSV infection usually include:

- Runny nose
- Decrease in appetite
- Coughing

- Sneezing

- Fever

- Wheezing

These symptoms usually appear in stages and not all at once. In very young infants with RSV, the only symptoms may be irritability, decreased activity, and breathing difficulties.

Respiratory syncytial virus can also cause more severe infections, such as bronchiolitis, an inflammation of the small airways in the lung, and pneumonia, an infection of the lungs. It is the most common cause of bronchiolitis and pneumonia in children younger than one year of age.

Almost all children will have had an RSV infection by their second birthday. People infected with RSV usually show symptoms within four to six days after getting infected.

Respiratory Syncytial Virus Care

Most RSV infections go away on their own in a week or two. You can manage fever and pain with over-the-counter (OTC) fever reducers and pain relievers, such as acetaminophen or ibuprofen. Talk to your healthcare provider before giving your child nonprescription cold medicines, since some medicines contain ingredients that are not recommended for children. It is important for people with RSV infection to drink enough fluids to prevent dehydration (loss of body fluids).

Healthy infants and adults infected with RSV do not usually need to be hospitalized. But some people with RSV infection, especially infants younger than six months of age and older adults, may need to be hospitalized if they are having trouble breathing or are dehydrated. In most of these cases, hospitalization only lasts a few days.

Visits to a healthcare provider for an RSV infection are very common. During such visits, the healthcare provider will evaluate how severe the person's RSV infection is to determine if the patient should be hospitalized. In the most severe cases, a person may require additional oxygen or intubation (have a breathing tube inserted through the mouth and down to the airway) with mechanical ventilation (a machine to help a person breathe).

There is no specific treatment for RSV infection, though researchers are working to develop vaccines and antivirals (medicines that fight viruses).

Respiratory Syncytial Virus Transmission

Respiratory syncytial virus can spread when an infected person coughs or sneezes. You can get infected if you get droplets from the cough or sneeze in your eyes, nose, or mouth, or if you touch a surface that has the virus on it, like a doorknob, and then touch your face before washing your hands. Additionally, it can spread through direct contact with the virus, like kissing the face of a child with RSV.

People infected with RSV are usually contagious for three to eight days. However, some infants, and people with weakened immune systems can continue to spread the virus even after they stop showing symptoms, for as long as four weeks. Children are often exposed to and infected with RSV outside the home, such as in school or child-care centers. They can then transmit the virus to other members of the family.

Respiratory syncytial virus can survive for many hours on hard surfaces, such as tables and crib rails. It typically lives on soft surfaces, such as tissues and hands for shorter amounts of time.

People of any age can get another RSV infection, but infections later in life are generally less severe. People at highest risk for severe disease include:

- Premature infants

- Young children with congenital (from birth) heart or chronic lung disease

- Young children with compromised (weakened) immune systems due to a medical condition or medical treatment

- Adults with compromised immune systems

- Older adults, especially those with underlying heart or lung disease

In the United States and other areas with similar climates, RSV infections generally occur during fall, winter, and spring. The timing and severity of RSV circulation in a given community can vary from year to year.

Respiratory Syncytial Virus Prevention

There are steps you can take to help prevent the spread of RSV. Specifically, if you have cold-like symptoms you should:

- Cover your coughs and sneezes with a tissue or your upper shirt sleeve, not your hands

- Wash your hands often with soap and water for 20 seconds

- Avoid close contact, such as kissing, shaking hands, and sharing cups and eating utensils, with others

In addition, cleaning contaminated surfaces (such as doorknobs) may help stop the spread of RSV.

Ideally, people with cold-like symptoms should not interact with children at high risk for severe RSV disease, including premature infants, children younger than two years of age with chronic lung or heart conditions, and children with weakened immune systems. If this is not possible, they should carefully follow the prevention steps mentioned above and wash their hands before interacting with such children. They should also refrain from kissing high-risk children while they have cold-like symptoms.

Parents of children at high risk for developing severe RSV disease should help their child, when possible, do the following:

- Avoid close contact with sick people

- Wash their hands often with soap and water

- Avoid touching their face with unwashed hands

- Limit the time they spend in child care centers or other potentially contagious settings, especially during fall, winter, and spring. This may help prevent infection and spread of the virus during the RSV season.

There is no vaccine yet to prevent RSV infection, but scientists are working hard to develop one. And there is a medicine that can help protect some babies at high risk for severe RSV disease. Healthcare providers usually give this medicine called "palivizumab" to premature infants and young children with certain heart and lung conditions as a series of monthly shots during RSV season. If you are concerned about your child's risk for severe RSV infection, talk to your child's doctor.

Chapter 47

Sudden Infant Death Syndrome

Sudden infant death syndrome (SIDS) is the sudden, unexplained death of a baby younger than one year of age that does not have a known cause even after a complete investigation. This investigation includes performing a complete autopsy, examining the death scene, and reviewing the clinical history.

When a baby dies, healthcare providers, law enforcement personnel, and communities try to find out why. They ask questions, examine the baby, gather information, and run tests. If they cannot find a cause for the death, and if the baby was younger than one year old, the medical examiner or coroner will call the death "SIDS."

If there is still some uncertainty as to the cause after it is determined to be fully unexplained, then the medical examiner or coroner might leave the cause of death as "unknown."

Fast Facts about Sudden Infant Death Syndrome

- Sudden infant death syndrome is the leading cause of death among babies between 1 month and 1 year of age.

- More than 2,000 babies died of SIDS in 2010, the last year for which such statistics are available.

This chapter includes text excerpted from "About SIDS and Safe Infant Sleep," *Eunice Kennedy Shriver* National Institute of Child Health and Human Development (NICHD), December 30, 2017.

- Most SIDS deaths occur when babies between 1 month and 4 months of age, and the majority (90%) of SIDS deaths occur before a baby reaches 6 months of age. However, SIDS deaths can occur anytime during a baby's first year.

- Sudden infant death syndrome is a sudden and silent medical disorder that can happen to an infant who seems healthy.

- Sudden infant death syndrome is sometimes called "crib death" or "cot death" because it is associated with the timeframe when the baby is sleeping. Cribs themselves do not cause SIDS, but the baby's sleep environment can influence sleep-related causes of death.

- Slightly more boys die of SIDS than girls do.

- In the past, the number of SIDS deaths seemed to increase during the colder months of the year. At present, the numbers are more evenly spread throughout the calendar year.

- Sudden infant death syndrome rates for the United States have dropped steadily since 1994 in all racial and ethnic groups. Thousands of infant lives have been saved, but some ethnic groups are still at higher risk for SIDS.

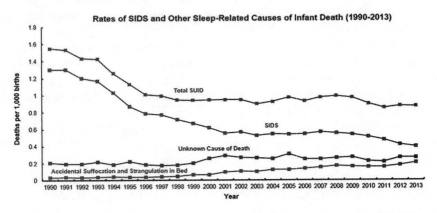

Figure 47.1. *U.S. Rates of SIDS and Other Sleep-Related Causes of Infant Death (1990–2013)*

What Sudden Infant Death Syndrome Is Not

Sudden infant death syndrome is not the cause of every sudden infant death.

Each year in the United States, thousands of babies die suddenly and unexpectedly. These deaths are called "SUID," which stands for "sudden unexpected infant death."

Sudden unexpected infant death includes all unexpected deaths: those without a clear cause, such as SIDS, and those from a known cause, such as suffocation. One-half of all SUID cases are SIDS. Many unexpected infant deaths are accidents, but a disease or something is done on purpose can also cause the baby to die suddenly and unexpectedly.

"Sleep-related causes of infant death" are those linked to how or where a baby sleeps or slept. These deaths are due to accidental causes, such as suffocation, entrapment, or strangulation. Entrapment is when the baby gets trapped between two objects, such as a mattress and a wall, and cannot breathe. Strangulation is when something presses on or wraps around the baby's neck, blocking the baby's airway. These deaths are not SIDS.

Other things that SIDS is not:

- Sudden infant death syndrome is not the same as suffocation and is not caused by suffocation.

- Sudden infant death syndrome is not caused by vaccines, immunizations, or shots.

- Sudden infant death syndrome is not contagious.

- Sudden infant death syndrome is not the result of neglect or child abuse.

- Sudden infant death syndrome is not caused by cribs.

- Sudden infant death syndrome is not caused by vomiting or choking.

- Sudden infant death syndrome is not completely preventable, but there are ways to reduce the risk.

What Causes Sudden Infant Death Syndrome

Scientists and healthcare providers are working very hard to find the cause or causes of SIDS. If we know the cause or causes, someday we might be able to prevent SIDS from happening at all.

More and more research evidence suggests that infants who die from SIDS are born with brain abnormalities or defects. These defects are typically found within a network of nerve cells that send signals to other nerve cells. The cells are located in the part of the brain that probably controls breathing, heart rate, blood pressure, temperature, and waking from sleep. At the present time, there is no way to identify babies who have these abnormalities, but researchers are working to develop specific screening tests.

But, scientists believe that brain defects alone may not be enough to cause a SIDS death. Evidence suggests that other events must also occur for an infant to die from SIDS. Researchers use the Triple-Risk Model to explain this concept. In this model, all three factors have to occur at the same time for an infant to die from SIDS. Having only one of these factors may not be enough to cause death from SIDS, but when all three combine, the chances of SIDS are high.

Even though the exact cause of SIDS is unknown, there are ways to reduce the risk of SIDS and other sleep-related causes of infant death.

What Is Known about Risk for Sudden Infant Death Syndrome and Other Sleep-Related Causes of Infant Death

Even though the exact cause of SIDS is not known, it is found that some things can increase a baby's risk for SIDS and other sleep-related causes of infant death. The good news is that there are ways to reduce the risk.

Known Risk Factors for SIDS and Other Sleep-Related Causes of Infant Death

Research shows that several factors put babies at higher risk for SIDS and other sleep-related causes of infant death. Babies who usually sleep on their backs but who are then placed to sleep on their stomachs, such as for a nap, are at very high risk for SIDS.

Babies are at higher risk for SIDS if they:

- Sleep on their stomachs

- Sleep on soft surfaces, such as an adult mattress, couch, or chair or under soft coverings

- Sleep on or under soft or loose bedding

- Get too hot during sleep

- Are exposed to cigarette smoke in the womb or in their environment, such as at home, in the car, in the bedroom, or other areas

- Sleep in an adult bed with parents, other children, or pets; this situation is especially dangerous if:
  - The adult smokes, has recently had alcohol, or is tired
  - The baby is covered by a blanket or quilt
  - The baby sleeps with more than one bed-sharer
  - The baby is younger than 11 to 14 weeks of age

Ways to Reduce the Risk of Sudden Infant Death Syndrome and Other Sleep-Related Causes of Infant Death

Research shows that there are several ways to reduce the risk of SIDS and other sleep-related causes of infant death. Some of them are discussed below:

Always Place Baby on His or Her Back to Sleep for Naps and at Night to Reduce the Risk of Sudden Infant Death Syndrome

The back sleep position is the safest position for all babies, until they are one year old. Babies who are used to sleeping on their backs, but who are then placed to sleep on their stomachs, such as for a nap, are at very high risk for SIDS.

If baby rolls over on his or her own from back to stomach or stomach to back, there is no need to reposition the baby. Starting sleep on the back is most important for reducing SIDS risk.

Preemies (infants born preterm) should be placed on their backs to sleep as soon as possible after birth.

Can My Baby Choke If Placed on the Back to Sleep?

The short answer is no—babies are not more likely to choke when sleeping on their backs.

Use a Firm and Flat Sleep Surface, Such as a Mattress in a Safety-Approved Crib, Covered by a Fitted Sheet with No Other Bedding or Soft Items in the Sleep Area

Never place a baby to sleep on soft surfaces, such as on a couch, sofa, waterbed, pillow, quilt, sheepskin, or blanket. These surfaces can be very dangerous for babies. Do not use a car seat, stroller, swing, infant carrier, infant sling, or similar products as baby's regular sleep area. Following these recommendations reduces the risk of SIDS and death or injury from suffocation, entrapment, and strangulation.

A crib, bassinet, portable crib, or play yard that follows the safety standards of the Consumer Product Safety Commission (CPSC) is recommended.

Why Should I Not Use Crib Bumpers in My Baby's Sleep Area?

Evidence does not support using crib bumpers to prevent injury. In fact, crib bumpers can cause serious injuries and even death.

Breastfeed Your Baby to Reduce the Risk of Sudden Infant Death Syndrome

Breastfeeding has many health benefits for mother and baby. Babies who breastfeed, or are fed breastmilk, are at lower risk for SIDS than are babies who were never fed breastmilk. A longer duration of exclusive breastfeeding leads to lower risk.

If you bring baby into your bed for feeding, put her or him back in a separate sleep area when finished. This sleep area should be made for infants, such as a crib or bassinet, and close to your bed. If you fall asleep while feeding or comforting baby in an adult bed, place her or him back in a separate sleep area as soon as you wake up. Evidence shows that the longer a parent and an infant bed share, the higher the risk for sleep-related causes of infant death, such as suffocation.

What If I Fall Asleep While Feeding My Baby?

It is less dangerous to fall asleep with an infant in an adult bed than on a sofa or armchair. The latest safe sleep recommendations include precautions in case you fall asleep while feeding your baby.

Share Your Room with Your Baby. Keep Your Baby in Your Room Close to Your Bed, but on a Separate Surface Designed for Infants, Ideally for Your Baby's First Year, but at least for the First Six Months

Room-sharing reduces the risk of SIDS. Your baby should not sleep in an adult bed, on a couch, or on a chair alone, with you, or with anyone else, including siblings or pets. Having a separate safe sleep surface for the baby reduces the risk of SIDS and the chance of suffocation, strangulation, and entrapment.

If you bring your baby into your bed for feeding or comforting, remove all soft items and bedding from the area. When finished, put your baby back in a separate sleep area made for infants, such as a crib or bassinet, and close to your bed.

Couches and armchairs can also be very dangerous for babies if adults fall asleep as they feed, comfort, or bond with the baby while on these surfaces. Parents and other caregivers should be mindful of how tired they are during these times.

There is no evidence for or against devices or products that claim to make bed sharing "safer."

Can I Practice Skin-to-Skin Care as Soon as My Baby Is Born?

Yes, when mom is stable, awake, and able to respond to her baby.

Do Not Put Soft Objects, Toys, Crib Bumpers, or Loose Bedding under Baby, over Baby, or Anywhere in Baby's Sleep Area

Keeping these items out of your baby's sleep area reduces the risk of SIDS and suffocation, entrapment, and strangulation. Because evidence does not support using them to prevent injury, crib bumpers are not recommended. Crib bumpers are linked to serious injuries and deaths from suffocation, entrapment, and strangulation. Keeping these and other soft objects out of a baby's sleep area is the best way to avoid these dangers.

To reduce the risk of SIDS, women should:

- Get regular prenatal care during pregnancy

- Avoid smoking, drinking alcohol, and using marijuana or illegal drugs during pregnancy or after the baby is born

- Not smoke during pregnancy

- Not smoke or allow smoking around your baby

Think about Giving Your Baby a Pacifier for Naps and Nighttime Sleep to Reduce the Risk of Sudden Infant Death Syndrome

- Do not attach the pacifier to anything, such as a string, clothing, stuffed toy, or blanket—that carries a risk for suffocation, choking, or strangulation.

- Wait until breastfeeding is well established (often by three to four weeks) before offering a pacifier. Or, if you are not breastfeeding, offer the pacifier as soon as you want. Do not force the baby to use it.

- If the pacifier falls out of baby's mouth during sleep, there is no need to put the pacifier back in.

Pacifiers reduce the risk of SIDS for all babies, including breastfed babies.

Do Not Let Your Baby Get Too Hot during Sleep

Dress your baby in sleep clothing, such as a wearable blanket designed to keep her or him warm without the need for loose blankets in the sleeping area.

Dress your baby appropriately for the environment, and do not overbundle. Parents and caregivers should watch for signs of overheating, such as sweating or the baby's chest feeling hot to the touch.

Keep the baby's face and head uncovered during sleep.

Can I Swaddle My Baby to Reduce the Risk of Sudden Infant Death Syndrome?

There is no evidence that swaddling reduces SIDS risk. In fact, swaddling can increase the risk of SIDS and other sleep-related causes of infant death.

Follow Healthcare-Provider Guidance on Your Baby's Vaccines and Regular Health Checkups

Vaccines not only protect the baby's health, but research shows that vaccinated babies are at lower risk for SIDS.

Avoid Products That Go against Safe Sleep Recommendations, Especially Those That Claim to Prevent or Reduce the Risk for Sudden Infant Death Syndrome

There is currently no known way to prevent SIDS.

Evidence does not support the safety or effectiveness of wedges, positioners, or other products that claim to keep infants in a specific position or to reduce the risk of SIDS, suffocation, or reflux. In fact, many of these products are associated with injury and death, especially when used in the baby's sleep area.

Do Not Use Heart or Breathing Monitors in the Home to Reduce the Risk of Sudden Infant Death Syndrome

If you have questions about using these monitors for other health conditions, talk with your baby's healthcare provider, and always follow safe sleep recommendations.

Give Your Baby Plenty of Tummy Time When She or He Is Awake and Someone Is Watching

Supervised tummy time helps strengthen your baby's neck, shoulders, and arm muscles. It also helps to prevent flat spots on the back of your baby's head.

Limiting the time spent in car seats, once the baby is out of the car, and changing the direction the infant lays in the sleep area from week to week also can help to prevent these flat spots.

Part Six

Diagnosing and Treating Respiratory Disorders

Chapter 48

Working with Your Doctor

Partnering with your healthcare professional means staying in touch regularly to maintain control of your asthma. If your medicines work well, you should plan on seeing your doctor again in the next two to six weeks. If not, call to schedule another visit right away. Once your asthma is under control, you may be able to gradually cut back your doctor visits to once every one to six months.

Each visit with your doctor or other healthcare professional is a chance for you to find out if you are doing the right things to manage your asthma and to learn about things that may improve your asthma control.

To make sure you get the most out of each visit, bring the following items with you:

- Your peak flow meter and the record of your peak flows, if you use a peak flow meter

- Your inhaler and other medicines

- A record of recent asthma symptoms or attacks, medication use, and hospital visits

- Your written asthma action plan

This chapter includes text excerpted from "So You Have Asthma—A Guide for Patients and their Families," National Heart, Lung, and Blood Institute (NHLBI), March 2013. Reviewed August 2019.

Ask your doctor to make sure you are using your inhalers and peak flow meter the right way. Also, ask your doctor to review and update your written asthma action plan. A list of sample questions for your doctor or other healthcare professional has been given below. Before you leave the doctor's office, be sure you have the answers to these and any other questions you have.

Just a few years ago, having asthma meant living a life filled with should nots and cannots. That is not the case anymore. As of now, most people who have asthma should be able to get their asthma under control—and keep it that way for a lifetime.

Managing your asthma sounds like a lot to do, and there certainly is a lot to learn, but you can do it—especially when it is a team effort! And over time, managing your asthma will become a routine part of your life.

Tips for Communicating with the Doctor

Proper communication with your doctor is very important. Here are a few tips for creating good, clear communication with your doctor or other healthcare professional.

Speak up. Tell your doctor or other healthcare professional about what you want to achieve by improving control of your asthma. Ask for her or his help in achieving those treatment goals.

Be open. When your doctor or other healthcare professional asks you questions, answer as honestly and completely as you can. Briefly describe your symptoms. Include when you started having each symptom, how often you have it, and whether it has been getting worse.

Keep it simple. If you do not understand something your doctor or other healthcare professional says, ask for a simple explanation. Be especially sure that you understand how to take any medicines you are given. If you are worried about understanding what the doctor or other healthcare professional says, or if you have trouble hearing, bring a friend or relative with you to your appointment. You may want to ask that person to write down instructions for you.

Questions to Ask Your Doctor or Other Healthcare Professional

Following is a list of sample questions that you can ask your doctor or a healthcare professional:

- Are you sure it is asthma?

- Do I need other tests to confirm the diagnosis?

- If I think my medicine is not working, is it OK to take more right away?

- What should I do if I miss a dose?

- Will my medicine cause me any problems, such as shakiness, sore throat, or upset stomach?

- What if I have problems taking my medicines or following my treatment plan?

- Is this the right way to use my inhaler? How do I use my inhaler with a spacer?

- Is this the right way to use my peak flow meter?

- How can I tell if I am having an asthma attack? What medicines should I take and how much of each should I take? When should I call you? When should I go to the emergency room?

- Once my asthma is under control, will I be able to reduce the amount of medicine I am taking?

- When should I see you again?

Chapter 49

Overview of Pulmonary Function Tests and Spirometry

Pulmonary Function Tests

Pulmonary function tests, or PFTs, measure how well your lungs work. The PFTs include tests that measure lung size and airflow, such as spirometry and lung volume tests. Other tests measure how well gases such as oxygen get in and out of your blood. These tests include pulse oximetry and arterial blood gas tests. Another pulmonary function test, called "fractional exhaled nitric oxide" (FeNO), measures nitric oxide, which is a marker for inflammation in the lungs. You may have one or more of these tests to diagnose lung and airway diseases, compare your lung function to expected levels of function, monitor if your disease is stable or worsening, and see if your treatment is working.

This chapter contains text excerpted from the following sources: Text under the heading "Pulmonary Function Tests" is excerpted from "Pulmonary Function Tests," National Heart, Lung, and Blood Institute (NHLBI), December 13, 2016; Text under the heading "Spirometry" is excerpted from "Spirometry," U.S. Department of Energy (DOE), February 27, 2010. Reviewed August 2019.

The purpose, procedure, discomfort, and risks of each test will vary.

- **Spirometry measures the rate of airflow and estimates lung size.** For this test, you will breathe multiple times, with regular and maximal effort, through a tube that is connected to a computer. Some people feel lightheaded or tired from the required breathing effort.

- **Lung volume tests are the most accurate way to measure how much air your lungs can hold.** The procedure is similar to spirometry, except that you will be in a small room with clear walls. Some people feel lightheaded or tired from the required breathing effort.

- **Lung diffusion capacity assesses how well oxygen gets into the blood from the air you breathe.** For this test, you will breathe in and out through a tube for several minutes without having to breathe intensely. You also may need to have blood drawn to measure the level of hemoglobin in your blood.

- **Pulse oximetry estimates oxygen levels in your blood.** For this test, a probe will be placed on your finger or another skin surface such as your ear. It causes no pain and has few or no risks.

- **Arterial blood gas tests directly measure the levels of gases, such as oxygen and carbon dioxide, in your blood.** Arterial blood gas tests are usually performed in a hospital, but may be done in a doctor's office. For this test, blood will be taken from an artery, usually in the wrist where your pulse is measured. You may feel brief pain when the needle is inserted or when a tube attached to the needle fills with blood. It is possible to have bleeding or infection where the needle was inserted.

- **Fractional exhaled nitric oxide tests measure how much nitric oxide is in the air that you exhale.** For this test, you will breathe out into a tube that is connected to the portable device. It requires steady but not intense breathing. It has few or no risks.

Other tests may be needed to assess lung function in infants, children, or patients who are not able to perform spirometry and lung volume tests. Before your tests, you may be asked to not eat some foods or take certain medicines that can affect some pulmonary function test results.

Spirometry

Spirometry, which is also known as "pulmonary function testing," is a tool for measuring lung function. Specifically, the test measures the volume (amount) and/or flow (speed) of air that can be inhaled or exhaled. Spirometry testing is a vital component for diagnosing occupational lung diseases and for assessing and monitoring such conditions as asthma and chronic obstructive pulmonary disease (COPD).

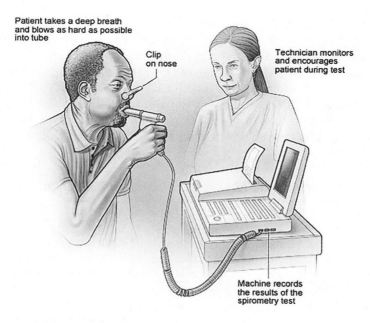

Figure 49.1. *Spirometry* (Source: "COPD," National Heart, Lung, and Blood Institute (NHLBI).)

The image shows how spirometry is done. The patient takes a deep breath and blows as hard as possible into a tube connected to a spirometer. The spirometer measures the amount of air breathed out. It also measures how fast the air was blown out.

The lung diseases detected by spirometry are mostly caused by smoking, respiratory infections, and breathing in hazardous dusts, fumes, or vapors. For workers, the spirometry test is used to measure lung function in individuals who have symptoms, such as chronic cough, shortness of breath, and/or wheezing to help determine whether they have lung diseases that may have resulted from occupational exposures during work at facilities. Workers with abnormal spirometry results are referred to their primary care physicians for further evaluation.

The test is performed by deeply inhaling and then forcefully exhaling into a spirometer (the machine that records the measurements). There are two measurements that are crucial in the interpretation of spirometry results.

The first measurement is the forced vital capacity (FVC), or total amount of air that can forcibly be blown out after a deep breath. The second measurement is the forced expiratory volume-one second (FEV1) or amount of air that an individual can forcibly blow out in one second. Another common value reported in a spirometry test is the ratio of FEV1 to FVC. In healthy middle-aged adults, the ratio should be above 70 percent; the normal value decreases with age. The table below shows normal and abnormal spirometry readings.

A reduction in FVC can be caused by restrictive lung disease (such as asbestosis). Abnormalities in the FEV1 and the FEV1/FVC result from a decrease in the airflow out of the lung. This decrease may be caused by obstructive lung diseases, such as silicosis, emphysema, and asthma. The table below provides an interpretation of spirometry results.

Table 49.1. Normal and Abnormal Spirometry Readings

Spirometry Test	Normal	Abnormal
FVC and FEV1	• Equal to or greater than 80%, or above the lower limit of normal using statistical testing	• Mild 70 to 79% • Moderate 60 to 69% • Severe less than 50%
FEV1/FVC	• Equal to or greater than 70%, or above the lower limit of normal using statistical testing	• Mild 60 to 69% • Moderate 50 to 59% • Severe less than 50%

Chapter 50

Blood Gases Test

A blood gas test is a method used to check and measure the presence of oxygen and carbon dioxide in a person's blood. This test is performed to check whether the lungs are working efficiently while exchanging the supply of oxygen and carbon dioxide and to determine acidity levels in the blood. This test is commonly known as "blood gas analysis."

Types of Blood Gas Test

The blood gas test can be classified into two types:

- **Arterial blood gas (ABG) test**—a test that is done with a blood sample taken from one's wrist
- **Capillary blood gas (CBG) test**—a test that is done with a blood sample taken from one's earlobe

Purpose of the Blood Gas Test

The blood gas test is used in determining the precise levels of oxygen and carbon dioxide in one's body, which helps a doctor to determine the normal functioning of the kidney and lungs. This test plays a vital role in the pulmonary function testing lab or clinic.

The symptoms that call for a blood gas test are an imbalance in oxygen, carbon dioxide, and pH levels, including shortness of breath,

"Blood Gases Test," © 2019 Omnigraphics. Reviewed August 2019.

difficulty in breathing, confusion, and nausea, as these conditions may be signs of certain medical conditions, such as:

- Kidney failure

- Heart failure

- Uncontrolled diabetes

- Hemorrhage

- Shock

- Chemical poisoning

- Drug overdose

A blood gas test might be ordered if the doctor suspects conditions that affect breathing. The blood gas test not only helps in detecting certain diseases but also helps in monitoring the treatment of certain lung and kidney diseases.

How Is the Blood Gas Test Performed?

Generally, blood samples are taken from the arteries and, in rare cases, blood samples from veins are taken.

Blood samples for ABG tests are taken from any of the arteries, such as radial artery in the wrist; femoral artery in the groin; or brachial artery in the arm, or are taken from the earlobe for CBG tests.

This procedure is safe and trouble-free and takes only a few minutes to complete. A small needle is inserted into the artery through the skin or pricked from the earlobe and the blood samples are quickly sent to the laboratory.

Interpreting the Results of a Blood Gas Test

The test measures the following:

- **Arterial blood pH.** A pH of 7 is neutral and any value above 7 indicates the basic or alkaline level, while a pH value of less than 7 indicates the acidic level in blood. A low pH indicates that the acidic level is high with higher carbon dioxide levels, and a high pH indicates that the blood is more basic and has a higher bicarbonate level.

- **Bicarbonate**, a chemical substance that helps in maintaining the pH level of the blood, preventing the blood from being too acidic or basic

- **Partial pressure of oxygen** determines how well oxygen is able to flow into the blood with the measure of the pressure of oxygen dissolved in the blood.

- **Partial pressure of carbon dioxide** determines how well carbon dioxide is able to flow into the blood with the measure of the pressure of carbon dioxide dissolved in the blood.

- **Oxygen saturation** is the measure of the pressure of oxygen being carried by the hemoglobin present in the red blood cells (RBCs).

Normal Results

Values at sea level:

- The partial pressure of oxygen (PaO_2): 75 to 100 millimeters of mercury (mm Hg), or 10.5 to 13.5 kilopascal (kPa)

- The partial pressure of carbon dioxide ($PaCO_2$); 38 to 42 mm Hg (5.1 to 5.6 kPa)

- Arterial blood pH: 7.38 to 7.42

- Oxygen saturation (SaO_2): 94 to 100 percent

- Bicarbonate (HCO_3): 22 to 28 milliequivalents per liter (mEq/L)

At altitudes of 900 meters and above, the oxygen value is lower.

The normal values may vary with respect to laboratories as each laboratory uses different measurements or different specimens for the test. Do consult your doctor to know about specific test results.

The values might also have a varied reference range if they are from a capillary or a venous sample and the oxygen levels may be low if one lives above sea level.

Risks Associated with the Blood Gas Test

The blood gas test requires only a small quantity of blood sample, and hence the procedure is very simple. However, one should always inform her or his doctor if they are prone to excessive bleeding or if one is taking an over-the-counter (OTC) prescription such as blood thinners, which might affect bleeding.

Other side effects associated with this test are:

- Feeling faint

- Infection at the punctured sight

- Accumulation of blood under the skin (hematoma)
- Bleeding or bruising at the punctured site

Do consult your doctor if you experience a prolonged or unexpected side effect.

References

1. Nall, Rachel, "Blood Gas Test," Healthline, July 1, 2019.

2. "Blood Gases," MedlinePlus, A.D.A.M Medical Encyclopedia, July 10, 2019.

3. "Blood Gases," American Association for Clinical Chemistry (AACC), May 1, 2019.

Chapter 51

Bronchoscopy

What Is Bronchoscopy?

Bronchoscopy is a procedure that looks inside the lung airways. It involves inserting a bronchoscope tube, with its light and small camera, through your nose or mouth, down your throat into your trachea, or windpipe, and to the bronchi and bronchioles of your lungs. This procedure is used to find the cause of a lung problem. It can detect tumors, signs of infection, excess mucus in the airways, bleeding, or blockages in the lungs. It also can allow your doctor to take samples of mucus or tissue for other laboratory tests, as well as to insert airway stents, or small tubes, to keep your airway open to treat some lung problems.

What Happens before, during, and after Bronchoscopy?
Before the Procedure

Before the procedure, you will be given medicine to relax you. A liquid medicine also will be given to numb your nose and throat. If you have low blood oxygen levels during the procedure, you will be treated with oxygen therapy. If you have a lot of bleeding in your lungs or a

This chapter includes text excerpted from "Bronchoscopy," National Heart, Lung, and Blood Institute (NHLBI), November 28, 2014. Reviewed August 2019.

large object is stuck in your airway, you may require rigid bronchoscopy in a hospital operating room under general anesthesia.

During the Procedure

The procedure is performed using a flexible bronchoscope or a rigid bronchoscope. Flexible bronchoscopy is more common than rigid bronchoscopy, and flexible bronchoscopy usually does not require general anesthesia.

After the Procedure

After the procedure, you will be monitored to make sure you do not have complications. You may experience a sore throat, cough, or hoarseness that will go away with time. If you had the procedure as an outpatient, you likely will be able to go home after a few hours, but you will need a ride home because of the medicines or anesthesia you received. You will need to follow up with your doctor after the procedure to get your results.

Complications Associated with Bronchoscopy

Bronchoscopy is usually safe, but there is a small risk for fever, minor bleeding, or pneumonia. Pneumothorax, or collapsed lung, is a rare but serious side effect that can be treated. Your doctor may do a chest x-ray after the procedure to check for lung problems.

Additional Complications*

Common complications of diagnostic bronchoscopy relate to the bronchoscope's irritation of the respiratory tract (cough, bronchospasm), sampling procedures (bleeding, pneumothorax), and sedation (desaturation, hypotension, loss of consciousness). Severe complications requiring intervention or resulting in increased mortality or morbidity are rare.

Text excerpted from "One Bronchoscopy, Two Errors," Agency for Healthcare Research and Quality (AHRQ), U.S. Department of Health and Human Services (HHS), January 7, 2019.

Chapter 52

Chest Scans and X-Rays

Chest Computed Tomography Scan

A chest computed tomography (CT) scan is a more detailed type of chest x-ray. This painless imaging test takes many detailed pictures, called "slices," of your lungs and the inside of your chest. Computers can combine these pictures to create three-dimensional (3D) models to help show the size, shape, and position of your lungs and structures in your chest. This imaging test is often done to follow up on abnormal findings from earlier chest x-rays. A chest CT scan also can help determine the cause of lung symptoms such as shortness of breath or chest pain, or check to see if you have certain lung problems such as tumors, excess fluid around the lungs that is known as "pleural effusion," "pulmonary embolism," "emphysema," "tuberculosis," and "pneumonia."

Your chest CT scan may be done in a medical imaging facility or hospital. The CT scanner is a large, tunnel-like machine that has a

This chapter contains text excerpted from the following sources: Text under the heading "Chest Computed Tomography Scan" is excerpted from "Chest CT Scan," National Heart, Lung, and Blood Institute (NHLBI), July 25, 2012. Reviewed August 2019; Text under the heading "Chest Magnetic Resonance Imaging" is excerpted from "Chest MRI," National Heart, Lung, and Blood Institute (NHLBI), December 10, 2016; Text under the heading "Chest X-Ray" is excerpted from "Chest X-Ray," National Heart, Lung, and Blood Institute (NHLBI), December 10, 2016; Text under the heading "Lung or Pulmonary Ventilation and Perfusion Scans " is excerpted from "Lung VQ Scan," National Heart, Lung, and Blood Institute (NHLBI), December 10, 2016.

table. You will lie still on the table and the table will slide into the scanner. Talk to your doctor if you are uncomfortable in tight or closed spaces to see if you need medicine to relax you during the test. You will hear soft buzzing or clicking sounds when you are inside the scanner and the scanner is taking pictures. You will be able to hear from and talk to the technician performing the test while you are inside the scanner. For some diagnoses, a contrast dye, often iodine-based, may be injected into a vein in your arm before the imaging test. This contrast dye highlights areas inside your chest and creates clearer pictures. You may feel some discomfort from the needle or, after the contrast dye is injected, you may feel warm briefly or have a temporary metallic taste in your mouth.

Chest CT scans have some risks. In rare instances, some people have an allergic reaction to the contrast dye. There is a slight risk of cancer, particularly in growing children, because the test uses radiation. Although the amount of radiation from one test is usually less than the amount of radiation you are naturally exposed to over three years, patients should not receive more CT scans than the number that clinical guidelines recommend. Another risk is that chest CT scans may detect an incidental finding, which is something that does not cause symptoms but now may require more tests after being found. Talk to your doctor and the technicians performing the test about whether you are or could be pregnant. If the test is not urgent, they may have you wait to do the test until after your pregnancy. If it is urgent, the technicians will take extra steps to protect your baby during this test. Let your doctor know if you are breastfeeding because contrast dye can pass into your breast milk. If you must have contrast dye injected, you may want to pump and save enough breast milk for one to two days after your test or you may bottle-feed your baby for that time.

Chest Magnetic Resonance Imaging

Chest magnetic resonance imaging (MRI) can provide detailed information to help your doctor diagnose lung problems, such as a tumor or pleural disorder, blood vessel problems, or abnormal lymph nodes. Chest MRI can help explain the results of other imaging tests, such as chest x-rays and chest CT scans.

Chest MRI may be done in a medical imaging facility or hospital. Before your test, a technician may inject a contrast dye into a vein in your arm to highlight your heart and blood vessels. You may feel some discomfort from the needle or have a cool feeling as the contrast dye is injected. The MRI machine is a large, tunnel-like machine that has a table. You will lie still on the table, and the table will slide into the machine. You will hear loud humming, tapping, and buzzing sounds when you are inside the machine as pictures of your chest are being taken. You will be able to hear from and talk to the technician performing the test while you are inside the machine. The technician may ask you to hold your breath for a few seconds during the test.

Chest MRI has few risks. In rare instances, the contrast dye may harm people who have kidney disease, or it may cause an allergic reaction. Researchers are studying whether multiple contrast dye injections, defined as four or more, may cause other adverse effects. Talk to your doctor and the technicians performing the test about whether you are or could be pregnant. Let your doctor know if you are breastfeeding because the contrast dye can pass into your breast milk. If you must have the contrast dye injected, you may want to pump and save enough breast milk for one to two days after your test or you may bottle-feed your baby for that time. Tell your doctor if you have:

- **A pacemaker or other implanted device** because the MRI machine can damage these devices

- **Metal inside your body** from previous surgeries because it can interfere with the MRI machine

- **Metal on your body** from piercings, jewelry, or some transdermal skin patches because they can interfere with the MRI machine or cause skin burns. Tattoos may cause a problem because older tattoo inks may contain small amounts of metal.

Chest X-Ray

This test can help diagnose and monitor conditions, such as pneumonia, heart failure, lung cancer, tuberculosis, sarcoidosis, and lung tissue scarring, called "fibrosis." Doctors may use chest x-rays to see how well certain treatments are working and to check for complications after certain procedures or surgeries.

The test may be done in the doctor's office, clinic, hospital, or other medical facility. Before having a chest x-ray, you will undress from the waist up, wear a gown, and remove jewelry and objects that could interfere with the test. You will stand, sit, or lie still for the test. A lead apron may be worn to protect your reproductive organs from the x-ray. The technician will operate the x-ray machine from behind a wall or in the next room. Usually, the technician takes two views, one from straight on and one from the side of your chest, but more views may be taken. A radiologist will analyze the images and send a report to your doctor.

Chest x-rays have few risks. The amount of radiation used in a chest x-ray is very small. Talk to your doctor and the technicians performing the test about whether you are or could be pregnant. If the procedure is not urgent, they may have you wait to do the test until after your pregnancy. If it is urgent, the technicians will take extra steps to protect your baby during this test.

Lung or Pulmonary Ventilation and Perfusion Scans

It uses special x-ray scanners outside of your body to create pictures of air and blood flow patterns in your lungs. This test can help diagnose or rule out a pulmonary embolism, or a blood clot in your lungs. A ventilation–perfusion (VQ) scan also can detect regional differences in lung blood flow and air distribution. Doctors may use VQ scans to examine the lungs before some surgeries.

Lung VQ scans are performed in radiology clinics or hospitals. There is no preparation for a VQ scan other than having had a recent chest x-ray. The test will take about an hour. For each scan, you will need to lie very still on a table as the table moves under the scanner and pictures are taken of your lungs. Before each scan, you will need to hold your breath for a few seconds. If you think you may have trouble staying still for the test, ask your doctor to suggest ways to avoid moving during the test. Before the ventilation scan, you will wear a breathing mask over your nose and mouth and will breathe in a small amount of a radioisotope gas mixed with oxygen. Before the perfusion scan, the technician will inject a small amount of radioisotope into a vein in your arm. You may feel discomfort from the injection. The scanner detects the energy that the radioisotopes released inside your body and uses the energy to make pictures of your lungs.

Lung VQ scans involve little pain or risk for most people. You may bruise at the injection site. In rare instances, some people have a treatable allergic reaction to the radioisotope. This test uses small amounts of radiation from the radioisotope that you breathe in and that is injected into your vein. Talk to your doctor and the technicians performing the test about whether you are or could be pregnant. If the test is not urgent, they may have you wait to do the test until after your pregnancy. If it is urgent, the technicians will take extra steps to protect your baby during this test. Let your doctor know if you are breastfeeding because radiation can pass into your breast milk. You may want to pump and save enough breast milk for one to two days after your test, or you may bottle-feed your baby for that time.

Chapter 53

Sweat Test for Cystic Fibrosis

What Is a Sweat Test?

A sweat test measures the amount of chloride, a part of salt, in sweat. It is used to diagnose cystic fibrosis (CF). People with CF have a high level of chloride in their sweat.

Cystic fibrosis is a disease that causes mucus buildup in the lungs and other organs. It damages the lungs and makes it hard to breathe. It can also lead to frequent infections and malnutrition. CF is an inherited disease, which means it is passed down from your parents, through genes.

Genes are parts of deoxyribonucleic acid (DNA) that carry information that determines your unique traits, such as height and eye color. Genes are also responsible for certain health problems. To have cystic fibrosis, you must have a *CF* gene from both your mother and your father. If only one parent has the gene, you will not get the disease.

Other names: sweat chloride test, cystic fibrosis sweat test, sweat electrolytes

This chapter includes text excerpted from "Sweat Test for Cystic Fibrosis," MedlinePlus, National Institutes of Health (NIH), July 24, 2018.

What Is Sweat Test Used For?

A sweat test is used to diagnose CF.

Why Do You Need a Sweat Test?

A sweat test can diagnose CF in people of all ages, but it is usually done on babies. Your baby may need a sweat test if she or he tested positive for CF on a routine newborn blood test. In the United States, new babies are usually tested for a variety of conditions including CF. Most sweat tests are done when babies are two to four weeks old.

An older child or adult who has never been tested for CF may need a cystic fibrosis sweat test if someone in the family has the disease and/or has symptoms of CF. These include:

- Salty-tasting skin

- Frequent coughing

- Frequent lung infections, such as pneumonia and bronchitis

- Trouble breathing

- Failure to gain weight, even with a good appetite

- Greasy, bulky stools

- In newborns, no stools made right after birth

What Happens during a Sweat Test

Your healthcare provider will need to collect a sample of sweat for testing. The entire procedure will take about an hour and will probably include the following steps:

- A healthcare provider will put pilocarpine, a medicine that causes sweating, on a small area of the forearm.

- Your provider will place an electrode on this area.

- A weak current will be sent through the electrode. This current makes the medicine seep into the skin. This may cause a little tingling or warmth.

- After removing the electrode, your provider will tape a piece of filter paper or gauze on the forearm to collect the sweat.

- Sweat will be collected for 30 minutes.

- The collected sweat will be sent to a lab for testing.

Will You Need to Do Anything to Prepare for the Sweat Test?

You do not need any special preparations for a sweat test, but you should avoid applying any creams or lotions to the skin for 24 hours before the procedure.

Are There Any Risks to the Sweat Test?

There is no known risk to a sweat test. Your child may have a tingling or tickling sensation from the electric current, but should not feel any pain.

What Do the Sweat Test Results Mean?

If the results show a high level of chloride, there is a good chance your child has cystic fibrosis. Your healthcare provider will probably order another sweat test and/or other tests to confirm or rule out a diagnosis. If you have questions about your child's results, talk to your healthcare provider.

Is There Anything Else You Need to Know about a Sweat Test?

While there is no cure for CF, there are treatments available that help reduce symptoms and improve quality of life (QOL). If your child was diagnosed with CF, talk with your healthcare provider about strategies and treatments to help manage the disease.

Chapter 54

Thoracentesis

Thoracentesis is a procedure in which a needle is inserted into the pleural space between the lungs and the chest wall. This procedure is done to remove excess fluid, known as a "pleural effusion," from the pleural space to help you breathe easier. It may be done to determine the cause of your pleural effusion. Some conditions, such as heart failure, lung infections, and tumors can cause pleural effusions.

Thoracentesis is performed in a doctor's office or hospital. The procedure usually takes 10 to 15 minutes, unless you have a lot of fluid in your pleural space. For the procedure, most patients sit quietly on the edge of a chair or bed with their head and arms resting on a table. Your doctor may use ultrasound to determine the best location to insert the needle. After cleaning the skin around the area where the needle will be inserted, your doctor will inject numbing medicine. A needle is inserted between your ribs into the pleural space. You may feel some discomfort or pressure when the needle is inserted. As your doctor draws out excess fluid from around your lungs, you may feel like coughing or have chest pain. The needle will be removed, and a small bandage will be applied to the site.

After the procedure, your blood pressure and breathing will be monitored to make sure you do not have complications. The fluid that was

This chapter contains text excerpted from the following sources: Text in this chapter begins with excerpts from "Thoracentesis," National Heart, Lung, and Blood Institute (NHLBI), December 10, 2016; Text beginning with the heading "Risks of Thoracentesis" is excerpted from "Thoracentesis/Pleural Biopsy," U.S. Department of Veterans Affairs (VA), July 2005. Reviewed August 2019.

removed from your chest will be sent for laboratory testing to determine the cause of your pleural effusion and to help plan your treatment. Your doctor may order a chest x-ray to check for lung problems.

The risks of thoracentesis include pneumothorax or collapsed lung, pain, bleeding, bruising, or infection. Liver or spleen injuries are rare complications.

Risks of Thoracentesis

These risks will be explained in greater detail when you go for your test.

- **Infection:** Sterile equipment is used.

- **Bleeding:** You will have blood tests that tell your provider how well your blood clots.

- **Pneumothorax or collapse of part of the lung:** You will have a chest x-ray after the test so the doctors can see how your lungs look after the test.

Before the Test

- In some cases, a chest ultrasound is done to locate the fluid pocket. This is done in the Radiology Department. This test will not cause any discomfort. Ultrasound uses sound waves to examine your lungs. A jelly is put on your chest and a plastic bulb is held against your skin. This picks up the sound waves in your chest. They form a picture on a television screen showing the size of the pocket of fluid or air and where it is.

- You can eat breakfast and take your medications the morning of the test.

- Arrange to have someone drive you to the medical center and take you home after the test. If possible, bring someone who can stay with you before and after the test.

During the Test

- You will change into a patient gown so the doctors can reach your back.

- You will sit in a comfortable position with your arms resting on a table in front of you. Part of your back will be wiped with a cool, cleaning solution.

- You will feel a needle prick and stinging when you are given medicine to numb a small area of your back.

- You may feel as if someone is pushing on your back as the catheter is put in place.

Try not to move suddenly while the catheter is in place. Tell the doctor if you feel any changes in your chest as the fluid is removed. You may feel like coughing or you may feel an ache. This probably means that enough fluid has been removed. The doctor may ask you to hum as the catheter is removed. The puncture spot is covered with a bandaid or a small dressing. Keep the band-aid or dressing on and keep your back clean and dry for the next 24 hours.

Chapter 55

Tuberculin Tests

What Is Tuberculin Skin Testing?

The Mantoux tuberculin skin test (TST) is the standard method of determining whether a person is infected with *Mycobacterium tuberculosis*. Reliable administration and reading of the TST requires a standardization of procedures, training, supervision, and practice.

How Is the Tuberculin Skin Testing Administered?

The TST is performed by injecting 0.1 ml of tuberculin purified protein derivative (PPD) into the inner surface of the forearm. The injection should be made with a tuberculin syringe, with the needle bevel facing upward. The TST is an intradermal injection. When placed correctly, the injection should produce a pale elevation of the skin (a wheal) 6 to 10 mm in diameter.

How Is the Tuberculin Skin Testing Read?

The skin test reaction should be read between 48 and 72 hours after administration. A patient who does not return within 72 hours will need to be rescheduled for another skin test.

This chapter includes text excerpted from "Tuberculosis (TB)," Centers for Disease Control and Prevention (CDC), May 4, 2016.

The reaction should be measured in millimeters of the induration (palpable, raised, hardened area or swelling). The reader should not measure erythema (redness). The diameter of the indurated area should be measured across the forearm (perpendicular to the long axis).

How Are Tuberculin Skin Testing Reactions Interpreted?

Skin test interpretation depends on two factors:

- Measurement in millimeters of the induration
- Person's risk of being infected with tuberculosis (TB) and of progression to disease if infected

What Are False-Positive Reactions?

Some people may react to the TST even though they are not infected with *M. tuberculosis*. The causes of these false-positive reactions may include, but are not limited to, the following:

- Infection with nontuberculosis mycobacteria
- Previous Bacillus Calmette–Guérin (BCG) vaccination
- Incorrect method of TST administration
- Incorrect interpretation of reaction
- Incorrect bottle of antigen used

What Are False-Negative Reactions?

Some people may not react to the TST even though they are infected with *Mycobacterium tuberculosis*. The reasons for these false-negative reactions may include, but are not limited to, the following:

- Cutaneous anergy (anergy is the inability to react to skin tests because of a weakened immune system)
- Recent TB infection (within 8 to 10 weeks of exposure)
- Very old TB infection (many years)
- Very young age (less than 6 months old)

- Recent live-virus vaccinations (e.g., measles and smallpox)
- Overwhelming TB disease
- Some viral illnesses (e.g., measles and chickenpox)
- Incorrect method of TST administration
- Incorrect interpretation of reaction

Who Can Receive a Tuberculin Skin Testing?

Most persons can receive a TST, but it is contraindicated for persons who have had a severe reaction (e.g., necrosis, blistering, anaphylactic shock, or ulcerations) to a previous TST. It is not contraindicated for any other people, including infants, children, pregnant women, people who are HIV-infected, or people who have been vaccinated with BCG.

How Often Can Tuberculin Skin Testings Be Repeated?

In general, there is no risk associated with repeated tuberculin skin test placements. If a patient does not return within 48 to 72 hours for a tuberculin skin test reading, a second test can be placed as soon as possible. There is no contraindication to repeating the TST, unless a previous TST was associated with a severe reaction.

What Is a Boosted Reaction?

In some people who are infected with *M. tuberculosis*, the ability to react to tuberculin may wane over time. When given a TST years after infection, these people may have a false-negative reaction. However, the TST may stimulate the immune system, causing a positive, or boosted, reaction to subsequent tests. Giving a second TST after an initial negative TST reaction is called "two-step testing."

Why Is Two-Step Testing Conducted?

Two-step testing is useful for the initial skin testing of adults who are going to be retested periodically, such as healthcare workers or nursing-home residents. This two-step approach can reduce the likelihood that a boosted reaction to a subsequent TST will be misinterpreted as a recent infection.

Can Tuberculin Skin Testings Be Given to People Receiving Vaccinations?

Vaccination with live viruses may interfere with TST reactions. For people scheduled to receive a TST, testing should be done as follows:

- Either on the same day as vaccination with live-virus vaccine or four to six weeks after the administration of the live-virus vaccine
- At least one month after smallpox vaccination

Chapter 56

Other Respiratory Disorder Tests

Chapter Contents

Section 56.1

Gallium Scan

This section includes text excerpted from "Procedures/Diagnostic
Tests—Gallium Scan," Clinical Center, National Institutes of
Health (NIH), February 1, 2001. Reviewed August 2019.

A gallium scan is a safe, effective, and painless scan. It uses a
compound that gives off a small amount of radiation (radioisotope).
This compound is received by injection. The compound is used only for
diagnostic purposes and helps your doctor locate specific sites of tumor,
abscess, inflammation, or other abnormalities within your body. The
scan takes place in the nuclear medicine department.

Preparing for Gallium Scan

Before you receive the injection, there is no preparation. You may
eat and drink whatever you like.

During Gallium Scan

After you receive the injection and before the pictures are taken,
be sure to have a good bowel movement. If you need a laxative to do
this, please ask for one.

A small amount of the radioisotope will be injected into a vein. You
will feel a pinprick as the injection is given.

Depending on the purpose of the scan, it may be done 24 or 48 hours
after the injection. Sometimes the scan is repeated daily, over 3 to 4
days, but no additional injection will be given. If your test takes place
over several days, please return to the diagnostic imaging section at
the time scheduled for you by the appointment clerk.

During the scan, you will lie on your back on a firm table with your
head flat. A very sensitive machine (scanner) that receives and records
radiation, will move over your body from your head to your toes. Many
pictures will be taken as the scanner moves.

Stay very still while pictures are being taken.

The scan lasts one to two hours.

After Gallium Scan

There are no side effects, but a small amount of radioisotope may
still be present in your body for up to four weeks.

You may urinate in the toilet as usual. Your urine and blood will be labeled "Radioactive" if sent to the laboratory during the first four weeks after the injection. Your body rids itself of the compound as it does the food you eat.

If you have questions about the procedure, please ask. Your nurse and doctor are ready to assist you at all times.

Special Instructions

Because it uses radioactivity, this scan is not performed on pregnant women. If you are pregnant or think you might be pregnant, please inform your doctor immediately so that a decision can be made about this scan. Also, please inform your doctor immediately if you are breast-feeding. Some scans can be performed in breast-feeding women if they are willing to stop breastfeeding for a while.

Section 56.2

Pleural Needle Biopsy

"Other Respiratory Disorder Tests—Pleural Needle Biopsy,"
© 2017 Omnigraphics. Reviewed August 2019.

Pleural needle biopsy, also known as "closed pleural biopsy," is a medical procedure that is usually performed to identify the cause of fluid accumulation in and around the lungs. This procedure is also used to check for diseases and infections in the chest, such as tuberculosis (TB) or cancer. During a pleural needle biopsy, a surgeon or other medical professional collects samples of the lungs, the tissue linings of the lungs, and the inside of the chest wall (also known as the "pleural cavity").

How Pleural Needle Biopsy Is Performed

Blood tests and chest x-rays are typically ordered prior to a pleural needle biopsy. Pleural needle biopsies are performed at a hospital, doctor's office, or other medical centers. The person receiving the biopsy will typically be in a sitting position. The healthcare provider cleans the skin at the biopsy site and administers anesthetic to numb the skin, the lining of the lungs, and the chest wall. A hollow needle is inserted through the skin into the chest cavity. In some cases, an ultrasound or other medical imaging system is used to guide the needle. A smaller needle is then inserted through the hollow needle. Tissue samples are collected using the smaller needle. Because samples are taken from the lungs, the person receiving the biopsy is often asked to sing, hum, or make the sound "eee" during the procedure, to minimize the risk of air entering the chest cavity and to keep the lungs inflated. After the tissue samples are collected, a bandage is placed over the biopsy site. Post-biopsy chest x-rays may also be ordered.

Results of Pleural Needle Biopsy

The results of a pleural needle biopsy can indicate the presence of a variety of health conditions including cancer, tumor, mesothelioma, TB or other infection, or vascular disease. A surgical pleural biopsy may be required if the results of a pleural needle biopsy are inconclusive.

Risks of Pleural Needle Biopsy

During a pleural needle biopsy, there is a small risk that the needle used for sample collection may puncture the wall of the lung. This can result in a collapsed lung. There is also a small risk of air entering the chest cavity during the procedure, which can also result in a collapsed lung. In most cases, a punctured or collapsed lung will heal without intervention. In some cases, the collapsed lung will need to be reinflated and any accumulated fluid will need to be drained.

Reference

1. "Pleural Needle Biopsy," MedlinePlus, A.D.A.M. Medical Encyclopedia, August 11, 2015.

Chapter 57

Medicines for Respiratory Symptoms

Chapter Contents

Section 57.1

Antibiotics for Respiratory Infections

This section includes text excerpted from "Improving Antibiotic Prescribing for Uncomplicated Acute Respiratory Tract Infections," Effective Health Care Program, Agency for Healthcare Research and Quality (AHRQ), January 2016.

Antibiotics transformed the practice of medicine in the last half of the 20th century. With antibiotics, common infections and injuries that would previously have caused death or debility can now be effectively treated and cured. With antibiotic use, however, some bacteria can adapt, which can result in the development of antibiotic resistance, a public-health problem that has grown substantially in the last several decades. In the United States, at least 2 million people acquire infections with antibiotic-resistant bacteria each year, causing approximately 23,000 deaths. Although reasons for higher rates of antibiotic resistance at a population level are multifactorial, including the use of antibiotics in livestock and underdevelopment of new antibiotics, a key factor is high outpatient consumption of antibiotics.

The problem of inappropriate antibiotic use may be biggest for uncomplicated acute respiratory tract infections (RTIs) because they account for approximately 70 percent of primary diagnoses in adults presenting for ambulatory care office visits with a chief symptom of cough. Acute RTIs include acute bronchitis, acute otitis media (AOM), pharyngitis/tonsillitis, rhinitis, sinusitis, and other viral syndromes, but not community-acquired pneumonia or acute exacerbations of chronic obstructive pulmonary disease (COPD), bronchiectasis, or other chronic underlying lung diseases. Despite guidelines recommending no antibiotic treatment for uncomplicated acute RTIs, the majority of outpatient antibiotic prescriptions in the United States are for acute RTIs. The National Ambulatory and National Hospital Ambulatory Medical Care Surveys (NAMCS/NHAMCS) found that in the period 2007 to 2009, antibiotics were prescribed during 101 million ambulatory visits for patients aged 18 years and above annually. Similarly, although the majority of bronchitis and pharyngitis is viral rather than bacterial, a 2013 report on healthy adults visiting outpatient offices and emergency departments (EDs) for acute bronchitis found that antibiotics were prescribed at 73 percent of visits from 1996 through 2010, and a 2014 analysis of data from the NAMCS/NHAMCS indicated that 60 percent of children diagnosed with pharyngitis from 1997 through 2010 were prescribed antibiotics.

The reasons for overuse of antibiotics for acute RTIs are numerous, diverse, and complex, with both internal and external factors, including geographic location; environment (e.g., clinic type); patient demographics (e.g., children versus. adults); availability of follow-up care; patient and clinician preferences, communication, and relationship; clinician specialty, knowledge, and experience; clinical inertia; peer group influence; and oversight or feedback from infectious disease experts. Consequently, strategies to reduce antibiotic use for acute RTIs have varied targets. Strategies may target clinicians who care for patients with acute RTIs in outpatient settings, adult and/or pediatric patients with acute RTIs, the parents of pediatric patients with acute RTIs, healthy adults and/or children in the general population without a current RTI, or organizations whose attendance policies may indirectly affect the use of antibiotics (e.g., employers, school officials). Intervention strategies have also varied in the ways they are designed to change antibiotic prescribing behavior, including education, strategies to improve communication between clinicians and patients, clinical strategies, such as delayed prescribing or use of point-of-care diagnostic tests, system-level strategies, such as clinician reminders or audit and feedback, or multifaceted approaches that incorporate various elements.

Interventions to improve antibiotic use are intended to achieve a variety of outcomes, including diminished antibiotic resistance, fewer adverse drug events, and decreased healthcare costs. However, long-term studies to evaluate these important impacts are largely yet to be done, and studies of antibiotic resistance would need to be conducted in large populations and over long time periods. In the absence of patient-centered outcomes, it has been suggested that the rate of "inappropriate" prescription of antibiotics would be the best surrogate outcome. But although a number of guidelines define when antibiotic use is warranted, defining and determining "appropriate" use for study purposes is difficult because determination of appropriateness is subjective and requires both access to adequate patient-level data and clinical knowledge. Similarly, while "prescription" and "use" are not synonymous, measuring actual use is much more difficult and resource intensive than counting prescriptions. Therefore, studies have generally evaluated the impact of interventions on overall antibiotic prescriptions, based on the understanding that for certain clinical conditions, the majority of antibiotic use is unnecessary and should be reduced. The usefulness of overall prescribing as a proxy for appropriate prescribing may vary because the rate of inappropriate prescribing ranges widely, from 50 to 80 percent, based on patient, provider, and setting factors.

A main concern with using a reduction in overall prescribing of antibiotics for RTIs as a measure of success is that it may increase the risk of undertreatment of patients for whom antibiotics would have been indicated and lead to increases in undesirable outcomes, such as hospitalization, medical complications, clinic visits, time off work and/or school, patient dissatisfaction, and longer symptom duration. In addition, the interventions may require substantial time and resources. Therefore, these negative outcomes must be assessed alongside the prescribing outcomes.

Section 57.2

Antihistamines

This section includes text excerpted from "Antihistamines," LiverTox®, National Institutes of Health (NIH), July 1, 2019.

Histamine is an important mediator of immediate hypersensitivity reactions acting locally and causing smooth muscle contraction, vasodilation, increased vascular permeability, edema, and inflammation. Histamine acts through specific cellular receptors which have been categorized into four types, H1 through H4. Antihistamines represent a class of medications that block the histamine type 1 (H1) receptors. Importantly, antihistamines do not block or decrease the release of histamine, but rather ameliorate its local actions. Agents that specially block other H2 receptors are generally referred to as H2 blockers rather than antihistamines.

Histamine type 1 receptors are widely distributed and are particularly common on smooth muscle of the bronchi, gastrointestinal tract, uterus, and large blood vessels. H1 receptors are also found in the central nervous system. The antihistamines are widely used to treat symptoms of allergic conditions, including itching, nasal stuffiness, runny nose, teary eyes, urticaria, dizziness, nausea, and cough. Their most common use alone or in combination with other agents is for symptoms of upper respiratory illnesses such as the common cold. The central nervous system effects of antihistamines include sedation and decrease in anxiety, tension and adventitious movements.

Antihistamines are typically separated into sedating (first generation) and nonsedating (second generation) forms, based upon their central nervous system effects, the nonsedating agents being less likely to cross the blood–brain barrier. In addition, some antihistamines have additional anticholinergic, antimuscarinic, or other actions. The antihistamines are some of the most commonly used drugs in medicine, and most are available in multiple forms, both by prescription and in over-the-counter (OTC) products, alone or combined with analgesics or sympathomimetic agents. Common uses include short-term treatment of symptoms of the common cold, seasonal allergic rhinitis (hay fever), motion sickness, nausea, vertigo, cough, urticaria, pruritus, and anaphylaxis. The sedating antihistamines are also used as mild sleeping aids and to alleviate tension and anxiety. Many antihistamines are also available in topical forms, as creams, nasal sprays, and eye drops for local use in alleviating allergic symptoms. The nonsedating antihistamines are typically used in extended or long-term treatment of allergic disorders, including allergic rhinitis (hay fever), sinusitis, atopic dermatitis, and chronic urticaria.

The antihistamines have several adverse side effects which are related to their antihistaminic actions. Side effects are, however, usually mild and rapidly reversed with stopping therapy or decreasing the dose. These common side effects include sedation, impaired motor function, dizziness, dry mouth and throat, blurred vision, urinary retention, and constipation. Antihistamines can worsen urinary retention and narrow angle glaucoma.

The antihistamines rarely cause liver injury. Their relative safety probably relates to their use in low doses for a short time only. The nonsedating antihistamines, however, are often used for an extended period and several forms have been linked to rare instances of clinically apparent acute liver injury which has generally been mild and self-limiting; the antihistamines most commonly linked to liver injury have been cyproheptadine, cetirizine, and terfenadine (which is no longer in clinical use).

First generation antihistamines includes:

- Brompheniramine

- Carbinoxamine

- Chlorcyclizine

- Chlorpheniramine
- Clemastine
- Cyclizine
- Cyproheptadine
- Dexbrompheniramine
- Dexchlorpheniramine
- Dimenhydrinate
- Diphenhydramine
- Doxylamine
- Hydroxyzine
- Meclizine
- Phenyltoloxamine
- Promethazine
- Triprolidine

Second generation antihistamines includes:

- Acrivastine
- Cetirizine
- Fexofenadine
- Levocetirizine
- Loratadine
- Desloratadine

Section 57.3

Cough and Cold Medicines for Respiratory Symptoms

This section includes text excerpted from "Symptom Relief,"
Centers for Disease Control and Prevention (CDC),
April 17, 2015. Reviewed August 2019.

While antibiotics cannot treat infections caused by viruses, there are still a number of things you or your child can do to relieve some symptoms and feel better while a viral illness runs its course. Over-the-counter (OTC) medicines may also help relieve some symptoms.

How to Feel Better
General Advice

For upper respiratory infections, such as sore throats, ear infections, sinus infections, colds, and bronchitis, try the following:

- Get plenty of rest

- Drink plenty of fluids

- Use a clean humidifier or cool mist vaporizer

- Avoid smoking, secondhand smoke, and other pollutants (airborne chemicals or irritants)

- Take acetaminophen, ibuprofen, or naproxen to relieve pain or fever

- Use saline nasal spray or drops

Sore Throat

Try the following tips if you or your child has a sore throat:

- Soothe a sore throat with ice chips, sore throat spray, popsicles, or lozenges (do not give lozenges to young children)

- Use a clean humidifier or cool mist vaporizer

- Gargle with salt water

- Drink warm beverages

- Take acetaminophen, ibuprofen, or naproxen to relieve pain or fever

Ear Pain

The following tips can be used to help ease the pain from earaches:

- Put a warm moist cloth over the ear that hurts
- Take acetaminophen, ibuprofen or naproxen to relieve pain or fever

Runny Nose

Stop a runny nose in its tracks by trying the following tips:

- Get plenty of rest
- Increase fluid intake
- Use a decongestant or saline nasal spray to help relieve nasal symptoms

Sinus Pain and Pressure

Try the following tips to help with sinus pain and pressure:

- Put a warm compress over the nose and forehead to help relieve sinus pressure
- Use a decongestant or saline nasal spray
- Breathe in steam from a bowl of hot water or shower
- Take acetaminophen, ibuprofen, or naproxen to relieve pain or fever

Cough

The following tips can be used to help with coughing:

- Use a clean humidifier or cool mist vaporizer
- Breathe in steam from a bowl of hot water or shower
- Use nonmedicated lozenges (do not give lozenges to young children)
- Use honey if your child is at least one year old

Over-the-Counter Medicines

For children and adults, OTC pain relievers, decongestants, and saline nasal sprays may help relieve some symptoms, such as runny nose, congestion, fever, and aches, but they do not shorten the length of time you or your child is sick. Remember to always use OTC products as directed. Not all products are recommended for children of certain ages.

Pain Relievers for Children

For babies six months of age or younger, parents should only give acetaminophen for pain relief. For a child six months of age or older, either acetaminophen or ibuprofen can be given for pain relief. Be sure to ask your child's healthcare professional for the right dosage for your child's age and size. Do not give aspirin to your child because of Reye syndrome, a rare but very serious illness that harms the liver and brain.

Cough and Cold Medicines for Children Younger Than Four Years of Age

Do not use cough and cold products in children younger than four years of age unless specifically told to do so by a healthcare professional. Overuse and misuse of OTC cough and cold medicines in young children can result in serious and potentially life-threatening side effects. Instead, parents can clear nasal congestion (snot) in infants with a rubber suction bulb. A stuffy nose can also be relieved with saline nose drops or a clean humidifier or cool-mist vaporizer.

Cough and Cold Medicines for Children Older Than Four Years of Age

Over-the-counter cough and cold medicines may give your child some temporary relief of symptoms even though they will not cure your child's illness. Parents should talk with their child's healthcare professional if they have any concerns or questions about giving their child an OTC medication. Parents should always tell their child's healthcare professional about all prescription and OTC medicines they are giving their child.

Chapter 58

Asthma Medications: Overview of Long-Term Control and Quick-Relief Medications

Medications for asthma are categorized into two general classes: long-term control medications used to achieve and maintain control of persistent asthma and quick-relief medications used to treat acute symptoms and exacerbations.

Long-Term-Control Medications

Corticosteroids: Block late-phase reaction to allergen, reduce airway hyperresponsiveness, and inhibit inflammatory cell migration and activation. They are the most potent and effective anti-inflammatory medication currently available. Inhaled corticosteroids (ICSs) are used in the long-term control of asthma. Short courses of oral systemic corticosteroids are often used to gain prompt control of the disease when initiating long-term therapy; long-term oral systemic corticosteroid is used for severe persistent asthma.

This chapter includes text excerpted from "Medications," National Heart, Lung, and Blood Institute (NHLBI), August 28, 2007. Reviewed August 2019.

Cromolyn sodium and nedocromil: Stabilize mast cells and interfere with chloride channel function. They are used as an alternative, but not preferred, medication for the treatment of mild persistent asthma. They can also be used as preventive treatment prior to exercise or unavoidable exposure to known allergens.

Immunomodulators: Omalizumab (anti-immunoglobulin E (Anti-IgE)) is a monoclonal antibody that prevents binding of IgE to the high-affinity receptors on basophils and mast cells. Omalizumab is used as adjunctive therapy for patients 12 years of age and above who have allergies and severe persistent asthma. Clinicians who administer omalizumab should be prepared and equipped to identify and treat anaphylaxis that may occur.

Leukotriene modifiers: Include leukotriene receptor antagonists (LTRAs) and a 5-lipoxygenase inhibitor. Two LTRAs are available—montelukast (for patients >1 year of age) and zafirlukast (for patients ≥7 years of age). The 5-lipoxygenase pathway inhibitor zileuton is available for patients 12 years of age and above; liver function monitoring is essential. LTRAs are alternative, but not preferred, therapy for the treatment of mild persistent asthma. LTRAs can also be used as adjunctive therapy with ICSs, but for youths of 12 years of age and above and adults they are not the preferred adjunctive therapy compared to the addition of long-acting beta-agonists (LABAs). Zileuton can be used as an alternative but not preferred adjunctive therapy in adults.

Long-acting beta-agonists: Salmeterol and formoterol are bronchodilators that have a duration of bronchodilation of at least 12 hours after a single dose.

- LABAs are not to be used as monotherapy for long-term control of asthma.

- LABAs are used in combination with ICSs for long-term control and prevention of symptoms in moderate or severe persistent asthma.

- Of the adjunctive therapies available, LABA is the preferred therapy to combine with ICS in youth of 12 years of age and above and adults.

- The beneficial effects of LABA in combination therapy for the great majority of patients who require more therapy than low-dose ICS alone to control asthma (i.e., require step 3 care or higher) should be weighed against the increased risk of severe exacerbations, although uncommon, associated with the daily use of LABAs.

- For patients of five years of age and older who have moderate persistent asthma or asthma inadequately controlled on low-dose ICS, the option to increase the ICS dose should be given equal weight to the option of adding LABA.

- For patients five years of age and older who have severe persistent asthma or asthma inadequately controlled on step 3 care, the combination of LABA and ICS is the preferred therapy.

- LABA may be used before exercise to prevent EIB, but the duration of action does not exceed five hours with chronic regular use. Frequent and chronic use of LABA for EIB is discouraged, because this use may disguise poorly controlled persistent asthma.

- The use of LABA for the treatment of acute symptoms or exacerbations as of now is not recommended.

Methylxanthines: Sustained-release theophylline is a mild to moderate bronchodilator used as alternative, not preferred, adjunctive therapy with ICS. Theophylline may have mild anti-inflammatory effects. Monitoring of serum theophylline concentration is essential.

Quick-Relief Medications

Anticholinergics: Inhibit muscarinic cholinergic receptors and reduce the intrinsic vagal tone of the airway. Ipratropium bromide provides additive benefit to short-acting beta-agonists (SABAs) in moderate-to-severe asthma exacerbations. May be used as an alternative bronchodilator for patients who do not tolerate SABA.

SABAs: Albuterol, levalbuterol, and pirbuterol are bronchodilators that relax smooth muscle. Therapy of choice for relief of acute symptoms and prevention of exercise-induced bronchospasm (EIB).

Systemic corticosteroids: Although not short-acting, oral systemic corticosteroids are used for moderate and severe exacerbations as adjunct to SABAs to speed recovery and prevent recurrence of exacerbations.

Chapter 59

Corticosteroids for Asthma Treatment

The corticosteroids are a group of chemically related natural hormones and synthetic agents that resemble the human adrenal hormone cortisol and have potent anti-inflammatory and immunosuppressive properties and are widely used in medicine. Corticosteroid therapy is associated with several forms of liver injury, some due to exacerbation of an underlying liver disease and some that appear to be caused directly by corticosteroid therapy. This discussion will cover eight agents: betamethasone, cortisone, dexamethasone, hydrocortisone, methylprednisolone, prednisolone, prednisone, and triamcinolone.

Background

The corticosteroids are hormones that have glucocorticoid (cortisol-like) and/or mineralocorticoid (aldosterone-like) activities and which are synthesized predominantly by the adrenal cortex. In clinical practice, the term "corticosteroids" usually refers to the glucocorticoids

This chapter contains text excerpted from the following sources: Text in this chapter begins with excerpts from "Corticosteroids," LiverTox®, National Institutes of Health (NIH), July 1, 2019; Text under the heading "Inhaled Corticosteroids: Keep Airways Open" is excerpted from "Inhaled Corticosteroids: Keep Airways Open," National Heart, Lung, and Blood Institute (NHLBI), January 2013. Reviewed August 2019.

and are represented by a large group of natural or synthetic steroid compounds that have varying potency, durations of action, and relative glucocorticoid (measured by anti-inflammatory activity) vs. mineralocorticoid (measured by sodium retention) activities. Cortisol and the corticosteroids act by engagement of the intracellular glucocorticoid receptor, which then is translocated to the cell nucleus where the receptor-ligand complex binds to specific glucocorticoid-response elements on DNA, thus activating genes that mediate glucocorticoid responses. The number of genes modulated by corticosteroids are many and the effects are multiple and interactive with other intracellular pathways. Thus, the effects of corticosteroids on inflammation and the immune system cannot be attributed to a single gene or pathway. The potent anti-inflammatory and immunosuppressive qualities of the corticosteroids have made them important agents in the therapy of many diseases. Corticosteroids are available in multiple forms, including oral tablets and capsules; powders and solutions for parenteral administration; topical creams and lotions for skin disease; eye, ear, and nose liquid drop for local application; aerosol solutions for inhalation and liquids or foams for rectal application. Representative corticosteroids (and the year of their approval for use in the United States) include cortisone (1950), prednisone (1955), prednisolone (1955), methylprednisolone (1957), dexamethasone (1958), betamethasone (1961), and hydrocortisone (1983). All are available in generic forms.

The corticosteroids are used widely in medicine largely for their potent anti-inflammatory and immunosuppressive activities. The clinical conditions for which corticosteroids are used include, but are not limited to: asthma, systemic lupus erythematosus, rheumatoid arthritis, psoriasis, inflammatory bowel disease, nephritic syndrome, cancer, leukemia, organ transplantation, autoimmune hepatitis, hypersensitivity reactions, cardiogenic and septic shock, and, of course, glucocorticoid deficiency diseases such as in Addison disease and panhypopituitarism.

Inhaled Corticosteroids: Keep Airways Open

Inhaled corticosteroids are the most effective medications for long-term management of persistent asthma.

Use Inhaled Corticosteroids for Better Asthma Control and Fewer Flare-Ups

Because asthma is a chronic inflammatory disorder, persistent asthma is most effectively controlled with daily long-term control

medication directed toward suppressing inflammation. Inhaled corticosteroids (ICS) are the most effective long-term therapy available for
mild, moderate, or severe persistent asthma. ICS are anti-inflammatory
medications that reduce airway hyperresponsiveness, inhibit inflammatory cell migration and activation, and block late-phase reaction
to allergen. In general, ICS are well tolerated and safe at the recommended dosages.

Generally, ICS improve asthma control more effectively, in both
children and adults, than any other single long-term control medication. However, alternative options for medications are available to
tailor treatment to individual patient circumstances, needs, and preferences. The benefits of ICS outweigh the concerns about the potential
risk of a small, nonprogressive reduction in growth velocity in children,
or other possible adverse effects.

Educate Patients on the Role of Inhaled Corticosteroids in Long-Term Asthma Management

Communicating the effectiveness, safety, and the importance of
ICS for asthma control and addressing concerns about their long-term
use should occur at all levels of healthcare. It is also important for
clinicians and educators to tailor their communications based on consideration of the patient's health literacy level. As well, it is crucial
to develop a heightened awareness of health disparities and cultural
barriers that facilitate more effective communication with minority
(ethnic or racial) or economically disadvantaged patients regarding
the use of asthma medications that may improve asthma outcomes.

Chapter 60

Oxygen Therapy

You can receive oxygen therapy from tubes resting in your nose, a face mask, or a tube placed in your trachea, or windpipe. This treatment increases the amount of oxygen your lungs receive and deliver to your blood. Oxygen therapy may be prescribed for you when you have a condition that causes your blood oxygen levels to be too low. Low blood oxygen may make you feel short of breath, tired, or confused, and can damage your body.

Oxygen therapy can be given for a short or long period of time in the hospital, another medical setting, or at home. Oxygen is stored as a gas or liquid in special tanks. These tanks can be delivered to your home and contain a certain amount of oxygen that will require refills. Another device for use at home is an oxygen concentrator, which pulls oxygen out of the air for immediate use. Because oxygen concentrators do not require refills, they will not run out of oxygen. Portable tanks and oxygen concentrators may make it easier for you to move around while using your therapy.

Oxygen poses a fire risk, so you should never smoke or use flammable materials when using oxygen. You may experience side effects from

This chapter contains text excerpted from the following sources: Text in this chapter begins with excerpts from "Oxygen Therapy," National Heart, Lung, and Blood Institute (NHLBI), December 26, 2012. Reviewed August 2019; Text under the heading "Oxygen Therapy for Patients with Chronic Obstructive Pulmonary Disease" is excerpted from "Oxygen Therapy for Patients with COPD," *NIH News in Health*, National Institutes of Health (NIH), December 2016.

this treatment, such as a dry or bloody nose, tiredness, and morning headaches. Oxygen therapy is generally safe.

Oxygen Therapy for Patients with Chronic Obstructive Pulmonary Disease

Certain people with the lung disease known "as chronic obstructive pulmonary disease" (COPD) will not benefit from long-term oxygen therapy, a new study reports. The finding will help doctors and patients choose among different treatment options for this common condition, which makes it hard to breathe.

Chronic obstructive pulmonary disease is the third-leading cause of death in the United States. The disease damages the lung's airways, so less air can be breathed in and out. As a result, less oxygen can pass through the lungs and into the blood, and blood oxygen levels drop.

Chronic obstructive pulmonary disease symptoms—such as coughing, wheezing, and breathlessness—get worse over time. Treatment options include lifestyle changes, such as quitting smoking, and medicines that help open the airways.

Long-term oxygen therapy has been shown to help COPD patients who have severely low blood oxygen. This therapy involves breathing in oxygen through a nasal tube or mask.

National Institutes of Health (NIH)-funded scientists set out to determine if this same treatment would also help COPD patients who had moderately low blood oxygen. More than 700 such patients enrolled in the study. They were randomly divided into two groups: one received the oxygen treatment; the other did not.

Participants were followed for one to six years. The researchers saw no differences between the treated and untreated groups in terms of their survival, symptoms, or quality of life.

"These results provide insight into a long-standing question about oxygen use in patients with COPD and moderately low levels of blood oxygen," says Dr. James Kiley, a lung disease expert at NIH. "For the most part, this treatment did not improve or prolong life in study participants."

Chapter 61

Pulmonary Rehabilitation

What Is Pulmonary Rehabilitation?

Pulmonary rehabilitation, or PR, is a program for people who have chronic (ongoing) breathing problems. It can help improve your quality of life (QOL) and ability to function. PR does not replace your medical treatment. Instead, you use them together.

Pulmonary rehabilitation is often an outpatient program that you do in a hospital or clinic. Some people have PR in their homes. You work with a team of healthcare providers to find ways to lessen your symptoms, increase your ability to exercise, and make it easier to do your daily activities.

Who Needs Pulmonary Rehabilitation

Your healthcare provider may recommend PR if you have a chronic lung disease (CLD) or another condition that makes it hard for you to breathe and limits your activities. For example, PR may help you if you:

- **Have chronic obstructive pulmonary disease (COPD).** The two main types are emphysema and chronic bronchitis. In COPD, your airways (tubes that carry air in and out of your lungs) are partially blocked. This makes it hard to get air in and out.

This chapter includes text excerpted from "Pulmonary Rehabilitation," MedlinePlus, National Institutes of Health (NIH), July 13, 2018.

- **Have an interstitial lung disease**, such as sarcoidosis and pulmonary fibrosis. These diseases cause scarring of the lungs over time. This makes it hard to get enough oxygen.

- **Have cystic fibrosis (CF).** CF is an inherited disease that causes thick, sticky mucus to collect in the lungs and block the airways.

- **Need lung surgery.** You may have PR before and after lung surgery to help you prepare for and recover from the surgery.

- **Have a muscle-wasting disorder** that affects the muscles used for breathing. An example is muscular dystrophy.

Pulmonary rehabilitation works best if you start it before your disease is severe. However, even people who have advanced lung disease can benefit from PR.

What Does Pulmonary Rehabilitation Include?

When you first start PR, your team of healthcare providers will want to learn more about your health. You will have lung function, exercise, and possibly blood tests. Your team will go over your medical history and current treatments. They may check on your mental health and ask about your diet. Then they will work together to create a plan that is right for you. It may include:

- **Exercise training.** Your team will come up with an exercise plan to improve your endurance and muscle strength. You will likely have exercises for both your arms and legs. You might use a treadmill, stationary bike, or weights. You may need to start slowly and increase your exercise as you get stronger.

- **Nutritional counseling.** Being either overweight or underweight can affect your breathing. A nutritious eating plan can help you work towards a healthy weight.

- **Education about your disease and how to manage it.** This includes learning how to avoid situations that make your symptoms worse, how to avoid infections, and how/when to take your medicines.

- **Techniques you can use to save your energy.** Your team may teach you easier ways to do daily tasks. For example, you may learn ways to avoid reaching, lifting, or bending. Those movements make it harder to breathe, since they use up energy and make you tighten your abdominal muscles. You may also learn how to better deal with stress, since stress can also take up energy and affect your breathing.

- **Breathing strategies.** You will learn techniques to improve your breathing. These techniques may increase your oxygen levels, decrease how often you take breaths, and keep your airways open longer.

- **Psychological counseling and/or group support.** It can feel scary to have trouble breathing. If you have a CLD, you are more likely to have depression, anxiety, or other emotional problems. Many PR programs include counseling and/or support groups. If not, your PR team may be able to refer you to an organization that offers them.

Chapter 62

Lung Transplant Surgery

Lung transplants are used to improve the quality of life (QOL) and extend the lifespan of people who have severe or advanced chronic lung conditions. In rare instances, a lung transplant may be performed at the same time as a heart transplant in patients who have severe heart and lung disease.

You may be eligible for lung transplant surgery if you have severe lung disease that does not respond to other treatments. If you are otherwise healthy enough for surgery, you will be placed on the National Organ Procurement and Transplantation Network's (OPTN) waiting list. This network handles the nation's organ-sharing process. If a match is found, you will need to have your lung transplant surgery right away.

This surgery will be performed in a hospital. You will have general anesthesia and will not be awake for the surgery. Tubes will help you breathe, give you medicine, and help with other bodily functions. A surgeon will open your chest, cut the main airway and blood vessels, and remove your diseased lung. The surgeon will connect the healthy donor lung, reconnect the blood vessels, and close your chest.

After the surgery, you will recover in the hospital's intensive care unit (ICU) before moving to a hospital room for one to three weeks. Your doctor may recommend pulmonary rehabilitation (PR) after your lung transplant surgery to help you regain and improve your breathing. PR may include exercise training, education, and counseling.

This chapter includes text excerpted from "Lung Transplant," National Heart, Lung, and Blood Institute (NHLBI), January 23, 2019.

Pulmonary function tests will help doctors monitor your breathing and recovery. After leaving the hospital, you will visit your doctor often to check for infection or rejection of your new lung, to test your lung function, and to make sure that you are recovering well.

The first year after lung transplant surgery is when you are most at risk for possibly life-threatening complications, such as rejection and infection. To help prevent rejection, you will need to take medicines for the rest of your life that suppress your immune system and help prevent your body from rejecting your new lungs. These important medicines weaken your immune system and increase your chance for infections, and over time they can increase your risk for cancer, diabetes, osteoporosis, and kidney damage. Practicing good hygiene, obtaining routine vaccines, and adopting healthy lifestyle choices, such as heart-healthy eating and not smoking are very important. Getting emotional support and following your doctor's advice will help you recover and stay as healthy as possible.

Part Seven

Living with Chronic Respiratory Problems

Chapter 63

Living with Acute Respiratory Distress Syndrome

Some people fully recover from acute respiratory distress syndrome (ARDS). Others continue to have health problems. After you go home from the hospital, you may have one or more of the following problems:

- **Shortness of breath.** After treatment, many people who have ARDS recover close-to-normal lung function within six months. For others, it may take longer. Some people have breathing problems for the rest of their lives.

- **Tiredness and muscle weakness.** Being in the hospital and on a ventilator can cause your muscles to weaken. You also may feel very tired following treatment.

- **Depression.** Many people who have had ARDS feel depressed for a while after treatment.

- **Problems with memory and thinking clearly.** Certain medicines and a low blood oxygen level can cause these problems.

This chapter includes text excerpted from "ARDS," National Heart, Lung, and Blood Institute (NHLBI), May 18, 2014, Reviewed August 2019.

- **These health problems may go away within a few weeks, or they may last longer.** Talk with your doctor about how to deal with these issues.

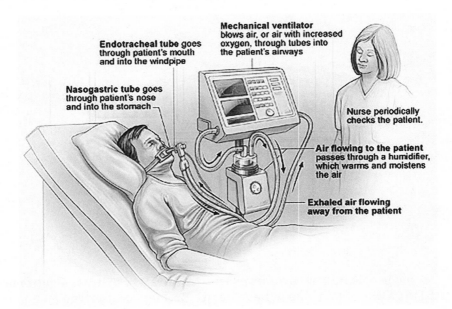

Figure 63.1. *Patient on a Ventilator* (Source: "Ventilator/Ventilator Support," National Heart, Lung, and Blood Institute (NHLBI).)

Getting Help

You can take steps to recover from ARDS and improve your quality of life. For example, ask your family and friends for help with everyday activities.

If you smoke, quit. Smoking can worsen lung problems. Talk to your doctor about programs and products that can help you quit. Also, try to avoid secondhand smoke and other lung irritants, such as harmful fumes. If you have trouble quitting smoking on your own, consider joining a support group. Many hospitals, workplaces, and community groups offer classes to help people quit smoking.

Go to pulmonary rehabilitation (rehab) if your doctor recommends it. Rehab might include exercise training, education, and counseling. Rehab can teach you how to return to normal activities and stay active. Your rehab team might include doctors, nurses, and other specialists. They will work with you to create a program that meets your needs.

Emotional Issues and Support

Living with ARDS may cause fear, anxiety, depression, and stress. Talk about how you feel with your healthcare team. Talking with a professional counselor also can help. If you are very depressed, your doctor may recommend medicines or other treatments that can improve your quality of life.

Joining a patient support group may help you adjust to living with ARDS. You can see how other people who have the same symptoms have coped with them. Talk to your doctor about local support groups or check with an area medical center.

Support from family and friends also can help relieve stress and anxiety. Let your loved ones know how you feel and what they can do to help you.

Chapter 64

Living with Asthma

Chapter Contents

Section 64.1

What You Should Do If You Have Asthma

This section includes text excerpted from "Asthma," National Heart, Lung, and Blood Institute (NHLBI), May 19, 2019.

If you or your child has been diagnosed with asthma, work with your doctor to learn how to manage it yourself. Because asthma symptoms may be different at different times, it is important to know which medicines to use to prevent and relieve symptoms. You can work with your doctor to develop a treatment plan, called an "asthma action plan." Follow-up care will help to make sure your or your child's asthma is well-controlled. Staying healthy also includes avoiding asthma triggers and maintaining a healthy lifestyle.

Follow Your Asthma Action Plan

Work with your doctor to create an asthma action plan that works for you. An asthma action plan is a written treatment plan document that describes the following:

- How to identify allergens or irritants to avoid
- How to recognize and handle asthma attacks
- Which medicines to take and when to take them
- When to call your doctor or go to the emergency room
- Who to contact in case of an emergency

If your child has asthma, then all of your child's caretakers and school staff should know about the asthma action plan.

Receive Routine Medical Care

Regular checkups are important to help your doctor determine how well you are controlling the asthma and adjust treatment if needed. Your doctor will also do regular tests to see how well your lungs are working and how well air is flowing.

Your asthma is well-controlled if you have reached these markers:

- You can do all of your normal activities.
- You do not have symptoms more than twice a week.

- You do not have more than one asthma attack a year requiring corticosteroids by mouth.

- You do not take quick-relief medicines more than two days a week.

- You do not wake from sleep more than one or two times a month because of symptoms.

Symptoms in young children who do not have their asthma controlled include fatigue, irritability, and mood changes.

Your doctor will also make sure you are using your inhaler correctly. There are different types of inhalers. Review the way you use your inhaler at every medical visit. Sometimes asthma may get worse because of incorrect inhaler use.

Medical care is also important for managing conditions that can make it harder to treat asthma, such as gastroesophageal reflux disease (GERD) or sinus infections. Work with your doctor to help keep them under control.

Your medicines or dosages may change over time, based on changes in your condition or in your life, such as:

- **Age.** Older adults may need different treatments because of other conditions they may have and the medicines they take. Beta-blockers, pain relievers, and anti-inflammatory medicines can affect asthma.

- **Pregnancy.** Your asthma symptoms may change during pregnancy. You are also at increased risk of asthma attacks. Your doctor will continue to treat you with long-term medicines such as inhaled corticosteroids. Controlling your asthma is important to prevent complications, such as preeclampsia, preterm delivery, and low birth weight of the baby.

- **Surgery.** Asthma may increase your risk of complications during and after surgery. For instance, having a tube put into your throat may cause an asthma attack. Talk to your doctor and surgeon about how to prepare for surgery.

Monitor Your Asthma at Home

Monitoring and managing your asthma at home is important for your health. Ask your doctor about asthma training or support groups. Education can help you understand your asthma, the purpose of your medicines, how to prevent symptoms, how to recognize asthma attacks early, and when to seek medical attention.

Your doctor may show you how to monitor your asthma using a peak flow meter. You can compare your numbers over time to make sure your asthma is controlled. A low number can help warn you of an asthma attack, even before you notice symptoms.

Keeping a diary may help if you find it hard to follow your asthma action plan or the plan is not working well. If you have any of the following experiences, record them in the diary and make an appointment to see your doctor. Bring the diary with you to your appointment.

- You are limiting normal activities and missing school or work.

- You have to use your quick-relief inhaler more than two days a week.

- Your asthma medicines do not seem to work well anymore.

- Your peak flow number is low or varies a lot from day to day.

- Your symptoms occur more often, are more severe, or cause you to lose sleep.

Adopt Healthy Lifestyle Changes

Your doctor may recommend one or more of the following lifestyle changes to help keep asthma symptoms in check:

- **Aiming for a healthy weight.** Obesity can make asthma harder to manage. Talk to your doctor about programs that can help. Even a 5 to 10 percent weight loss can help symptoms.

- **Being physically active.** Even though exercise is an asthma trigger for some people, you should not avoid it. Physical activity is an important part of a healthy lifestyle. Talk with your doctor about what level of physical activity is right for you. Ask about medicines that can help you stay active.

- **Heart-healthy eating.** Eating more fruits and vegetables, and getting enough vitamin D, can provide important health benefits that may help you with asthma control.

- **Managing stress.** Learn breathing and relaxation techniques, which can help symptoms. Meet with a mental-health professional if you have anxiety, depression, or panic attacks.

- **Quitting smoking or avoiding secondhand smoke.** Smoking tobacco and smoke from secondhand smoke make asthma harder to treat.

Prevent Worsening of Asthma Symptoms and Attacks

Certain things can set off or worsen asthma symptoms. These are called "asthma triggers." Once you know what these triggers are, you can take steps to control many of them.

A common trigger for asthma is exposure to allergens.

- If animal fur triggers asthma symptoms, keep pets with fur out of your home or bedrooms.

- Keep your house as dust-free and mold-free as possible.

- Remove yourself from what is triggering your symptoms in the workplace. If you have occupational asthma, even low levels of the substance to which you are sensitive can trigger symptoms.

- Try to limit time outdoors if allergen levels are high.

Other asthma triggers include:

- **Emotional stress.** Emotional stress, such as intense anger, crying, or laughing can cause hyperventilation and airway narrowing, triggering an asthma attack.

- **Influenza (flu).** Get the flu vaccine each year to help prevent the flu, which can increase the risk of an asthma attack.

- **Medicines.** Some people who have severe asthma may be sensitive to medicines, such as aspirin, and may experience serious respiratory problems. Tell your doctor about all the medicines you or your child currently take.

- **Poor air quality or very cold air.** Pollution or certain kinds of weather, such as thunderstorms, can affect air quality. Pollution can include indoor pollution caused by gases from inefficient cooking or heating devices that are not vented. Outdoor air pollution may be hard to avoid, but you can keep windows closed and avoid strenuous outdoor activity when air quality is low.

- **Tobacco smoke,** including secondhand smoke.

Prevent and Treat Complications over Your Lifetime

To help you prevent complications, your doctor may recommend the following:

- **Keeping your medicine dose as low as possible to prevent long-term side effects.** High doses over time can increase your risk of cataracts and osteoporosis. A cataract is the clouding of the lens in your eye. Osteoporosis is a disorder that makes your bones weak and more likely to break.

- **Monitoring your asthma and contacting your doctor if anything changes.** When asthma is unmanaged, it can lead to potentially life-threatening asthma attacks. If you are pregnant, it can put the health of your baby at risk.

Learn the Warning Signs of Serious Complications and Have a Plan

Ask your doctor about when to call 911 for emergency care. This information should be written in your asthma action plan.

Call your doctor in these cases:

- Your medicines do not relieve an asthma attack.

- Your peak flow number is low.

Section 64.2

Asthma Medication Delivery Mechanisms

This section includes text excerpted from "So You
Have Asthma," National Heart, Lung, and Blood
Institute (NHLBI), March 2013, Reviewed August 2019.

Inhalers

Many asthma medicines—both quick-relief and long-term control
medicines—come as sprays and powders in an inhaler. An inhaler is
a handheld device that delivers the medicine right to the airways in
your lungs where it is needed. There are several kinds of inhalers—just
a few examples are pictured.

Quick-relief medicine is very good at stopping asthma symptoms,
but it does nothing to control the inflammation in your airways that
produces these symptoms. If you need to use your quick-relief inhaler
more often than usual, or if you need to use it more than two days a
week, it may be a sign that you also need to take a long-term control
medicine to reduce the inflammation in your airways. Discuss this
with your doctor as soon as possible

The metered-dose inhaler (MDI) is a small canister that
delivers a measured dose of medicine through your mouth to your
airways.

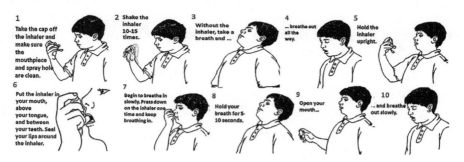

Figure 64.1. *Using a Metered Dose Inhaler with a Spacer (Inhaler in Mouth)* (Source: "Know How to Use Your Asthma Inhaler," Centers for Disease Control and Prevention (CDC).)

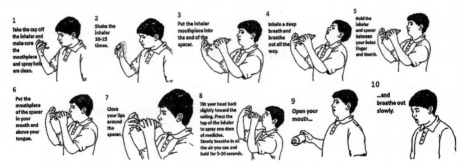

Figure 64.2. *Using a Metered Dose Inhaler with a Spacer* (Source: "Know How to Use Your Asthma Inhaler," Centers for Disease Control and Prevention (CDC).)

A dry powder inhaler delivers a preset amount of asthma medication in powder form.

Different types of inhalers require different ways to use them. It is important for you to learn how to use your inhaler correctly. Read the instructions that come with it. Also, ask your doctor, pharmacist, or other healthcare professionals to show you how to use it. Then try it yourself and ask her or him to make sure you are using it the right way.

Spacers and Valved Holding Chambers

A spacer or valved holding chamber can make using an MDI a lot easier. It can also decrease the amount of medicine that lands on your tongue or in the back of your mouth. This reduces irritation to your throat and increases the amount of medicine that gets down into your lungs where it belongs.

- There are many kinds of spacers that can be chosen to fit your needs.

- Some have a mouthpiece.

- Some have a face mask that comes in different sizes to fit infants, children, and adults.

- Many spacers fit on the end of an inhaler; for some, the canister of medicine fits into the device.

- Some MDIs come with built-in spacers.

Spacers are not needed for dry powder devices.

Spacers also come with instructions on how to use them and keep them clean. It is important to ask your doctor, pharmacist, or other healthcare professionals to show you how to use a spacer with your MDI. Then try it yourself and ask her or him to make sure you are doing it correctly.

Nebulizers

A nebulizer is another device for taking inhaled medicines. It provides the medicine in a fine, steady mist. Using a nebulizer is usually easy; you simply breathe in and out normally through a mask or mouthpiece connected to the nebulizer. But it takes more time to use than an inhaler. It is also more expensive and requires more maintenance. Instructions for using different nebulizers vary, so follow the instructions on the package insert. Nebulized asthma medicine may be especially useful for infants, young children, and adults who have trouble using an inhaler. Regardless of which of these devices you use, you have to use them the right way, or you will not get all the medicine into your lungs. The best way to learn to use these devices correctly is to ask your doctor, pharmacist, or other healthcare professionals to show you how. Then demonstrate it back to her or him to make sure you have it right.

What Medicines Do You Need?

Your doctor is likely to consider a number of factors when deciding which medicines and how much of each you need. Your medicines should:

- Prevent your ongoing symptoms (you should not need to use your quick-relief medicine more than two days a week)

- Help maintain your normal lung function

- Help you be as active as you want to be, whether at work or at school

- Prevent your having repeated asthma attacks

- Help do all of this without causing major side effects

Each time you see your doctor, she or he will weigh all these things before recommending any changes in your medicines. Usually, if you have been doing well for several months, your doctor may consider reducing the number or doses of medicines you are taking. But if your asthma is still not under control, she or he may recommend adding some medicines or increasing the doses of some of those you are already taking. The goal is to achieve the best asthma control possible with the least amount of medicine.

Section 64.3

Asthma Care before, during, and after a Hurricane or Other Tropical Storm

This section includes text excerpted from "Natural Disasters and Severe Weather," Centers for Disease Control and Prevention (CDC), November 8, 2017.

Before a Hurricane or Other Tropical Storm

During and after a hurricane, you may need supplies to keep your family safe and healthy. Remember that a hurricane could cut off your power and water supply. You also may not be able to drive because of damage to your car. Roads may be flooded or blocked.

That is why it is best to be prepared—stock up on everything you might need, including:

- At least a three-day supply of asthma medications

- Copies of important documents, such as insurance cards and immunization records (and asthma action plans, if available)

- Equipment you may need to use when cleaning up after the storm, including N95 respirators, goggles, protective gloves, and waterproof boots

Remember that certain items, such as medications and paper documents, need to be kept in waterproof containers.

Avoiding Common Asthma Triggers during and after a Hurricane or Other Tropical Storm

Flu vaccination can be received as soon as the vaccine is available, usually by October.

- **People with asthma should get a flu shot every year.** Influenza, commonly called "the flu," can trigger an asthma attack. Everyone six months of age and older should get a flu vaccine every year. It is particularly important for people with asthma to be vaccinated against the flu every year because they are more likely to have serious health problems from getting the flu.

- **Personal hygiene and handwashing after a disaster or emergency.** Illnesses such as colds or the flu can trigger an asthma attack. Keeping hands clean helps prevent the spread of these germs.

- **Coping with a disaster or traumatic event.** During and after a disaster it is natural to experience different and strong emotions. Strong emotions can trigger an asthma attack. If your home was flooded and you were not able to dry your home (including furniture and other items) within 24 to 48 hours, you should assume you have mold growth. Breathing in mold can trigger an asthma attack. If possible, people with asthma should stay away from moldy sites.

Using Asthma Medications or Devices during and after a Hurricane or Other Tropical Storm

Asthma can be controlled by taking asthma medication exactly as directed by a doctor or other medical professional.

- Know how to use your asthma inhaler.

- Prevent carbon monoxide poisoning when using generators for breathing treatments during power outages.

When a power outage occurs after a storm, some people may use generators as a backup power source. These generators provide power to appliances, lights, and other vital items in the home, including "breathing treatments" for asthma (also known as "nebulizer machines"). Using generators improperly can cause poisonous gas (carbon monoxide) to build up in a home, garage, or camper. Never use a generator indoors or less than 20 feet from any window, door, or vent. When using a generator, use a battery-powered or battery backup carbon monoxide detector.

Chapter 65

Living with Chronic Obstructive Pulmonary Disease

Chapter Contents

Section 65.1

What You Should Do If You Have Chronic Obstructive Pulmonary Disease

This section includes text excerpted from "Living with COPD,"
Centers for Disease Control and Prevention (CDC), April 26, 2018.

Fighting for each breath is only part of the struggle for those living with chronic obstructive pulmonary disease (COPD), which includes emphysema and chronic bronchitis.

Chronic obstructive pulmonary disease makes breathing hard for the 16 million Americans who have been diagnosed with COPD. Millions more have COPD but have not been diagnosed and are not being treated. Some symptoms of COPD are frequent coughing or wheezing, excess phlegm or sputum, and shortness of breath. Adults with COPD are more likely to be unable to work and have trouble with daily activities. These problems are even worse for those who smoke and who are not physically active. If you have COPD, there are things you can do to make life easier.

The Impact of Chronic Obstructive Pulmonary Disease

Having COPD can greatly affect your day-to-day life:

- Every one in four adults with COPD say they are not able to work.

- Among adults who are employed, COPD may cause them to miss work.

- Half of adults with COPD say they limit their activities because of health problems.

- More than one in three adults with COPD have trouble walking or climbing stairs.

- Nearly one in four adults with COPD say they need to use special equipment for health problems.

- Medical costs, such as visits to the doctor or hospital, are higher for adults with COPD than those without COPD.

What You Can Do

There are things you can do to make living with COPD easier:

- **Quit smoking.** If you smoke, the most important part of your treatment is to quit smoking.

- **Ask about pulmonary rehabilitation.** Pulmonary rehabilitation (or "pulmonary rehab") is a personalized treatment program that teaches you how to manage your COPD symptoms to improve your quality of life (QOL). Plans may include learning to breathe better, how to conserve your energy, and advice on food and exercise.

- **Take your medications.** Symptoms such as coughing or wheezing can be treated with medication.

- **Avoid lung infections.** Lung infections can cause serious problems in people with COPD. Certain vaccines, such as flu and pneumonia vaccines, are especially important for people with COPD to get.

Section 65.2

Managing Dyspnea and Other Complications

This section includes text excerpted from "Controlled Breathing and Dyspnea in Patients with Chronic Obstructive Pulmonary Disease," Rehabilitation Research and Development Service (RR&D), U.S. Department of Veterans Affairs (VA), June 17, 2003. Reviewed August 2019.

Dyspnea is an important and debilitating symptom in patients with chronic obstructive pulmonary disease (COPD). Some pathophysiological factors known to contribute to dyspnea include:

- Increased intrinsic mechanical loading of the inspiratory muscles

- Increased mechanical restriction of the chest wall

- Functional inspiratory muscle weakness
- Increased ventilatory demand related to capacity
- Gas exchange abnormalities
- Dynamic airway compression
- Cardiovascular effects

The relief of dyspnea is an important goal of the treatment of COPD, an irreversible airway disease. In addition to some conventional treatments, such as bronchodilator therapy, exercise training, and oxygen therapy, controlled breathing is also applied to alleviate dyspnea.

"Controlled breathing" is an all-embracing term for a range of exercises, such as active expiration, slow and deep breathing, pursed-lips breathing (PLB), relaxation therapy, specific body positions, inspiratory muscle training, and diaphragmatic breathing. The aims of these exercises vary considerably and include improvement of (regional) ventilation and gas exchange, amelioration of such debilitating effects on the ventilatory pump as dynamic hyperinflation, improvement of respiratory muscle function, decrease in dyspnea, and improvement of exercise tolerance and quality of life (QOL).

In patients with COPD, controlled breathing is used to relieve dyspnea by:

- Reducing dynamic hyperinflation of the rib cage and improving gas exchange
- Increasing strength and endurance of the respiratory muscles
- Optimizing the pattern of thoracoabdominal motion

In addition, psychological effects (such as controlling respiration) might contribute to the effectiveness of controlled breathing.

Controlled-Breathing Techniques to Reduce Dynamic Hyperinflation

Hyperinflation is due to altered static lung mechanics (loss of elastic recoil pressure, static hyperinflation) and/or dynamic factors (air trapping and increased activity of inspiratory muscles during expiration, dynamic hyperinflation). The idea behind decreasing dynamic hyperinflation of the rib cage is that this intervention will presumably result in the inspiratory muscles working over a more advantageous part of their length–tension relationship. Moreover, it is expected to decrease the elastic work of breathing, because the chest wall moves over a more favorable part of its pressure volume curve. In this way, the workload on the inspiratory muscles should diminish, along with the sensation of dyspnea. In addition, breathing at a lower functional residual capacity (FRC) will result in an increase in alveolar gas refreshment, while tidal volume remains constant. Several treatment strategies are aimed at reducing dynamic hyperinflation.

Relaxation Exercises

The rationale for relaxation exercises arises from the observation that hyperinflation in reversible (partial) airway obstruction is, at least in part, caused by an increased activity of the inspiratory muscles during expiration. This increased activity may continue even after recovery from an acute episode of airway obstruction and hence contributes to the dynamic hyperinflation. However, hyperinflation in COPD is mainly due to altered lung mechanics (loss of elastic recoil pressure and air trapping) and is not associated with increased activity of inspiratory muscles during expiration. Relaxation is also meant to reduce the respiratory rate and increase tidal volume, thus improving breathing efficiency.

Pursed-Lips Breathing

Pursed-lips breathing works to improve expiration, both by requiring active and prolonged expiration and by preventing airway collapse. Relaxed expiration causes less "air trapping," which results in a reduction of hyperinflation. Compared to spontaneous breathing, PLB reduces respiratory rate, dyspnea, and arterial partial pressure of carbon dioxide (PCO_2), and improves tidal volume and oxygen saturation in resting conditions.

Active Expiration

Contraction of the abdominal muscles results in increased abdominal pressure during active expiration. This lengthens the diaphragm and contributes to operating the diaphragm close to its optimal length. Indeed, diaphragm displacement and its contribution to tidal volume during resting breathing was not different in COPD patients than in healthy subjects. In addition, active expiration will increase elastic recoil pressure of the diaphragm and the rib cage. The release of this pressure after relaxation of the expiratory muscles will assist the next inspiration. In patients with severe COPD, contraction of abdominal muscles becomes often invariably linked to resting breathing.

Chapter 66

Living with Cystic Fibrosis

If you or your child has been diagnosed with cystic fibrosis (CF), it is important that you continue your treatments, follow up with your doctor, and learn how to manage the condition. The goal of CF care is to control symptoms and prevent complications.

Receive Routine Follow-Up Care

Regular checkups with your doctor may be part of your follow-up and treatment. How often your regular checkups take place will depend on your age. Younger patients, and those who have just been diagnosed, will have more frequent visits. As adults, you may see your doctor less often, perhaps every three months and then once a year for an evaluation.

Regular checkups may include:

- Education about airway clearance, infection control, energy, and nutrition goals

- Height and weight measurement, and calculation of body mass index (BMI)

- Physical activity guidance

- Physical exam, including examination of the heart, lungs, and abdomen to check the liver and for abdominal pain

This chapter includes text excerpted from "Cystic Fibrosis," National Heart, Lung, and Blood Institute (NHLBI), March 13, 2019.

- Physical therapy evaluation and needs

- Psychological assessment and support

Monitor Your Condition

In addition to more frequent regular checkups, you may need to see your doctor for additional tests and evaluations, which may include the following:

- **Abdominal ultrasound** or computerized tomography (CT) scan to look for the cause of abdominal pain, check the pancreas and liver, and look for distal intestinal obstruction

- **Blood tests** to check for diabetes, infection, liver disease, side effects of medicines such as damage to the kidneys, nutritional status, including complete blood count, and vitamin levels

- **Bone mineral density tests** to check for osteopenia or osteoporosis in those who are at risk. You may be at risk if you are taking corticosteroids long term, have severe lung disease, or do not get adequate nutrition. Testing of bone mineral density may be done with an x-ray test called a "dual-energy x-ray absorptiometry" (DEXA or DXA) scans.

- **Chest CT scan** to look for changes in lung function or lung infection

- **Chest x-ray** to look for lung abnormalities and infections. Early changes may be seen on an x-ray before you notice symptoms. In younger children this may be done every other year to decrease radiation exposure.

- **Colonoscopy** to monitor for colorectal cancer because of increased risk

- **Glucose monitoring** and testing to check for CF-related diabetes

- **Lung biopsy** to test for specific bacteria

- **Pancreas function testing,** which may include looking at an enzyme called "pancreatic elastase-1" in your stool

- **Pulmonary function tests,** which includes checking oxygen levels in your blood and spirometry, which is the most important and widely used tool to assess lung function in CF. Regular spirometry is used to monitor lung function in people age six and older and may be done in children as young as age three.

- **Respiratory sample smear and culture,** which involves taking airway secretion or mucus samples every three months to look for microorganisms in the respiratory tract, and if necessary, treat them

- **Review of caloric intake,** and pancreatic enzyme replacement

- **Review of treatments and medicines,** including a pharmacist's assessment

Healthy Lifestyle Changes

Staying healthy is an extremely important part of CF care. Your medical team will work with you to develop a plan for lifestyle changes that can become part of your everyday life. These include the following:

- **Avoiding tobacco smoke,** including secondhand smoke

- **Being physically active** to improve lung function. Physical activity helps with airway clearance and improves bone mineral density, muscle strength, flexibility, and posture. Before starting any exercise program, ask your doctor about what level of physical activity is right for you.

- **Healthy eating** to improve overall health. Healthy eating is also important for normal growth in children who have CF. You may need to increase your food or calorie intake by eating more foods or by eating high-energy foods. A high-sodium eating plan or supplementation with sodium may be recommended at times.

Prevent or Reduce Complications over Your Lifetime

To help you prevent complications and reduce the risk of infections, your doctor may recommend the following:

- **Continue your treatments,** including medicines, supplements, and daily airway clearance techniques. Treating infections and pulmonary exacerbations is important to preserve lung function and slow the progression of disease. Lung disease is the major source of CF-related complications.

- **Practice good hand hygiene** whenever it is appropriate, such as before and after taking medicines and breathing treatments, before you eat, after you use the bathroom, and after blowing your nose. Wash your hands often with soap or use an alcohol-based hand sanitizer.

- **Receive recommended vaccines,** which includes routine immunizations, vaccine for pneumococcus, and an influenza shot every year at the start of flu season. Anyone who lives with you or whom you see often should also get regular vaccines.

Treatments for Complications

Your doctor may recommend medicines to treat complications of CF, including:

- **Antibiotics** to prevent or treat lung infections and pulmonary exacerbations

- **Insulin** to treat diabetes caused by destruction of the pancreas, if needed

- **Medicine** to help unclog ducts in the liver and improve bile flow. This includes ursodeoxycholic acid. This may improve abnormal liver function blood tests.

- **Nutritional supplements** when healthy eating is not enough. Your doctor may recommend supplements such as calcium, multivitamins, oral pancreatic enzymes, sodium, or vitamin A, D, E, and K.

- **Oxygen therapy** to treat low levels of oxygen in the blood. This may improve the ability to be physically active and attend school or work.

- **Surgeries** such as lung transplant may help people with advanced lung disease and respiratory failure. Liver transplant may be an option for advanced liver disease such as cirrhosis. A person who undergoes a lung transplant will also need pulmonary rehabilitation after the surgery.

Learn the Warning Signs of Serious Complications and Have a Plan

Cystic fibrosis may have serious complications. Call your doctor if you believe you have any of the following:

- **Pulmonary exacerbation,** which involves a worsening of lung symptoms, such as more coughing or wheezing, chest congestion, and a change in mucus color. You may also have weight loss, poor appetite, or fever.

- **Hemoptysis,** which may be a sign that an artery has broken and is bleeding into the airway

- **Sudden shortness of breath or chest pain,** which may be a sign of a pneumothorax, or collapsed lung

Chapter 67

Living with Idiopathic Pulmonary Fibrosis

If you have been diagnosed with idiopathic pulmonary fibrosis (IPF), it is important to continue your treatment plan. Talk to your doctor about how often to schedule follow-up care and how to monitor and understand your condition so you know when to get medical help. Your doctor may also recommend lifestyle changes and pulmonary rehabilitation to help you manage the disease.

It is important to know that the progression of IPF is different for each person and cannot be predicted. Managing your condition is best done with the help of a healthcare team that can help improve your quality of life (QOL).

Receive Routine Follow-Up Care

Regular checkups with your doctor may be part of your follow-up and treatment. Tell your doctor if you suddenly experience a worsening of symptoms over a period of days or weeks. This event is called an "exacerbation." Sometimes a trigger or other factors may trigger it, but often there is no obvious cause. Exacerbations from IPF can be life threatening and are more common in advanced stages of IPF. People who have an exacerbation from IPF may have repeat episodes.

This chapter includes text excerpted from "Idiopathic Pulmonary Fibrosis," National Heart, Lung, and Blood Institute (NHLBI), May 13, 2015. Reviewed August 2019.

If your condition worsens, you may benefit from full-time oxygen therapy. Some people who have IPF carry portable oxygen when they go out.

Monitor Your Condition

Patients who have IPF can have other conditions as well, so it may be necessary to see multiple doctors who specialize in different areas of medical care.

Your doctor may use the following tests and procedures to monitor your condition, and also to determine whether to recommend a lung transplant.

- **Chest computed tomography (CT) scan** to look for lung cancer, or to see how you are responding to treatment or if your condition is getting worse

- **Liver function tests** to monitor possible side effects from medicines.

- **Pulmonary function tests,** which your doctor may recommend every few months

Adopt Healthy Lifestyle Changes

Your doctor may recommend that you adopt healthy lifestyle changes to increase your overall health and prevent other conditions. This includes:

- **Quitting smoking.** If you smoke, quit. Also, try to avoid other lung irritants, such as dust, chemicals, and secondhand smoke.

- **Being physically active.** Physical activity can help you maintain your strength and lung function and reduce stress. Try moderate exercise, such as walking or riding a stationary bike. Ask your doctor about using oxygen while exercising.

- **Aiming for a healthy weight**

- **Heart-healthy eating.** Also, eating smaller meals more often may relieve stomach fullness, which can make it hard to breathe.

Your doctor may recommend these lifestyle changes as part of a pulmonary rehabilitation program.

Take Care of Your Mental Health

Living with IPF may cause fear, anxiety, depression, and stress. Talking about how you feel with your healthcare team may help. Your doctor may recommend:

- **Counseling,** particularly cognitive behavioral therapy (CBT)

- **Medicines or other treatments,** such as antidepressants, or other treatments that can improve your QOL

- **Joining a patient support group,** which may help you adjust to living with IPF. You can see how other patients manage similar symptoms and their condition. Talk with your doctor about local support groups or check with an area medical center.

- **Getting support from family and friends,** which can help relieve stress and anxiety. Let your loved ones know how you feel and what they can do to help you.

- **Discussing palliative care,** if the disease becomes very advanced. For people who have severe symptoms from IPF, palliative care doctors may help them have a better QOL with fewer symptoms.

Prevent Exacerbations

To prevent exacerbations, your doctor may recommend avoiding situations where breathing is more difficult, such as in high altitudes, or when the air quality outside is poor from dust or pollution. Your doctor may treat exacerbations with medicines, such as glucocorticoids, or increased levels of supplemental oxygen.

Chapter 68

Living with Sarcoidosis

If you have been diagnosed with sarcoidosis, it is important that you continue your medicine, follow up with your doctor when directed, make healthy lifestyle changes, and prevent complications. Some people may achieve total, or life-long, remission. Other people may achieve temporary remission and go on to experience a relapse, or return of the disease. If you are pregnant, talk to your doctor about the medicines you take to avoid problems for you and your baby.

Receive Routine Follow-Up Care

How often you need to see your doctor will depend on the severity of your symptoms, which organs are affected, which treatments you are using, and whether you have any side effects from treatment. Even if you do not have symptoms, you should see your doctor for ongoing care.

Monitor Your Condition

If the disease is not worsening, your doctor may watch you closely to see whether the disease goes away on its own. If the disease does start to get worse, your doctor can prescribe treatment.

Some people have sarcoidosis that persists, or recurs, for many years after diagnosis. This may be called "chronic," "severe,"

This chapter includes text excerpted from "Sarcoidosis," National Heart, Lung, and Blood Institute (NHLBI), March 29, 2018.

"advanced," "refractory," or "progressive sarcoidosis." To monitor your condition, your doctor may recommend the following tests at regular intervals.

- **A chest x-ray** to monitor your lungs for permanent scarring, also known as pulmonary fibrosis

- **An eye exam** to detect eye damage. See an eye doctor every year. Sarcoidosis can cause permanent eye damage without symptoms.

- **Heart tests** to monitor how well your heart is working. Sarcoidosis only rarely affects the heart, but cardiac sarcoidosis may be life-threatening. Tests may include electrocardiography (ECG or EKG), echocardiography, or cardiac magnetic resonance imaging (MRI).

- **Liver function tests** to determine if your liver is working the way that it should. These tests are particularly important if you have liver sarcoidosis. You may need treatment for cholestasis, which is a type of liver disease that causes severe itching without a rash.

- **Pulmonary function tests** to monitor how sarcoidosis is affecting your lungs over time. If your lung function worsens, you may need different treatment.

Your doctor may perform other tests based on which organs are involved and what medicine is prescribed. For example, your doctor will monitor you for side effects of corticosteroids, such as osteoporosis, if used long term.

Adopt Healthy Lifestyle Changes

Your doctor may recommend that you adopt lifelong lifestyle changes to help prevent sarcoidosis from worsening if you do not need medicine. These may include:

- **Heart-healthy eating**

- **Aiming for a healthy weight**

- **Being physically active.** Even though fatigue can make it hard to exercise if you have sarcoidosis, physical activity can actually improve energy and help with other symptoms, such as shortness of breath and muscle weakness. Try to stay as active as you can, but talk to your doctor first about an exercise that is appropriate for you.

- **Managing stress**

- **Quitting smoking.** If you smoke, quit. Also, try to avoid other lung irritants, such as dust, chemicals, and secondhand smoke.

Prevent a Relapse

If your sarcoidosis goes into remission, your doctor may carefully stop your medicines. However, she or he will still need to monitor you for a relapse, also called a "flare," of the disease.

Relapses can be hard to predict. Most people who relapse do so in the first six months after stopping treatment. The longer you go without symptoms, the less likely you are to have a relapse.

See your doctor if you have a relapse. You may need a second round of treatment.

Prevent and Treat Complications over Your Lifetime

To help prevent some of the complications of sarcoidosis, your doctor may recommend the following:

- **An implantable cardioverter-defibrillator** that may help prevent sudden cardiac arrest

- **Surgery** if sarcoidosis has damaged organs or you are at risk for serious or life-threatening health problems. Surgery can include a heart, lung, or liver transplant, or treatment for complications in the brain.

- **Lifestyle changes** if you have hypercalcemia, which means your body has problems absorbing calcium. This can lead to high levels of calcium in your blood and urine. Your doctor may recommend avoiding sunlight, drinking plenty of fluids, and eating fewer foods with calcium.

Other treatments may be used to treat organs that are less commonly affected.

- **Anti-epileptic medicines** if sarcoidosis affects your brain and causes seizures

- **Eye drops**

- **Hormone replacement therapy** if sarcoidosis causes endocrine problems

- **Medicines for nerve pain**

- **Nonsteroidal anti-inflammatory drugs (NSAIDs)**

- **Physical therapy**

- **Radiation**

- **Vasodilator therapy** to relax your blood vessels. This may be necessary if your sarcoidosis causes pulmonary hypertension.

Learn the Warning Signs of Serious Complications and Have a Plan

Watch for the warning signs of complications that may require emergency medical treatment. These include signs of blindness or brain tumors, such as changes in your vision or if you cannot see clearly or see color. Other complications that require immediate medical attention include kidney failure, sudden cardiac arrest, and sudden shortness of breath or muscle weakness.

Emotional Issues

Sarcoidosis may make you feel socially isolated, anxious, or depressed, and you may continue to feel fatigued even after your treatment has ended. But certain activities or treatments may help improve your emotional health.

- **Counseling,** particularly cognitive therapy, can be helpful.

- **Joining a patient support group,** which may help you adjust to living with sarcoidosis. You can see how other people who have the same symptoms have coped with them. Talk with your doctor about local support groups or check with an area medical center.

- **Medicines or other treatments.** Your doctor may recommend medicines such as antidepressants or other treatments that can improve your quality of life.

- **Support from family and friends** can help relieve stress and anxiety. Let your loved ones know how you feel and what they can do to help you.

Pregnancy

If you have sarcoidosis and are pregnant or planning to become pregnant, talk with your doctor about the risks involved. Also, if you become pregnant, it is important to get good prenatal care and regular sarcoidosis checkups during and after pregnancy.

Most women who have sarcoidosis give birth to healthy babies. Women with sarcoidosis are at risk for some complications related to pregnancy, including:

- Hemorrhaging after giving birth

- Preterm delivery

- Preeclampsia

- Venous thromboembolism, such as pulmonary embolism and deep vein thrombosis

Talk to your doctor about any medicines you take. Some medicines prescribed to adults with sarcoidosis are not safe to take during pregnancy.

Part Eight

Additional Help and Information

Chapter 69

Glossary of Terms Related to Respiratory Disorders

acute respiratory distress syndrome: A lung condition that leads to low oxygen levels in the blood.

airways: Pipes that carry oxygen-rich air to the lungs. They also carry carbon dioxide, a waste gas, out of the lungs.

allergens: Allergens are a type of asthma trigger, which cause symptoms through an allergic reaction rather than by irritation.

allergy: A type of excessive immune system reaction to a substance in a person's environment. Allergies can be triggered by eating, touching, or breathing in an allergen.

alpha-1 antitrypsin deficiency: A condition that raises the risk for lung disease (especially if you smoke) and other diseases.

alveoli: The millions of tiny compartments within the lungs at the ends of the airways. Alveoli are where gas exchange takes place—that is, where the blood picks up oxygen (from the air a person has breathed in) and releases carbon dioxide (to be breathed out).

anticholinergics: This type of medicine relaxes the muscle bands that tighten around the airways. This action opens the airways, letting

---

This glossary contains terms excerpted from documents produced by several sources deemed reliable.

more air out of the lungs to improve breathing. Anticholinergics also help clear mucus from the lungs.

asbestos: A mineral that, in the past, was widely used in many industries. Asbestos is made up of tiny fibers that can escape into the air. When breathed in, these fibers can stay in your lungs for a long time.

asthma: A chronic disease of the lungs. Symptoms include cough, wheezing, a tight feeling in the chest, and trouble breathing.

breathing pattern: A general term designating the characteristics of the ventilatory activity, e.g., frequency of breathing.

breathing rate: The number of breaths per minute.

bronchi: The airways that lead from the trachea to each lung, and then subdivide into smaller and smaller branches.

bronchiectasis: A condition in which damage to the airways causes them to widen and become flabby and scarred.

bronchitis: Inflammation of the main air passages to your lungs. It causes cough, shortness of breath, and chest tightness.

bronchoalveolar lavage: A clinical technique which removes cell samples from the lower lungs to allow assessment of inflammation and other respiratory conditions.

bronchoconstriction: The reduction in the diameter of the bronchi, usually due to squeezing of the smooth muscle in the walls. This reduces the space for air to go through and can make breathing difficult.

bronchodilator: A medicine that relaxes the smooth muscles of the airways. This allows the airway to open up (to dilate) since the muscles are not squeezing it shut.

bronchopulmonary dysplasia (BPD): A serious lung condition that affects infants.

bronchoscopy: A procedure that allows your doctor to look inside your lungs' airways, called the bronchi and bronchioles.

capillaries: Small blood vessels that run through the walls of the air sacs of the lungs.

chronic obstructive pulmonary disease (COPD): It is a progressive disease that makes it hard to breathe. COPD can cause coughing that produces large amounts of mucus, wheezing, shortness of breath, chest tightness, and other symptoms.

cilia: Tiny hairs coated with sticky mucus that trap germs and other foreign particles that enter the airways during breathing.

corticosteroids: A type of medicine used to reduce inflammation. Corticosteroid drugs mimic a substance produced naturally by the body. In asthma, corticosteroids are often taken through an inhaler for long-term control. They may also be taken orally or given intravenously for a short time if asthma symptoms get out of control.

cystic fibrosis (CF): One of the most common serious genetic diseases. Cystic fibrosis (CF) causes the body to make abnormal secretions leading to mucus buildup. CF mucus buildup can impair organs such as the pancreas, the intestine, and the lungs.

deep vein thrombosis: A blood clot that forms in a vein deep in the body.

diaphragm: A dome-shaped muscle located below the lungs. It separates the chest cavity from the abdominal cavity. The diaphragm is the main muscle used for breathing.

dust mites: Very tiny creatures that live in the dust in people's homes. They thrive especially when the air is humid. Many people are allergic to dust mites, and trying to reduce the number of them in the home is part of many asthma control plans.

emphysema: Condition caused by damage to the air sacs in the lungs. This damage keeps the body from getting enough oxygen. Emphysema is usually caused by smoking.

expectorant: A drug that stimulates the flow of saliva and promotes coughing to eliminate phlegm from the respiratory tract.

gas exchange: The lungs' intake of oxygen and removal of carbon dioxide.

Haemophilus influenzae type b: A bacterial infection that may result in severe respiratory infections, including pneumonia, and other diseases such as meningitis.

inflammation: Used to describe an area on the body that is swollen, red, hot, and in pain.

influenza: It is a respiratory infection caused by multiple viruses. The viruses pass through the air and enter the body through the nose or mouth. The flu can be serious or even deadly for elderly people, newborn babies and people with certain chronic illnesses.

inhalation: The process of breathing in.

inhaled corticosteroid: Anti-inflammatory medicine breathed directly into the lungs. The advantage to this is that the medicine goes directly to where the inflammation is, and has minimal effects on the rest of the body (and, therefore, fewer side effects than corticosteroids taken orally).

irritant: A substance that triggers asthma symptoms by irritating the airway when breathed in. Examples include cigarette smoke, fumes from a harsh cleaning fluid, or strong perfume.

larynx: The voice box.

lung transplant: Surgery to remove a person's diseased lung and replace it with a healthy lung from a deceased donor.

lungs: The organs that lie on either side of the breastbone and fill the inside of the chest cavity. The left lung is slightly smaller than the right lung to allow room for the heart.

mucus: A thick, slippery fluid made by the membranes that line certain organs of the body, including the nose, mouth, and throat.

obesity hypoventilation syndrome (OHS): A breathing disorder that affects some obese people.

otitis media: A viral or bacterial infection that leads to inflammation of the middle ear. This condition usually occurs along with an upper respiratory infection. Symptoms include earache, high fever, nausea, vomiting and diarrhea.

pleurisy: A condition in which the pleura is inflamed. The pleura are membranes that consist of two large, thin layers of tissue. One layer wraps around the outside of your lungs. The other layer lines the inside of your chest cavity.

pneumonia: An infection in one or both of the lungs. Many germs— such as bacteria, viruses, and fungi—can cause pneumonia. The infection inflames your lungs' air sacs, which are called alveoli. The air sacs may fill up with fluid or pus, causing symptoms such as a cough with phlegm, fever, chills, and trouble breathing.

pulmonary artery: This artery and its branches deliver blood rich in carbon dioxide (and lacking in oxygen) to the capillaries that surround the air sacs of the lungs.

pulmonary embolism (PE): A sudden blockage in a lung artery. The blockage usually is caused by a blood clot that travels to the lung from a vein in the leg.

pulmonary function tests: A series of tests done to determine whether a person has breathing problems, and precisely what those problems are. These are used to differentiate among different diseases and disorders. It is sometimes hard for a doctor to tell just by a regular exam whether a person has asthma or another condition, and pulmonary function tests can help clarify the diagnosis.

pulmonary hypertension: Increased pressure in the pulmonary arteries.

pulmonary rehabilitation: A broad program that helps improve the well-being of people who have chronic (ongoing) breathing problems.

respiratory failure: A condition in which not enough oxygen passes from the lungs into the blood.

respiratory system: Organs and tissues that help breathing. The main parts of this system are the airways, the lungs and linked blood vessels, and the muscles that enable breathing.

sarcoidosis: An inflammatory disease marked by the formation of granulomas (small nodules of immune cells) in the lungs, lymph nodes, and other organs. Sarcoidosis may be acute and go away by itself, or it may be chronic and progressive.

sputum: Mucus and other matter brought up from the lungs by coughing.

thoracentesis: A procedure to remove excess fluid in the space between the lungs and the chest wall.

trachea: The largest breathing tube in the body, passing from the throat down to the chest (where it connects to the two bronchi leading to the lungs).

tracheostomy: A surgically made hole that goes through the front of your neck and into your trachea. The hole is made to help you breathe.

upper respiratory tract: Area of the body that includes the nasal passages, mouth, and throat.

vaccine: A product made from very small amounts of weak or dead germs that can cause diseases — for example, viruses, bacteria, or toxins. It prepares your body to fight the disease faster and more effectively so you won't get sick. Vaccines are administered through needle injections, by mouth, and by aerosol.

ventilation: Physiological process by which gas is renewed in the lungs.

ventilator: A machine that supports breathing. These machines mainly are used in hospitals.

wheezing: Breathing with difficulty, with a whistling noise. Wheezing is a symptom of asthma.

x-ray: A type of high-energy radiation. In low doses, x-rays are used to diagnose diseases by making pictures of the inside of the body.

yoga: An ancient system of practices used to balance the mind and body through exercise, meditation (focusing thoughts), and control of breathing and emotions.

Chapter 70

Directory of Organizations That Help People with Respiratory Disorders

Government Organizations That Provide Information about Respiratory Disorders

Agency for Healthcare Research and Quality (AHRQ)
Office of Communications
5600 Fishers Ln.
Seventh Fl.
Rockville, MD 20847
Phone: 301-427-1104
Website: www.ahrq.gov

Centers for Disease Control and Prevention (CDC)
1600 Clifton Rd.
Atlanta, GA 30329-4027
Toll-Free: 800-CDC-INFO
(800-232-4636)
Phone: 404-639-3311
Toll-Free TTY: 888-232-6348
Website: www.cdc.gov
E-mail: cdcinfo@cdc.gov

Resources in this chapter were compiled from several sources deemed reliable; all contact information was verified and updated in August 2019.

Eunice Kennedy Shriver
National Institute of
Child Health and Human
Development (NICHD)
Information Resource Center
(IRC)
P.O. Box 3006
Rockville, MD 20847
Toll-Free: 800-370-2943
Toll-Free Fax: 866-760-5947
Website: www.nichd.nih.gov
E-mail: NICHDInformation
ResourceCenter@mail.nih.gov

healthfinder.gov
National Health Information
Center (NHIC)
200 Independence Ave.
Washington, DC 20201
Website: www.healthfinder.gov
E-mail: healthfinder@hhs.gov

National Cancer Institute
(NCI)
9609 Medical Center Dr.
BG 9609 MSC 9760
Bethesda, MD 20892-9760
Toll-Free: 800-4-CANCER
(800-422-6237)
Website: www.cancer.gov
E-mail: NCIinfo@nih.gov

National Center for
Complementary and
Integrative Health (NCCIH)
9000 Rockville Pike
Bethesda, MD 20892
Toll-Free: 888-644-6226
Toll-Free TTY: 866-464-3615
Website: nccih.nih.gov
E-mail: info@nccih.nih.gov

National Center for Health
Statistics (NCHS)
3311 Toledo Rd.
Hyattsville, MD 20782-2064
Toll-Free: 800-CDC-INFO
(800-232-4636)
Toll-Free TTY: 888-232-6348
Phone: 301-458-4000
Website: www.cdc.gov/nchs/
index.htm
E-mail: cdcinfo@cdc.gov

National Health Information
Center (NHIC)
U.S. Department of Health and
Human Services (HHS)
1101 Wootton Pkwy, Ste. LL100
Rockville, MD 20852
Fax: 240-453-8281
Website: www.health.gov/
about-us/contact-us
E-mail: nhic@hhs.gov

National Heart, Lung, and
Blood Institute (NHLBI)
31 Center Dr.
Bldg. 31
Bethesda, MD 20892
Website: www.nhlbi.nih.gov

National Institute of Allergy
and Infectious Diseases (NIAID)
Office of Communications and
Government Relations (OCGR)
5601 Fishers Ln.
MSC 9806
Bethesda, MD 20892-9806
Toll-Free: 866-284-4107
Phone: 301-496-5717
Toll-Free TDD: 800-877-8339
Fax: 301-402-3573
Website: www.niaid.nih.gov
E-mail: ocpostoffice@niaid.nih.
gov

National Institute of Environmental Health Sciences (NIEHS)
P.O. Box 12233
MD K3-16
Research Triangle Park, NC 27709
Phone: 919-541-3345
Fax: 919-541-4395
Website: www.niehs.nih.gov
E-mail: webcenter@niehs.nih.gov

National Institute of Neurological Disorders and Stroke (NINDS)
P.O. Box 5801
Bethesda, MD 20824
Toll-Free: 800-352-9424
Website: www.ninds.nih.gov

National Institute on Aging (NIA)
31 Center Dr., MSC 2292
Bldg. 31, Rm. 5C27
Bethesda, MD 20892
Toll-Free: 800-222-2225
Toll-Free TTY: 800-222-4225
Website: www.nia.nih.gov
E-mail: niaic@nia.nih.gov

National Institutes of Health (NIH)
9000 Rockville Pike
Bethesda, MD 20892
Phone: 301-496-4000
TTY: 301-402-9612
Website: www.nih.gov

Office on Women's Health (OWH)
U.S. Department of Health and Human Services (HHS)
200 Independence Ave. S.W.
Rm. 712E
Washington, DC 20201
Toll-Free: 800-994-9662
Phone: 202-690-7650
Fax: 202-205-2631
Website: www.womenshealth.gov

Occupational Safety and Health Administration (OSHA)
U.S. Department of Labor (DOL)
200 Constitution Ave. N.W.
Rm. N3626
Washington, DC 20210
Toll-Free: 800-321-OSHA (800-321-6742)
Website: www.osha.gov

U.S. Bureau of Labor Statistics (BLS)
2 Massachusetts Ave. N.E.
Postal Square Bldg.
Washington, DC 20212-0001
Phone: 202-691-5200
Toll-Free TDD: 800-877-8339
Website: www.bls.gov

U.S. Department of Health and Human Services (HHS)
200 Independence Ave. S.W.
Washington, DC 20201
Toll-Free: 877-696-6775
Website: www.hhs.gov

U.S. Environmental Protection Agency (EPA)
1200 Pennsylvania Ave. N.W.
Washington, DC 20460
Phone: 202-564-4700
TTY: 202-272-0165
Fax: 202-501-1450
Website: www.epa.gov

U.S. Food and Drug Administration (FDA)
10903 New Hampshire Ave.
Silver Spring, MD 20993-0002
Toll-Free: 888-INFO-FDA
(888-463-6332)
Website: www.fda.gov

U.S. National Library of Medicine (NLM)
8600 Rockville Pike
Bethesda, MD 20894
Toll-Free: 888-FIND-NLM
(888-346-3656)
Phone: 301-594-5983
Website: www.nlm.nih.gov
E-mail: custserv@nlm.nih.gov

Private Organizations That Provide Information about Respiratory Disorders

Action on Smoking and Health (ASH)
1250 Connecticut Ave. N.W.
Seventh Fl.
Washington, DC 20036
Phone: 202-659-4310
Website: www.ash.org
E-mail: info@ash.org

Allergy and Asthma Network Mothers of Asthmatics (AANMA)
8229 Boone Blvd.
Ste. 260
Vienna, VA 22182
Toll-Free: 800-878-4403
Fax: 703-288-5271
Website: www.
allergyasthmanetwork.org

American Academy of Allergy, Asthma, and Immunology (AAAAI)
555 E. Wells St.
Ste. 1100
Milwaukee, WI 53202-3823
Phone: 414-272-6071
Website: www.aaaai.org
E-mail: info@aaaai.org

American Academy of Otolaryngology—Head and Neck Surgery (AAO—HNS)
1650 Diagonal Rd.
Alexandria, VA 22314-2857
Phone: 703-836-4444
Website: www.entnet.org

American Association for Respiratory Care (AARC)
9425 N. MacArthur Blvd.
Ste. 100
Irving, TX 75063-4706
Phone: 972-243-2272
Fax: 972-484-2720
Website: www.aarc.org
E-mail: info@aarc.org

American College of Chest Physicians
CHEST Global Headquarters
2595 Patriot Blvd.
Glenview, IL 60026
Toll-Free: 800-343-2227
Phone: 224-521-9800
Fax: 224-521-9801
Website: www.chestnet.org

American College of Physicians (ACP)
190 N. Independence Mall W.
Philadelphia, PA 19106-1572
Toll-Free: 800-523-1546
Phone: 215-351-2400
Website: www.acponline.org

American College of Radiology (ACR)
1891 Preston White Dr.
Reston, VA 20191
Toll-Free: 800-227-5463
Phone: 703-648-8900
Website: www.acr.org
E-mail: info@acr.org

American Lung Association (ALA)
55 W. Wacker Dr.
Ste. 1150
Chicago, IL 60601
Toll-Free: 800-LUNG-USA
(800-586-4872)
Website: www.lung.org
E-mail: info@lung.org

American Medical Association (AMA)
AMA Plaza
330 N. Wabash Ave.
Ste. 39300
Chicago, IL 60611-5885
Toll-Free: 800-262-3211
Website: www.ama-assn.org

American Thoracic Society (ATS)
25 Bdwy.
18th Fl.
New York, NY 10004
Phone: 212-315-8600
Fax: 212-315-6498
Website: www.thoracic.org
E-mail: atsinfo@thoracic.org

Asthma and Allergy Foundation of America (AAFA)
1235 S. Clark St.
Ste. 305
Arlington, VA 22202
Toll-Free: 800-7-ASTHMA
(800-727-8462)
Website: www.aafa.org
E-mail: info@aafa.org

Cleveland Clinic
9500 Euclid Ave.
Cleveland, OH 44195
Toll-Free: 800-223-2273
Phone: 216-444-2200
Website: my.clevelandclinic.org

COPD Foundation
3300 Ponce de Leon Blvd.
Miami, FL 33134
Toll-Free: 866-731-COPD
(866-731-2673)
Website: www.copdfoundation.org
E-mail: INFO@
COPDFOUNDATION.ORG

**Cystic Fibrosis Foundation
(CFF)**
4550 Montgomery Ave., Ste. 1100 N
Bethesda, MD 20814
Toll-Free: 800-FIGHT-CF
(800-344-4823)
Phone: 301-951-4422
Website: www.cff.org
E-mail: info@cff.org

March of Dimes
1550 Crystal Dr., Ste. 1300
Arlington, VA 22202
Toll-Free: 888-MODIMES
(888-663-4637)
Website: www.marchofdimes.com

**National Emphysema
Foundation (NEF)**
128 E. Ave.
Norwalk, CT 06851
Phone: 203-866-5000
Website: www.
emphysemafoundation.org
E-mail: info@
emphysemafoundation.org

**National Environmental
Education Foundation
(NEEF)**
4301 Connecticut Ave. N.W.
Ste. 160
Washington, DC 20008-2326
Phone: 202-833-2933
Website: www.neefusa.org

**National Jewish Health
(NJH)**
1400 Jackson St.
Denver, CO 80206
Toll-Free: 877-CALL-NJH
(877-225-5654)
Phone: 303-388-4461
Website: www.nationaljewish.
org

**Nemours Foundation /
KidsHealth®**
Website: www.kidshealth.org

Ontario Lung Association
18 Wynford Dr.
Ste. 401
Toronto, Ontario M3C 0K8
Fax: 416-864-9911
Website: www.lungontario.ca
E-mail: info@lungontario.ca

**Pan American Health
Organization (PAHO)**
World Health Organization
(WHO)
525 Twenty-third St. N.W.
Washington, DC 20037
Phone: 202-974-3000
Fax: 202-974-3663
Website: www.paho.org

Pulmonary Hypertension Association (PHA)
801 Roeder Rd.
Ste. 1000
Silver Spring, MD 20910
Toll-Free: 800-748-7274
Phone: 301-565-3004
Fax: 301-565-3994
Website: www.phassociation.org
E-mail: PHA@PHAssociation.org

Respiratory Health Association (RHA)
1440 W. Washington Blvd.
Chicago, IL 60607
Toll-Free: 888-880-LUNG
(888-880-5864)
Phone: 312-243-2000
Fax: 312-243-3954
Website: www.resphealth.org
E-mail: info@resphealth.org

University of Chicago Asthma and COPD Center
5841 S. Maryland Ave.
MC 6076
Chicago, IL 60637
Phone: 773-702-1016
Website: asthma.bsd.uchicago.edu
E-mail: asthma@medicine.bsd.uchicago.edu

Index

Index

639

Respiratory Disorders Sourcebook, Fifth Edition